TRAUMA IN PREGNANCY

HERBERT J. BUCHSBAUM, M.D.

Professor of Obstetrics and Gynecology and
Director, Division of Gynecologic Oncology,
University of Texas–Southwestern Medical School,
Dallas, Texas; Senior Attending Staff,
Parkland Memorial Hospital, Dallas, Texas

1979

W. B. SAUNDERS COMPANY   Philadelphia / London / Toronto

W. B. Saunders Company: West Washington Square
Philadelphia, PA   19105

1 St. Anne's Road
Eastbourne, East Sussex BN 21 3UN England

1 Goldthorne Avenue
Toronto, Ontario M8Z 5T9, Canada

Trauma in Pregnancy

ISBN   0-7216-2177-5

Last digit is the print number: 9   8   7   6   5   4   3   2   1

To my wife, Linda

CONTRIBUTORS

JOHN ALBRIGHT, M.D.

Associate Professor of Orthopaedics, Department of Orthopaedics, University of Iowa Hospitals and Clinics, Iowa City, Iowa

Fractures in Pregnancy

RICHARD A. BRAND, M.D.

Associate Professor of Orthopaedic Surgery and Engineering, University of Iowa Hospitals and Clinics, Iowa City, Iowa

Fractures in Pregnancy

CHARLES R. BRINKMAN, III, M.D.

Professor of Obstetrics and Gynecology, University of California at Los Angeles; Attending Obstetrician and Gynecologist, University of California at Los Angeles Center for Health Sciences Hospitals and Clinics, Los Angeles, California

Hypovolemia and Hypoxia

HERBERT J. BUCHSBAUM, M.D.

Department of Obstetrics and Gynecology, University of Texas Health Sciences Center at Dallas; Senior Attending Staff, Parkland Memorial Hospital, Dallas, Texas

Diagnosis; Penetrating Injury; Cesarean Section

WARREN MELVILLE CROSBY, M.D.

Professor and Vice Chairman, Department of Gynecology and Obstetrics, University of Oklahoma College of Medicine, University of Oklahoma Health Sciences Center, Oklahoma City, Oklahoma

Automobile Injuries and Blunt Trauma

DWIGHT P. CRUIKSHANK, M.D.

Assistant Professor of Obstetrics and Gynecology, University of Iowa College of Medicine; Attending Staff, University of Iowa Hospitals and Clinics, Iowa City, Iowa

Anatomy and Physiology; Cesarean Section

GEORGE EL-KHOURY, M.D.

Assistant Professor of Radiology-Orthopaedics, Department of Radiology, University of Iowa Hospitals and Clinics, Iowa City, Iowa

Fractures in Pregnancy

FRANCIS C. JACKSON, M.D.

Professor and Chairperson, Department of Surgery, Texas Tech University School of Medicine, Lubbock; Chief of Surgery, Health Sciences Center Hospital, Lubbock; Consultant,

Veterans Administration Hospitals, Amarillo and Big Spring; Consultant, R. E. Thomason General Hospital, El Paso, Texas
Accidental Injury

DAVID KADER, B.A., J.D., LL.M.

Associate Professor, University of Iowa College of Law, Iowa City, Iowa
Liability for Prenatal Harm

JAMES A. NICHOLAS, M.D., F.A.C.S.

Professor of Orthopaedic Surgery, Cornell Medical College; Director, Institute of Sports Medicine and Athletic Trauma, Lenox Hill Hospital; Director, Department of Orthopaedic Surgery, Lenox Hill Hospital; Consultant, Hospital for Special Surgery, New York, New York
Sports Injuries

ANNE M. SEIDEN, M.D.

Chairperson, Department of Psychiatry, Cook County Hospital; Associate Professor of Psychiatry and Preventive Medicine, University of Illinois—Abraham Lincoln School of Medicine and School of Public Health; Attending Psychiatrist, Michael Reese Hospital, Chicago, Illinois
Psychologic Trauma

BRUCE SPRAGUE, M.D.

Associate Professor of Orthopaedics, Department of Orthopaedics, University of Iowa Hospitals and Clinics, Iowa City, Iowa

Fractures in Pregnancy

JAMES W. TAYLOR, M.D.

Clinical Instructor, University of Tennessee Memorial Research Center and Hospital; Active Staff, St. Mary's Medical Center and Park West Hospital, Knoxville, Tennessee
Burns

ROBERT B. WALLACE, M.D., M.Sc.

Associate Professor, Department of Preventive Medicine and Environmental Health and Department of Internal Medicine, University of Iowa; Attending Physician, University of Iowa Hospitals and Clinics, Iowa City, Iowa
Occupational Hazards

VALERIE A. WILK, B.A.

Graduate Student in Epidemiology, Department of Preventive Medicine and Environmental Health, University of Iowa, Iowa City, Iowa
Occupational Hazards

JAMES R. WOODS, Jr., M.D.

Chief of Maternal-Fetal Medicine, Letterman Army Medical Center, Presidio of San Francisco, California
Hypovolemia and Hypoxia

PREFACE

Accidental injury and death, in spite of its shocking cost in lives and dollars, is now part of the American scene. Over 50 million Americans are injured annually and 130,000 killed in vehicular, occupational, and home accidents. Accidental death and injury has appropriately been called "the most neglected disease of modern society."

Accidents are the leading cause of death of Americans between the ages of 15 and 44, the period in a woman's life when most of her children are conceived and born. As a result of changing social mores, the gravid American woman is continuing to participate in the social, occupational, and even sports aspects of our society. She is therefore exposed to the same home, occupational, vehicular, and sports injuries as the rest of the population.

Although the incidence of accidental injury is difficult to assess, it has been reported that 7 per cent of women sustain some form of injury during pregnancy. With over 3 million live births per year (and nearly 1 million abortions), this represents over 200,000 injuries annually. The increasing number of accidents during pregnancy is beginning to be reflected in maternal mortality statistics. In one state, trauma was the most important cause of nonobstetric maternal deaths, accounting for 26 per cent of the deaths in this group (Minnesota Mortality Study).

The injured pregnant woman is unique in that two lives are involved, mother and fetus, whose sensitivities and responses to trauma differ. The effects of external maternal trauma on pregnancy outcome have been the source of much speculation. Reference was made to trauma as a cause of pregnancy wastage as early as the 15th Century B.C. in the code of Hammurabi. The Hebrew sages addressed themselves to this problem in Exodus 21:22.

> If a man strive, and hurt a woman with child, so that her fruit depart from her, and yet no mischief follow: he shall surely be punished according as the woman's husband will lay upon him; and he shall pay as the judges determine.

A causal relationship between external trauma and pregnancy interruption can no longer be accepted *a priori*. A pathologic defect in the conceptus or in implantation must first be ruled out. There is no exact correlation between severity of maternal injury and abortion, intrauterine fetal death, and premature labor. Yet, maternal injury can alter the course of pregnancy if maternal death, fetal injury, or fetal death in utero occurs, or as a result of alterations in maternal homeostasis that adversely and irrevocably affect the fetus.

The increasing role of traumatic injury as a complication of pregnancy, and the recent heightened interest in emergency medicine were the stimuli for this book. It is directed to all physicians who deal with women in the course of normal pregnancy, and to emergency room physicians, orthopedic surgeons, and traumatologists, who may see the injured gravida. It was my goal to bring to the trauma specialist information regarding the physiologic alterations of pregnancy and how these alterations modify the type of injury the mother sustains, the interpretation of clinical and laboratory studies, and the management of the injury. And for the obstetrician, I hope the book will present material on diagnosis and management of injuries during pregnancy that is not available elsewhere. The ultimate goal was improved care for the injured gravida and her child.

The variety of specialties represented by the contributing authors points to the importance of a multidisciplinary approach to the care of the injured gravida. The team should include the physician caring for the mother during her pregnancy, the trauma specialist, and a neonatologist.

I would like to acknowledge the help given by Marie Low, Medical Editor at W. B. Saunders Company. Her suggestions helped expand the scope of the book. Particular credit must be given to my secretary, Joyce Perry, for her efforts in the preparation of the manuscript, for maintaining correspondence with the contributors, and for the multitude of details involved in preparing a book.

HERBERT J. BUCHSBAUM, M.D.

CONTENTS

ix

Chapter 1

ACCIDENTAL INJURY — THE PROBLEM AND THE INITIATIVES

Francis C. Jackson

INTRODUCTION

During the past two decades accidental injury has been variously described as "the fashionable killer" (Kennedy, 1955), "a major challenge to medicine" (Yarborough, 1970), "the neglected disease of modern society" (National Academy of Sciences, 1966), and the "leading cause of death" in the American population between the ages of one and 38 years (National Safety Council, 1975).

The socioeconomic effects of trauma are also quite real. In 1969, the Georgia State Health Department calculated that the death rate from accidents was actually producing a loss of revenue of $56 million annually, basing these estimates upon lost taxes resulting from the interruption of the productive lives of its taxpayers. But the problem went much deeper than the effects of accidental injuries; it extended to the care of all medical emergencies.

The Assistant Secretary for Health and Scientific Affairs, Dr. Merlin K. DuVal, speaking in 1971 before a National Conference on Emergency Health Services was forced to confess that "Any description of our Emergency Medical Services becomes a litany of inadequacy and neglect" (Du Val, 1972). Dr. DuVal's remarks were based, in part, upon the National Academy of Sciences–National Research Council report entitled "Accidental Death and Disability: The Neglected Disease of Modern Society" (1966). This pamphlet resulted from a series of studies conducted by the Academy's Committees on Shock and Trauma. These efforts by the Academy to establish a new initiative in medicine's role in care of the acutely ill and injured had extended over a number of years. This document and other landmarks in the efforts to reduce deaths and disabilities from trauma will be discussed later in this chapter.

ACCIDENTAL DEATHS, INJURIES, AND
DISABILITIES: THE SCOPE

Trauma continues to be the fourth leading cause of death in the United States after heart disease, cancer, and strokes. On the average, there are 12 accidental deaths and about 1300 disabling injuries every hour of the day; this amounts to one death every 5 minutes and one injury every 3 seconds (National Safety Council, 1975). The total cost from accidents resulting in human injury and death, health care, compensation, lost wages, and property damage was estimated at over $5 million for every hour in the year of 1974 (National Safety Council, 1975) (Table 1–1).

Morbidity and Mortality

The National Health Survey reported that 60 million injuries were occurring annually among the more than 200 million Americans between 1971 and 1973. Twenty-three per cent were sufficient to be "bed disabling," while 77 per cent required medical attention or loss of activity (at work or at home) for at least one full day. The National Safety Council concluded that in 1974, 380,000 *permanent* injuries occurred following the 11 million disabling injuries which the Council identified in that year* (National Safety Council, 1975).

For Americans of ages 24 to 44 years accidents are the leading cause of death, exceeding cancer and heart disease (Table 1–2).

In terms of total morbidity, trauma has been seriously affecting nearly 250 of every 1000 Americans each year — one of every three males and one of every 10 females. Among the elderly, the injury rate for females approximates that for males, and females over 65 years of age are, apparently, more vulnerable since their rate of accidental injury actually exceeds that for males of the same age; i.e., 190 versus 115 per 1000 (U.S. Public Health Service, 1972).

When classified by location, accidents in the home account for *more than twice* the injuries from motor vehicle accidents and *nearly twice* those occurring at

---

*The differences between the National Health Survey and National Safety Council figures are due to differences in the definition of an injury. The National Survey includes crime-related and nonaccidental injuries.

**TABLE 1–1 Total Deaths (All Ages) in the United States
for the Four Leading Causes***

Cause	Number	Rate†
Heart disease	757,075	361
Cancer	351,055	167
Stroke	214,313	102
Accidents	115,821	55
Other	534,739	—
TOTALS	1,973,003	940

*National Safety Council: Accident Facts. 1975 Edition. Chicago, National Safety Council, 1975.
†Deaths per 100,000 population.

TABLE 1–2   Four Leading Causes of Death by Age Group (Both Sexes)*

CLASS	ALL-AGES	RATE†	AGES 25–44	RATE†
Heart disease	757,075	361	16,614	32
Cancer	351,055	167	17,184	34
Stroke	241,313	102	–	–
Accidents	115,821	55	24,750	48
TOTALS	1,438,264 (100%)	685	111,004 (8%)	217

*National Safety Council: Accident Facts. 1975 Edition. Chicago, National Safety Council, 1975. When all causes were included the total deaths were 1,973,003 and rate was 940.

†Deaths per 100,000 population for both males and females.

work. Occupational accidents account for about 21 per cent of all disabling injuries, whereas 36 per cent occur at home (Table 1–3).

The death toll, as well as morbidity from injuries, has fluctuated in recent years with a slow trend downward. The death rate from injuries per 100,000 population dropped 10 per cent between 1973 and 1974. The trend is primarily related to a reduction in highway accidents following the lowering of speed limits, the effectiveness of safety programs in industry, and a relative decline in home related accidents. The number of disabling accidents in the home has remained the same despite the increase in the total population. Nevertheless, one person in 52 is disabled by a home accident each year. Even though 95 per cent of these accidents occur in urban dwellings, the highest rate for accidents in the home is in rural dwellings.

Falls account for 35 per cent of the home deaths, with fire and poisonings being the next most common causes. In the age groups from 15 to 44 years, deaths from poisonings and drugs were the major cause. The rise occurred primarily between 1970 and 1974, possibly a reflection of increasing drug use (National Safety Council, 1975).

The Cost of Health Care and the Economic Impact of Injuries

The cost of accidental injury and its impact on the medical system are enormous. More hospital bed-days (17,544,000) were needed in 1965 for the

TABLE 1–3   Accidental Deaths and Injuries in 1974*

CLASS OF ACCIDENT	DEATHS	DISABLING INJURIES
Motor vehicle	46,200	1,800,000
Home	25,500	4,000,000
Work	13,400	2,300,000
Public†	24,000	3,000,000
TOTALS‡	105,000	11,000,000

*National Safety Council: Accident Facts. 1975 Edition. Chicago, National Safety Council, 1975.

†Includes recreation, transportation, public building accidents, etc.

‡Some deaths and injuries are included in more than one class so that subtotals contain duplications of injuries and deaths.

care of injuries than for cancer (14,829,000) or arteriosclerotic heart disease (11,492,000). In that year, the 16 per cent of all hospital bed-days for all conditions expended in the care of injuries (both male and female) was almost equal to the bed utilization for obstetric conditions, which traditionally is the major cause of hospital bed occupancy in short-stay facilities. It is estimated that 65,000 beds (8 per cent) among the 859,327 beds in short-term general hospitals are required for the management of trauma (Artz, 1976; Schlaeter, 1970). The total treatment costs for the treatment of trauma in these short-stay hospitals is over $1.2 billion annually (Stiffman, 1976).

Patient services by private physicians caring for injuries not requiring hospital care now necessitate 100 million office visits per year. This represents a treatment setting wherein 80 per cent of all injuries are managed and contributes $600 million to the total cost of health care annually. It is noteworthy that medical specialists actually treat fewer than half of all those injured (45 per cent); the balance are cared for by private care physicians and osteopaths (Stiffman, 1976).

The measurable total dollar loss from accidents in 1974 (including property damage, insurance, and other indirect costs) was estimated at over $43 billion; lost earnings accounted for 30 per cent and medical expenses for 13 per cent. The cost of motor vehicle accidents, alone, is nearly $20 billion (National Safety Council, 1975).

ACCIDENTAL DEATHS AND INJURIES AMONG FEMALES

Injury Rates

The National Center for Health Statistics reported that the overall injury rate for Americans of all ages and sexes was 249 per 1000. For males the rate was 314 and for females 189. The rates for both sexes were highest in the group under 17 years of age. Every year, in each group, one of three males and one of five females sustained an injury which required medical attention or caused a loss of at least one day of normal activity (U.S. Public Health Service, 1972).

The Center has noted that between 1964 and 1969 the number of injuries to women decreased every year, so that by 1969 there were 40 fewer injuries than in 1964. The survey suggested this decline was due to fewer accidents in the home. Whatever the reason for the drop in the number of injuries occurring in the home, there was a similar decline among males, whose injury rate for these accidents dropped by 35 during the same period. On the basis of the National Health Survey, it was estimated that over 20 million of the 62 million accidental injuries reported in 1974 involved females.

Deaths from Injury

The number of fatal injuries sustained by females was 33 per 100,000 population and 79 for men. The four most common causes of death among various age groups of women are listed in Table 1–4. As with men, accidental death is the leading cause among women in the younger age groups, and it

TABLE 1–4   Most Common Causes of Death by Age Group Among Females*

AGE	RANK			
	First	*Second*	*Third*	*Fourth*
All ages	Heart disease	Cancer	Stroke	Accidents
1–14	Accidents	Cancer	Congenital anomalies	Pneumonia
15–24	Accidents	Homicide	Cancer	Suicide
75 +	Heart disease	Stroke	Cancer	Arteriosclerosis

*National Safety Council: Accident Facts. 1975 Edition. Chicago, National Safety Council, 1975.
Note: Accidents ranked sixth as cause of death in 1974 among females over 75 years of age.

remains a threat through most of their lives. Death from homicide is the second and suicide the fourth major cause of death in the age group between 15 and 24 years (U.S. Public Health Service, 1972, 1974).

Motor Vehicle Injuries

The injury rates among women have been particularly affected by their increasing use of the automobile. Despite the fact that women drivers generally are involved in only somewhat fewer accidents than men (177 per 100 million miles driven versus 204 for men, in 1974) the men drivers are involved in twice as many of the fatal accidents. Increasing usage of motor vehicles has had a most dramatic effect on injuries to females, particularly since 1950. Between 1950 and 1969, the average increase in percentage of change in the death rate for females in vehicle accidents was an estimated 37 per cent, versus 24 per cent for males (U.S. Public Health Service, 1972) (see Chapter 6). The death rate, particularly for white females, following automotive accidents in this period increased a remarkable 83 per cent for ages 15 to 24, 44 per cent for ages 25 to 43 years, and 63 per cent for ages 35 through 44 years. The numbers of deaths for white males in the same period and age groups increased at a slower rate, i.e., 41 per cent, 27 per cent, and 15 per cent, respectively (U.S. Public Health Service, 1972).

Alcoholism

The use of alcohol, and more recently drugs, has become a part of the American culture, affecting to a considerable degree the frequency of accidental injury as well as the socioeconomic structure. Since appreciable impairment of body function occurs whether the individual is a "problem" drinker or user or a "social" drinker or user, the likelihood of accidental injury is markedly increased (Haddon and Baker, 1978).

In most instances of alcohol ingestion particularly with regard to highway accidents, a blood concentration between 50 and 100 mg per 100 ml is considered presumptive evidence of intoxication. A 150 pound individual drinking after a meal would have to consume 5 ounces of 80 proof (U.S.) spirits to achieve a concentration of 50 mg per 100 ml. But concentrations of 100 to 250 mg per 100 ml are the most frequently encountered levels among people involved in vehicular accidents and even other injury events! (Haddon and Baker, 1978.)

The role of alcohol in motor vehicle accidents has been well established. The use of an alcoholic beverage is directly implicated in one half of all motor vehicle accidents fatal to the occupants, in more than one fifth of such accidents in which occupants experience serious injury, and in one third or more of crashes that are fatal to adult pedestrians (Haddon and Baker, 1978).

Positive blood alcohol concentrations have also been found in 42 per cent of adults dying in *nonhighway accidents,* such as falls, poisoning, and burns. Large amounts of alcohol have also been found in the blood of adults who drown and in victims of homicide and suicide (Waller, 1972).

Although the numbers of heavy drinkers among men exceed similar numbers among women by a ratio of three to one, the sex ratio of deaths from chronic drinkers, i.e., alcoholic cirrhosis, is two to one (Greenblatt and Schuckit, 1976).

Women, in general, obtain higher peaks of blood alcohol and demonstrate greater variability in these peak blood levels than men. It has been suggested that this may be related to the menstrual cycle and changing levels of sex hormones. The metabolism of alcohol is slowed by oral contraceptives and hormone supplements, and after hysterectomy. Usually this results in lower consumption rates for women (Greenblatt and Schuckit, 1976).

Alcoholism has always been a problem in industry, affecting the frequency of work accidents, time off, and the quality of job performance. In 1970, 43 per cent of the female population was employed in some form of work activity. In one report, 66 per cent of women alcoholics were employed at regular jobs (Greenblatt and Schuckit, 1976). Alcoholism is a critical health problem for both sexes in the "labor force and is the major contributing factor in most major injuries."

Injuries in the Home

Injuries that occur in the home are an obvious threat to many women. There is much data to confirm this assumption. The World Health Organization reported that home accidents accounted for 50 per cent of accidental deaths among females versus only 20 per cent among males (World Health Organization, 1972). Nearly one third of all injuries and one third of all bed disabling injuries reported for males and females by the National Health Survey occurred in the home from 1971 to 1973 (U.S. Public Health Service, 1972). In one major city, a study of 950 deaths from trauma revealed that 56 per cent occurred in the home and over one third of these were among females (Fitts, et al. 1964).

The National Electronics Injury Surveillance System (NEISS), operated by the U.S. Public Health Service, receives daily reports from 119 hospitals. (This will be increased to 130 hospitals by 1980.) In 1977 NEISS reported that eight household products, in particular, produced injuries to women twice as frequently as they did to males. Kitchen appliances, housewares, furnishings, and personal items such as sun lamps were identified (NEISS Data Highlights, 1977).

Accidents at Work

Women have been joining the American work force at an increasing rate. In 1933, there were 39 million workers, 8 per cent of whom were women. By 1974, the total number of people at work had more than doubled (87 million) and now one third were women (National Safety Council, 1975).

Most women are employed in the service industries (hotels, hospitals, schools, and clerical services) and the wholesale and retail trades (foodstores, apparel and accessory stores, eating places, and retail stores). Forty-six per cent of working women are in these professions, versus only 13 per cent of working males (Doublin, 1965). The Bureau of Labor Statistics indicates that the number of recorded injuries in each of these trades was 1,190,000 and 596,000, respectively, in 1973. The injury frequency rates* in these professions were not necessarily low, being 10.02 for service industries and 7.64 for the wholesale and retail trade industry. These can be compared with rates of 6.16 in the machinery industry and 4.21 for the chemical industry (National Safety Council, 1975). For all industries the frequency rate is 10.2, and it is highest in the mining industry (35.1) where there are few women workers (National Safety Council, 1975).

According to the National Safety Council, work injuries are primarily sprains and strains (40 per cent), lacerations and abrasions (16 per cent), and contusions (12 per cent). Twenty-seven per cent involve the trunk and 44 per cent the extremities. Usually these are due to "overexertion," striking an object, or falling.

However, three of four deaths and more than one half of the injuries suffered by workers are said by the Council to have occurred *away from work*. Since such injuries affect operating costs, such as disability wages, off-the-job accidents, as may occur to the working woman in the home, are tabulated as affecting the work force as a whole.

One especially susceptible group of working women seems to be unmarried women over 30 years of age who are involved in assembly work requiring speed and dexterity. The incidence of hand and arm injuries is high among these women, who are apparently concerned over the loss of their precision (Haddon and Baker, 1978).

Besides increased exposure to industrial and other hazards in recent years, women, as they age biologically, present a sex-associated shift in injury thresholds. This is said to account, for example, for the greater frequency of fracture of the distal forearm in postmenopausal years when compared with men or younger women. There are substantial variations in age and sex differences among the different bones (Alfranc and Bauer, 1962). This is related not only to frequency and severity of trauma but to differences in the degree to which various bones change with age among the sexes (Fork and Harlin, 1970). As has been previously noted, elderly women are much more vulnerable to the falling injury in the home and sustain a high frequency of hip injuries.

INJURIES AMONG FEMALES IN THE CHILDBEARING YEARS

For the purpose of this discussion, the age group from the mid-teens to 44 years of age will be considered the childbearing period. Fifty-three per cent of the population are women, and 42 per cent of women are between the ages of 14 and 44 years.

---

*Number of disabling work injuries per 1 million man-hours of exposure.

TABLE 1–5   Causes of Accidental Deaths Among Women of
Childbearing Age*

CLASS	TOTAL FEMALE DEATHS PER CLASS	AGE GROUP 15–44 YEARS	
		Number	*Per Cent*
Motor vehicle	15,570	6624	43
Falls	8199	335	4
Fires/Burns	2608	329	13
Drowning	1299	915	70
Firearms	349	317	91
Other (poisoning, etc.)	7327	787	11
TOTAL DEATHS	35,352	9307	26

*Estimated from 1973 data, *in* Accident Facts, 1975 Edition, p. 14. Chicago, National Safety Council, 1975.

In general, as persons advance in age, injuries tend to decrease. The highest injury rate for women occurs under 17 years of age, with 223 injuries per 1000 per year in this group, reported by the National Center for Health Statistics. In the age group of 17 to 44 years, the injury rate becomes 158 per 1000, and for women over the age of 65 years, 189 per 1000.

From data presented by the National Safety Council in 1975, it is estimated that 26 per cent of female deaths from the various classes of injury occur in the age group between 15 and 44 years, when the likelihood of pregnancy is greatest (Table 1–5). The vast majority of deaths, particularly from drowning and firearms, occur in this age span. Forty-three per cent of all deaths following motor vehicle accidents also fall into this age group. The fewest female accidental deaths in this period result from falls (4 per cent) and fire or burn injuries (13 per cent) (National Safety Council, 1975).

As previously noted, between 1950 and 1969, there was a dramatic increase in female deaths following motor vehicle accidents, particularly for white females between the ages of 15 and 24 years, when the death rate increased 83 per cent. Possibly because the opportunity to ride or drive motor vehicles was less for nonwhite females in this age group, their rate of increase in the same period was one half that for white women (National Safety Council, 1975).

With further changes in social habits and more active roles for women in the post World War II period, women were and are being increasingly exposed to the hazards of accidental injuries traditionally associated with the male population. This exposure has primarily occurred in the childbearing years. It naturally follows that the vast majority of such active women do not curtail their lifestyles solely because of the possibility of pregnancy, and they continue to drive and remain active until late in the third trimester.

THE IMPORTANCE OF INJURIES PRIOR TO PREGNANCY

A natural concern is whether any pregestational trauma will affect labor, the birth process, or the life of the fetus. Injuries to the bony pelvis, uterus, adnexae, and vagina have the potential to influence a normal labor and a vaginal delivery.

Injuries to Reproductive Organs

Trauma to the normal nongravid female pelvic viscera, particularly blunt trauma, is exceedingly rare. It was reported in 1961 that no textbook up to that time had recorded a nonpenetrating injury to the nonpregnant uterus, and this record apparently continues (Dyer and Barclay, 1962). The uterus, tubes, and ovaries remain well protected in the true pelvis from all but the penetrating injury, and even these are uncommon. In one major trauma center with over 100,000 Emergency Room visits annually, only 17 penetrating injuries in non-pregnant females were seen in a 10 year period. All were gunshot wounds. The uterus was the most frequently involved organ. However, some extragenital pathology was present in 70 per cent of the patients. Injuries to other abdominal organs occurred in two thirds of these patients, most commonly involving the small bowel. Eight of 14 patients later become pregnant, the majority having live birth deliveries via the vaginal route (Quast and Jordan, 1964).

Pelvic Fractures

The only traumatic injury prior to pregnancy and the onset of labor that is likely to be a problem is one that involves the bony elements of the pelvis. While the female pelvis has been considered more fragile than the male pelvis and is fractured with less force, it is reported that forces between 400 and 2600 pounds are required to disrupt it. Simple nondisplaced fractures are no threat to sub-sequent normal labor. It is the distortion of the pelvic inlet and outlet that is critical. Lateral crushing injuries distort the inlet while fractures of the pubis and ischial rami, from anteroposterior forces, compromise the outlet (Buchsbaum, 1974). Disruption of the sacroiliac joints is invariably followed by distortion and serious compromise of the inlet and outlet. Anatomic realignment of pelvic bones in such instances is most difficult and usually unsuccessful. Devastating pelvic fractures are usually seen among pedestrians struck by moving vehicles. In one large study 25 per cent of pelvic fractures were sustained by pedestrians and 40 per cent of these were associated with multiple fractures. The frequency of related lower urinary tract injuries varies from 3 to 21 per cent, but vaginal and uterine injuries are exceedingly rare from the pelvic injuries alone.

The ultimate effect of pelvic fractures upon subsequent labor and survival varies considerably (Levine and Crampton, 1963). In one review, live births followed pelvic fractures in 78 per cent of women, with 52 per cent having vaginal deliveries. However, cesarean sections were necessary more often when the injury occurred prior to pregnancy (Speer and Peltier, 1972). Apparently only 10 per cent of women who sustain pelvic fractures will require a later cesarean section by reason of the fracture alone (Dyer and Barclay, 1962).

Other Injuries

Pregestational injuries to the perineum rarely affect subsequent pregnan-cy and normal birth. Lacerations to the vagina or urethra from straddle acci-dents, sexual activity, and foreign bodies rarely interfere with fertility or birth.

INJURIES DURING THE COURSE OF
PREGNANCY

Spontaneous Visceral Injuries

While controversial, spontaneous ruptures of abdominal organs, particularly the spleen and liver, have been described by numerous authors. Generally the suggestion of a spontaneous rupture is based on the inability of the patient to recall any traumatic episode. Predisposing factors have been suggested. The following have been implicated in splenic rupture: multiparity, hypertension, angiitis, hypervolemia, and splenomegaly. The vascular lesions of toxemia and eclampsia are suggested as predisposing factors in ruptures of these livers. Probably fewer than 100 instances have been found in the world literature in each instance (Buchsbaum, 1974).

Frequency of Accidental Injury

The accident rate for a large group of women followed in one prenatal clinic during a three month period before pregnancy through delivery was 9.6 per cent. The rate for the same group during the gestation period itself dropped to 6.9 per cent. The three major causes of these injuries were vehicular accidents, falls, and piercing instruments. Surprisingly, there was no greater frequency of injuries in any trimester (see below). The majority of injuries sustained were sprains, lacerations, and fractures or dislocations (Peckham and King, 1963). Importantly, deaths from such accidental injuries during pregnancy account for the majority (22 per cent) of nonobstetric deaths and are at least equal in frequency to deaths from toxemia. Despite this high rate, the true incidence of injuries among pregnant women is actually unknown (Stiffman, 1976).

Early in the first trimester, trauma probably has no adverse effect on the course of pregnancy. The association of external trauma with abortion has long been debated but undoubtedly is rare; probably the rate is as low as 0.007 per cent. The weight of clinical evidence suggests pathology in the ovum or in implantation as a cause for the abortion in the vast majority of instances, not external injury (Buchsbaum, 1968).

Although the gravid uterus emerging from the pelvis becomes a greater target for blunt and penetrating injuries, it still serves as a protective shield against damage to the bowel and great vessels of the mother. Similarly, the fluid-filled amniotic sac acts as a shock absorber against injury to the fetus. Nevertheless, as the pregnancy progresses into the last trimester, the likelihood of some type of injury, usually minor and frequently not involving the uterus and its contents, increases. The pregnant woman finds ambulation awkward and her body unstable. Her inability at times to see obstructions, imbalance caused by a shift in her center of gravity, and slowness in taking evasive action all make the threat of an accident quite real. A major factor in this setting is the even greater vulnerability of the infant, particularly to injuries which disrupt the urine wall or penetrate the uterine cavity.

The occurrence rate for minor trauma tends to increase in each succeeding trimester. In one study 9 per cent of accidents occurred in the first, 40 per cent in the second, and over 50 per cent in the third trimester. However, these authors suggested that noncatastrophic trauma does not significantly increase perinatal mortality (Fork and Harlin, 1970).

Since one of the major threats to pregnant women is from blunt abdominal trauma during a motor vehicle accident, considerable attention has been directed at an evaluation of various mechanisms to protect the pregnant woman as a driver or as a passenger (see Chapter 6). The evidence seems to suggest that a majority of belted mothers could survive major collisons if properly restrained (American Medical Association, 1972). Irrespective of the type of restraint systems used (lap belt or shoulder harness) the fetal loss is apparently about the same if the mother is not ejected from the vehicle. It is noteworthy that in one report, unrestrained pregnant women sustained a 33 per cent mortality when ejection from the vehicle occurred, whereas the fatality rate was only 5 per cent in those who were not ejected (American Medical Association, 1972; Crosby et al., 1972).

ESTABLISHING AN INITIATIVE IN THE CARE OF ACCIDENTAL INJURIES

With some understanding of the scope of the problem of trauma and accidental injury in the United States, it is appropriate to explore briefly the status of the immediate care of the sick and injured as it existed in the late 1950's and to recount the initiatives taken by the health professions, the government, and the public to meet the challenge of this "neglected disease."

The two most important deficiencies seemed to exist with ambulance services and with care rendered in hospital emergency departments. The prehospital care of the acutely ill and injured had deteriorated dramatically during and following World War II. By the 1960's it was quite apparent that the medical profession had neglected this link in health care.

Ambulance Service

In the mid-1960's funeral homes were still operating nearly one half of the ambulance services. Volunteer groups managed 24 per cent of emergency vehicles and commercial organizations or Fire and Police Departments, 14 per cent and 13 per cent, respectively. Only 3 per cent of the ambulance services studied in 37 states were hospital-operated, which had been a common arrangement prior to World War II. The vehicles operated were station wagons (24 per cent) or hearses (21 per cent). Only 5 percent of these units were equipped to communicate directly with hospital emergency departments (Huntley, 1971).

The equipment carried by emergency vehicles was equally disturbing; only one third met the *minimal* equipment standards of the American College of Surgeons (American College of Surgeons, 1970; Huntley, 1971). Forty-six per cent of ambulance services could not guarantee that two attendants would service every emergency call.

Likewise, the training of the attendants seemed spotty and adequate only for limited emergencies. While 5 per cent of attendants had no training whatsoever, 62 per cent did have advanced Red Cross First Aid or more formal education and 33 per cent had standard Red Cross instruction. There were no accepted standards for competence or training of ambulance attendants. Certification or licensure was a rarity. In many cities and towns the only requirement to serve on ambulance duty was a driver's license.

The degree of application of even the limited skills of attendants was in serious doubt. One study reported that only 0.16 per cent of seriously injured survivors received any first aid when transported by ambulance following automobile accidents to one emergency room in a major city (Lougheed, 1965). Another assessment of 159 traffic deaths suggested that 18 per cent of victims were "salvageable" if proper resuscitation measures had been conducted at the scene or in transit (Frey et al., 1969). When questioned in the national survey, however, 78 per cent of ambulance services were stating that first aid was rendered routinely at the scene of the emergency! There was little evidence that the immediate care rendered at the scene of a medical emergency was either adequate or of suitable quality.

Emergency Department Services

By 1960 the hospital Emergency Department was becoming the community's center for outpatient care, but fewer than one third of cases seen were true emergencies. A major concern of many experts was the care available in the Emergency Departments. One leader in the field declared in 1955, "There is little doubt in my mind that the weakest link in the chain of hospital care in most hospitals in this country is the emergency room attention to the injured" (Kennedy, 1955). He pointed out that delays in management and lack of professional expertise were major problems. The average delay for admission to the hospital after arrival in the Emergency Room was two and one half hours in one study (Skudder et al., 1961). It was obvious that changes were also necessary in the Emergency Services rendered at the hospital door.

According to the 1971 survey report only 17 per cent of hospitals had a licensed physician in the Emergency Department or on duty and available within the hospital on a 24 hour basis (Huntley, 1971). Many facilities rotated Emergency Department call among all specialists, without considerations of training or experience. One experienced expert, after observing the care of casualties in Vietnam, was forced to admit that the injured combat soldier was getting better care under military physicians. "Were he hit on a highway near his hometown, even if he were struck immediately outside the Emergency Room of most United States hospitals, rarely would he be given such prompt. expert operative care as routinely as furnished from the site of combat wounding in Vietnam" (Eiseman, 1967).

The Initiative

Concerned over the increasing death rate from trauma and the lack of professional and public concern, several groups of distinguished physicians (mainly members of the American College of Surgeons and the American Academy of Orthopaedic Surgeons) began an effort during this period to focus more attention on the inadequate care of the injured

From these multiple origins a national movement developed in Emergency

Health Care which terminated not only in major Federal legislation but also in statutes and regulations at all levels of state and local government. Indeed, the health system of the country was altered extensively to accommodate new thrusts and technology in the provision of pre–hospital emergency health services. Acutely aware of the growing morbidity and mortality from accidental injury, the National Academy's original Committees of Trauma and Shock formed several task forces of experts, including engineers, ambulance operators, and physicians, to study (among other elements) ambulance design and services, voice radio communications, and the medical care in emergency departments. Seemingly at no other time in the recorded history of the care of the injured in the United States were the talents of so many professional experts continuously engaged in a more pragmatic national effort to influence government action.

Two conferences generated by these efforts can be singled out for their contributions to the movement for more governmental action. The first was the Airlie Conference of May 1969, sponsored by the American College of Surgeons and the American Academy of Orthopaedic Surgeons. The 52 attendees at this meeting voted unanimously to urge the establishment of a Presidential Commission to evaluate and recommend improvements in emergency health services (American College of Surgeons, 1969). The second of these efforts to influence high level (i.e., Presidential) action was a telegram to President Richard M. Nixon from the participants in the Second National Conference on Emergency Health Services sponsored by the Division of Emergency Health Services of the U.S. Public Health Service in December of 1971. President Nixon was asked to mobilize resources and stimulate support for Emergency Medical Care (Huntley, 1971).

President Nixon's response was a call for a new program in technological research and development in Emergency Health Services. This was contained in his State of the Union Message the following January. His only positive action was the establishment of five demonstration Emergency Medical Systems with $8 million as proposed by the Health Services and Mental Health Administration in the Department of Health, Education, and Welfare. These "pilot" emergency service projects developed in Illinois, Arkansas, Ohio, Florida (Jacksonville), and California (San Diego), and demonstrated the life-saving effectiveness of a systematized community service for the acutely ill and injured. However, it remained for the Congress to take the final productive action. Through the efforts of Congressman Paul G. Rogers (Fla.) and Senator Edward M. Kennedy (Mass.), the House and Senate held several hearings in 1972, and the 93rd Congress responded with Public Law 93–154 in the following year (U.S. House of Representatives, 1972).

With the recognition that immediate care in all medical emergencies was an even more basic national problem, the Academy of Sciences had, in 1967, formed a Committee on Emergency Medical Services to lay further groundwork for rules, regulations, and standards. This committee was to implement some of the recommendations contained in the 1966 report on "Accidental Death and Disability" (Howard, 1974). Contracts were signed with the Departments of Transportation and Health, Education, and Welfare to develop standards and guidelines for ambulance designs, equipment, and services. Within a few months a series of documents were developed (National Academy of Sciences, 1970*a, b, c*).

Three vehicle designs (including equipment) were ultimately proposed by the Department of Transportation for emergency ambulances in 1970. A training curriculum was also developed for Emergency Medical Technicians (the new designation for the former ambulance "attendants") and published by the Academy in 1970(*b*).

These and other documents were adopted (with some refinements) by the National Highway Safety Bureau of the Department of Transportation and the Division of Emergency Health Services of the U.S. Public Health Service.

Another major step in the attempt to improve the management of the injured during this period was the evolution of a "systems" concept for emergency medical care. This concept was ultimately embodied as the central theme of the Emergency Medical Services Act. The law identified 15 dimensions necessary for regional or area-wide emergency medical services (Table 1–6) and emphasized that for such federal funding, an area-wide or regional "system" was necessary. Important in the evolution of systematization of emergency care were a number of landmark developments during the preceding decade.

The first such landmark was the recognition that trauma, as an endemic health problem, was deserving of a concentration of clinical medical expertise, i.e., of special facilities, with physicians, nurses, and technicians especially trained in the care of the injured. Usually coupled with these clinical programs were basic scientific investigations. Not surprisingly, the stimulus for this modernized approach to the injured had its origin in the military setting.

The first of several such modern "trauma units" was the Burn Unit established by the U.S. Army at Brooke Army Medical Center (Texas) in 1950. This was a natural outgrowth of the military's experience in World War II; general hospitals were established for the care of vascular injuries, hand problems, and major fractures. The burn center quickly demonstrated the effectiveness in the "clinical unit" approach to the care of such catastrophic injuries. The roles of wound infection and renal failure as threats to the survival of these patients were studied extensively, and gradual reductions in morbidity and mortality followed.

Ultimately, considerable interest in clinical research in the civilian sector was also generated, principally by the ever-increasing rate of major and multiple systems injuries incurred in high-speed automobile accidents.

The first of these non-military trauma centers was a "pilot" clinical Shock-Trauma Unit established at the University of Maryland in 1961 (Cowley, 1970). This was followed by the first federally financed Trauma Research Center at

TABLE 1–6   Elements in an Emergency Medical Service System*

1. Professional resources	9. Policies regarding ability to pay
2. Professional training	10. Critical care and rehabilitation
3. Communications	11. Record keeping
4. Transportation	12. Public education
5. Categorization of medical facilities	13. Evaluation
6. A patient referral pattern	14. Disaster program
7. Utilization of agencies	15. Reciprocity agreements
8. Consumer representation	

*Emergency Medical Service Systems Act (P.L. 93–154) of 1973.

Columbia–Presbyterian Medical Center in New York in 1966. By 1971, the National Institute of General Medical Sciences, in the Department of Health, Education, and Welfare, had funded eight such research centers in selected teaching hospitals throughout the country (Black and Deming, 1974). This was to lead to a multidisciplinary approach to the care of the injured within strategically located community hospitals.

The "center" concept was subsequently to evolve further into a categorization of all emergency capabilities of Community Hospitals; an effort formalized by a conference and a publication by the American Medical Association in 1971 (American Medical Association, 1971). Ultimately the well publicized "Illinois" plan for a statewide system of trauma centers became a natural outgrowth of this concept (Boyd, 1973). Within one year of its establishment Illinois authorities noted that despite a 27 per cent increase in highway accidents and 16 per cent increase in the number of injured, the ratio of deaths per injuries declined from 2.8 per cent to 2.1 per cent. The percentage of accident victims dying in the first hours also was reported to have decreased by 14 per cent.

A second major development was the recognition that coordination of many existing community agencies was necessary to provide more effective pre–hospital emergency services.

From this need grew the obvious political necessity of establishing Community Councils or Committees on Emergency Medical and Health Services with appropriate representatives from Governmental Agencies, hospitals, county medical societies, ambulance organizations, and other agencies. The American Medical Association in 1966 published a set of guidelines for such councils (American Medical Association, 1966). The Community Council became a requirement for funding under the Emergency Medical Services Act of 1973, and by 1976 there were 500 such councils throughout the country (Farrington, 1977).

A third step in the evolution of systems approach to Emergency Medical Care was the final publication by federal agencies of standards suggested by the committees of the National Academy of Sciences. These included criteria for Emergency Medical Service vehicles, their equipment, the training of EMT's, and communications requirements. Adoption of certain standards was made mandatory within the National Highway Act and issued as a regulation for Federal Funding of State Highway programs by the Department of Transportation in 1967.

These rules required that states receiving such federal monies develop regional plans for Emergency Medical Services using the published standards. Hospitals were to be selected on the basis of their capabilities in handling highway accidents. The penalty for failing to develop such a program was the loss of 10 per cent of the federal subsidy for a state's Highway Safety program. While such penalties were not evoked, the threat had a desirable stimulus.

The requirement of voice radio communications equipment under the Highway Safety Standards was further reinforced by the establishment by the Federal Communications Commission of "dedicated" radio frequencies for Emergency Medical Services in 1972. (These are contained in Subpart P, "Special Emergency Radio Service," Section 89,503, of the Commission's rules.) Thus, ambulance and hospital services were fully recognized, along with the police and fire departments, as significant elements in a community's emergency response. Subsequently, new VHF and UHF frequencies were assigned in several scattered bands to hospitals, emergency vehicles, physician paging systems, and biological telemetry systems.

A fourth landmark was the recognition that a Regional Communications or Operations Center for Medical Emergencies was required to permit a continuous interface with all elements meeting community emergency needs (American Medical Association, 1966). A direct outgrowth of the multipurpose Emergency Operations Center concept was the "911" telephone number as proposed by the American Telephone and Telegraph Company in 1968. Slow to evolve, despite worldwide usage, a toll-free, easily remembered code number such as "911" has still to improve the response of Emergency Services nationwide despite its inclusion in the Emergency Medical Services System Act of 1973.

The dispatching of emergency ambulances and the provision of professional guidance by radio by hospital-based physicians to Emergency Medical Technicians enroute to their emergency departments became a recognized need in rural as well as many urban areas.

A final step in the evolution of Emergency Medical Systems, as proposed under the Federal legislation, was the success of the previously mentioned demonstration systems established by the Health Services and Mental Health Administration in 1972. Despite many problems, the Illinois Trauma Program ("a systems approach to the care of the critically injured") was the most outstanding of these demonstrations, particularly as it had the enthusiastic support of a concerned and interested governor (Boyd. 1973).

Importantly, considerable clinical information supporting the establishment of regionalized Emergency Medical Care Systems was already beginning to evolve by 1972 when the House and Senate Subcommittees of the Congress began the hearings that were to lead to the Emergency Medical Services Act of 1973. Such legislation was to provide, according to Congressman Paul Rogers, "the missing link in the nation's total health system" (U.S. House of Representatives, 1972).

EPILOGUE

The National Academy's nine recommendations for improvements in the care of accidental deaths and disabilities, as expressed in 1966, were comprehensive and far reaching (National Academy of Sciences, 1966). Many have yet to be implemented. Nevertheless, it seems appropriate to review briefly, in closing, their context and assess the 10 year results.

The original report urged the formation of a *National Council on Accident Prevention* to coordinate information and implementation of preventive measures. *Basic and advanced first aid training* was to be extended to the lay population. *Ambulance services* were to have standardized, well-equipped vehicles, regulated by laws, and coordinated among community agencies. Pilot programs to evaluate physician-staffed ambulances and helicopter services were suggested. It was advised that *communications* be improved by assignment of radiofrequency channels for interagency transmissions and a single nationwide telephone number established to summon emergency aid. *Emergency Departments* were to be surveyed and patterns of number, types, and locations were to be established for optimal care. Categorization and accreditation processes were to be initiated, with regular inspections. Funds were requested to design and construct model emergency facilities. *Trauma Registries* were suggested for selected hospitals to study the natural history of trauma supported by a national registry that designated certain injuries as reportable diseases. *Routine autopsies* were considered important in the analysis of the accidental deaths. *Trauma Committees* were urged on a pilot basis in selected hospitals and studies on rehabilitation and a plan for the quantitation of degrees of disability were proposed. Other suggestions were studies of *medico-legal problems*, the care of *casualties in natural disasters*, and the need for *research in trauma* (Jackson, 1967).

Looking back over the process since the Academy's report, the President of the American Association for the Surgery of Trauma, Dr. Joseph D. Farrington, declared in 1976 that "the war goes on." Dr. Farrington noted some progress in emergency medical services despite uncertain and "parsimonious" federal funding. Besides the many documents on ambulances, training of EMT's, equipment and communication, he commended the new guidelines and assessment of Emergency Services developed by the Department of Transportation as it tested the effectiveness of the eight demonstration projects (Farrington, 1977).

Farrington conducted a survey and received replies from 46 states, plus Puerto Rico and the District of Columbia, The majority of states had made some major efforts to reduce serious accidents on their highways, particularly with roadside improvements. However, while unsafe drivers were being refused licenses, the use of restraint systems and protections still was not legislated Only one state and the District of Columbia have 100 per cent of their populations covered by a single entry phone number but 43 per cent of the population in 37 states were covered by some form of an ambulance dispatch system number. While 46 states have Emergency Medical Service Councils, the effectiveness of local councils ("where the action is") was questioned. Ambulance legislation was now effective in 26 states but only 52 per cent of all ambulances operating met Federal Standards. However, the proportion of funeral homes in the ambulance business had dropped to 15 per cent (from 44 per cent), largely because of the minimum wage law and training requirements.

Dr. Farrington also noted that 200,000 persons had graduated from the 81 hour basic training course for EMT's, but could find no evidence that a majority of these were actively engaged in ambulance services. Seventeen of 28 states still had no regulations regarding training. Many did not require licensing of volunteer EMT's, though this is the largest single group of ambulance operators. While reportedly there were 9465 paramedics as well, most of their advanced training was in the management of heart attacks. The courses were finally altered to include the management of major injuries. Communications between ambulances and hospitals were still limited to 62 per cent of the services and were as infrequent as 15 per cent in one state.

Categorization of emergency capabilities among hospitals was never well received and was accomplished in only 27 states; allegedly the vast majority of facilities were still in the "Basic Category" on a scale of Basic, General, Major, and Comprehensive Emergency Service capabilities.

Farrington's major concern was the lack of solid evidence that accidental deaths were actually decreasing, particularly those resulting from motor vehicle accidents, which were still the major cause of deaths from injury in persons under 75 years of age.

In conclusion, Farrington emphasized the need for more public education, more involvement by physicians in EMS Systems, more physician interaction with Emergency Medical Technicians, and a general awareness that death and disability were both preventable and manageable.

There is no question that vast strides have been made in the care of the injured, and there is every evidence that the concept of a systems approach to emergency care of the injured is progressing. It is hoped that the management of injuries among pregnant women will benefit from this progress and that this book will prove of value to all who treat the injured.

REFERENCES

American College of Surgeons, Committee on Trauma: Minimal equipment for ambulances. Bull Am Coll Surg 57:92, 1967.

American College of Surgeons, Committee on Trauma: essential equipment for ambulances. Bull Am Coll Surg 55:7, 1970.

American College of Surgeons: Emergency Medical Services: Recommendations for an Approach to an Urgent National Problem. Proceedings of the Airlie Conference on Emergency Medical Services. Chicago, American Academy of Orthopaedic Surgeons, 1969.

American Medical Association, Commission on Emergency Medical Services: Developing Emergency Medical Services — Guidelines for Community Councils. Chicago, American Medical Association, 1966.

American Medical Association, Commission on Emergency Medical Services: Recommendations of the Conference on the Guidelines for the Categorization of Hospital Emergency Capabilities. Chicago, American Medical Association, 1971.

American Medical Association, Committee on the Medical Aspects of Automotive Safety: Automobile safety belts during pregnancy. JAMA 221:20, 1972.

Alffram PA, Bauer GCH: Epidemiology of fractures of the forearm: a biomechanical investigation of bone strength J Bone Joint Surg [Am] 44A:105, 1962.

Artz, CP: Acute illness and injury in the United States. *In* Jelenko C, Frey CF (Eds): Emergency Medical Services: An Overview. Bowie, Maryland, RJ Brady Company, 1976.

Black E, Deming PA: The Injured Patients: A Trauma Conference Report. Bethesda, Maryland, National Institute of General Medical Sciences, Department of Health, Education and Welfare Publication, No. (NIH) 74–603, 1974.

Boyd DR: A symposium on the Illinois Trauma Program: a systems approach to the care of the critically injured. J Trauma 13:275, 1973.

Buchsbaum HJ: Traumatic injury in pregnancy. *In* Barber HRK, Graber EA: Surgical Diseases in Pregnancy. Philadelphia, WB Saunders Company, 1974.

Buchsbaum HJ: Accidental injury complicating pregnancy. Am J Obstet Gynecol 102:752, 1968.

Crowley RA: Today's Neglected Disease — Trauma. Center for Study of Trauma (Pamphlet). Baltimore, University of Maryland, 1970.

Crosby WM, King AI, Stout LC: Fetal survival following impact: improvement with shoulder harness restraint. Am J Obstet Gynecol 112:1101, 1972.

Doublin LI: Fact Book on Trauma. New York, Macmillan Company, 1965.

DuVal MK: The Hidden Crisis in Health Care. Proceedings of the Second National Conference on Emergency Health Services, Dec. 2–4, 1971. Washington DC, US Public Health Service, Division of Emergency Health Services, US Government Printing Office, 1972.

Dyer I, Barclay DL: Accidental trauma complicating pregnancy and delivery. Am J Obstet Gynecol 83:907, 1962.

Eiseman B: Battle casualty management in Vietnam. J Trauma 7:53, 1967.

Farrington JD: The war goes on. 1976 Presidential address: American Association for the Surgery of Trauma. J Trauma 17:655, 1977.

Fitts WJ, Jr: Men for the care of the injured: a crisis facing the 70's. Bull Am Coll Surg 55:9, 1970.

Fitts WT Jr, Lehr HB, Bitner RL, Spellman JW: An analysis of 950 fatal injuries. Surgery 56:663, 1964.

Fork AT, Harlin RS: Pregnancy outcome after noncatastrophic maternal trauma during pregnancy. Am J Obstet Gynecol 25:912, 1970.

Frey CF, Huelke DF, Gikas PW: Resuscitation and survival in motor accidents. J Trauma 9:292, 1969.

Gibson G, Bugbee G, Anderson OW: Emergency Medical Services in the Chicago Area. University of Chicago, Center for Health Administration Studies, 1970.

Greenblatt M, Schuckit MA: Alcoholism: Problems in Women and Children. New York, Grune & Stratton, 1976.

Haddon W, Jr, Baker SP: Injury Control. Washington DC, Insurance Institute for Highway Safety, 1978.

Hampton OP, Jr: Present status of ambulance services in the United States. Bull Am Coll Surg 50:177, 1965.

Hampton OP, Jr: Transportation of the injured: a report. Bull Am Coll Surg 45:55, 1960.

Howard JM: Definitive life support at the scene of an emergency. Para-Medical J 6:17, 1974.

Huntley HD: National status of emergency health services. In Ambulance Services and Hospital Emergency Departments: Digest of Surveys Conducted 1965 to 1971. Rockville, Maryland, US Department of Health, Education, and Welfare, US Public Health Service, Division of Emergency Health Services, 1971.

Jackson FC: Report on the Feasibility of Establishing a National Research and Informational Center for Emergency Disaster Medical Services. Task Force on Medical Disaster Surveys. Washington DC, Committee on Trauma, Division of Medical Sciences, National Academy of Sciences, National Research Council, 1967 (unpublished report).

Kennedy RH: Our fashionable killer, oration on Trauma. Bull Am Coll Surg 40:73, 1955.

Levine JI, Crampton RS: Major abdominal injuries associated with pelvic fractures. Surg Gynec Obstet 116:223, 1963.

Lougheed JC: Current status of emergency treatment in automobile accidents: with recommendations to professional and civilian personnel. South Med J 58:1083, 1965.

National Academy of Sciences, National Research Council, Commitee on Ambulance Design Criteria: Ambulance Design Criteria. A report to the National Highway Safety Bureau of Federal Highway Administration, US Department of Transportation. Washington DC, US Government Printing Office, 1970a.

National Academy of Sciences, National Research Council, Division of Medical Sciences, Committee on Emergency Medical Services: Advanced Training Program for Emergency Medical Technicians — Ambulance. US Department of Health, Education, and Welfare, HSM, 72–2007. Washington DC, National Academy of Sciences, 1970b.

National Academy of Sciences, National Research Council, Division of Medical Sciences, Committee on Emergency Medical Services: Medical Requirements for Ambulance Design and Equipment. US Public Health Service Publication 1071–C–3, Washington DC, US Government Printing Office, 1970c.

National Academy of Sciences, National Research Council: Accidental Death and Disability: The Neglected Disease of Modern Society. Washington DC, National Academy of Sciences, 1966.

National Safety Council: Accident Facts. 1975 Edition. Chicago, National Safety Council, 1975.

NEISS Data Highlights: Hazard Information and Analysis. US Consumer Product Safety Commission, March–May, 1977.

Peckman CH, King RW: A study of intercurrent conditions observed during pregnancy. Am J Obstet Gynecol 87:609, 1963.

Quast DC, Jordan GL: Traumatic wounds of the female reproductive organs. J Trauma 4:839, 1964.

Schlueter CF: Some economic dimensions of traumatic injuries. J Trauma 10:915, 1970.

Skudder PA, McCarroll JR, Wade PA: Hospital emergency facilities and services: a survey. Bull Am Coll Surg 46:44, 1961.

Skudder PA: An experiment in evaluating the management of trauma. Bull Am Coll Surg 46:42, 1961.

Speer DP, Peltier LF: Pelvis fractures and pregnancy. J Trauma 12:474, 1972.

Stiffman L: The impact of injuries on the medical system. In Frey CF (Ed): Initial Management of the Trauma Patient. Philadelphia, Lea & Febiger, 1976.

US Department of Commerce: Statistical Abstract of the United States 1974. 95th Annual Edition. Washington DC, US Department of Commerce, Bureau of the Census, 1974.

US House of Representatives: Hearings Before the Subcommittee on Public Health and Environment of the Committee on Interstate and Foreign Commerce. 92nd Congress, June 13–15, 1972, Serial No. 92–83. Washington DC, US Government Printing Office, 1972.

US Public Health Service: Age Patterns in Medical Care, Illness and Disability United States, 1968–69. Data from National Health Survey, Series 10, No. 70. Washington DC, US Public Health Service, Health Services and Mental Health Administration, National Center for Health Statistics, US Government Printing Office, 1972.

US Public Health Service: Mortality Trend for Leading Causes of Death United States, 1950–69. Vital and Health Statistics Data from the National Vital Statistics System, Series 20, No. 16. Washington DC, US Public Health Service, Health Services Administration, US Government Printing Office, 1974.

World Health Organization: The home environment. *In* Health Hazards of the Human Environment. Geneva, World Health Organization, 1972.

Waller JA: Non-highway injury fatalities. I. The roles of alcohol and problem drinking, drugs, and medical impairment. J Chronic Dis 25:33, 1972.

Yarborough RW: Accidental injury: a major challenge to medicine. J Trauma 10:1010. 1970.

Chapter 2

ANATOMIC AND PHYSIOLOGIC ALTERATIONS OF PREGNANCY THAT MODIFY THE RESPONSE TO TRAUMA

Dwight P. Cruikshank

Pregnancy is associated with marked physiologic and anatomic changes in nearly every organ system of the body. Although these alterations are normal and necessary to meet the needs of the developing fetus and prepare the mother for parturition, their manifestations may resemble changes that in the nonpregnant woman would be indicative of pathologic states. Furthermore, the altered physiologic and anatomic relationships may change the pattern of injury or disease, and in many instances necessitate modifications in therapy. Finally, many laboratory values are altered by the physiologic state of pregnancy.

Therefore, the physician attending a pregnant trauma victim must keep in mind several complicating factors, including the following:

1. The fact that the patient is pregnant may alter the pattern or severity of the injury.

2. The pregnancy may alter the signs and symptoms of the injury, and the results of laboratory tests used in diagnosis.

3. The management of the trauma victim needs to be modified to accommodate and preserve the physiologic changes induced by pregnancy.

4. The injury may have initiated or have been complicated by pathologic conditions peculiar to pregnancy (e.g., abruptio placentae, amniotic fluid embolism, ruptured uterus), or a pregnancy-related disease may occur coincidental to trauma and thus complicate the diagnosis and therapy (e.g., eclampsia complicating possible head trauma).

The purpose of this chapter is to review the anatomic and physiologic changes which the physician must understand to properly care for the traumatized pregnant woman.

CARDIOVASCULAR SYSTEM

Cardiac Output

Until recently it was thought that cardiac output increased gradually throughout pregnancy until 30 to 32 weeks, after which it declined to nearly nonpregnant levels at term (Burwell et al., 1938). Through the use of better techniques for measuring cardiac output, coupled with the recognition of the effects of maternal position (see below), it is now known that cardiac output rises by 1.0 to 1.5 L/min during the first 10 weeks of pregnancy to a level of 6.0 to 7.0 L/min, and this level is subsequently maintained until delivery (Walters et al., 1966; Lees et al., 1967; Ueland et al., 1969; Hytten and Lind, 1973).

With regard to the pregnant trauma victim, the crucial information on cardiac output is the effect of maternal position. It has been shown that when a woman in late pregnancy assumes the supine position, the inferior vena cava is almost completely occluded by the enlarged uterus (Kerr et al., 1964). Thus, venous return to the heart is diminished, and cardiac output falls. Ueland and co-workers (1969) have demonstrated that turning a pregnant woman from the supine to the lateral recumbent position will increase cardiac output 8 per cent at 20 to 24 weeks' gestation, 13.6 per cent at 28 to 32 weeks, and 28.5 per cent at term. Cardiac output is unchanged by the lateral recumbent position in nonpregnant women. The fall in cardiac output associated with the supine position occurs in all pregnant women, secondary to compression of the inferior vena cava. It is greater in some women than others, however, and is probably related to variations in the adequacy of collateral systems (azygos and vertebral veins) for maintaining venous return to the heart. Most pregnant women are able to maintain their blood pressure at normal levels in the supine position by increasing peripheral vascular resistance to compensate for lowered cardiac output (Lees et al., 1967), and in fact arterial blood pressure is usually slightly lower in the lateral recumbent than in the supine position (Schwarz, 1964; Trower and Walters, 1968). However, some women develop profound hypotension in the supine position (Lees et al., 1967), the "supine hypotensive syndrome," which is completely alleviated by turning to the lateral position.

There is evidence from animal studies that inferior vena cava occlusion may cause placental abruption by increasing the venous pressure in the intervillous space. Whether this can occur in humans as a result of lying in the supine position is controversial (Howard and Goodson, 1953; Mengert et al., 1953; Buchsbaum, 1968).

Nevertheless, it is apparent that in the pregnant trauma victim the supine position must be avoided. The patient should be kept on her left side whenever possible during diagnostic and therapeutic procedures. When this is not possible, as during laparotomy, the uterus should be displaced to the left, off the vena cava, with a uterine displacer bar attached to the operating table (Fig. 2–1). If this is not available, the table should be tilted 15 to 20 degrees to the left, or folded sheets should be placed under the patient's right hip and flank to rotate her body to this extent.

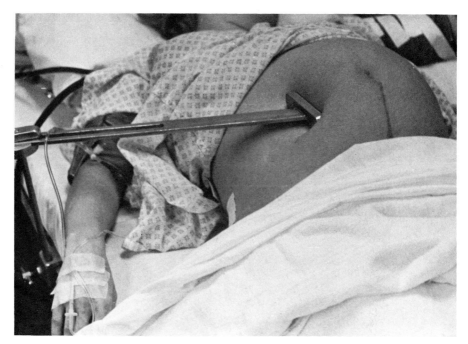

Figure 2-1   The uterine displacer in position during preparation for surgery.

Heart Rate

Tachycardia is a cardinal sign of diminished effective circulating blood volume, whether from hemorrhagic or from other types of shock. When measuring heart rate in the pregnant trauma victim for evaluation of blood loss or for monitoring fluid replacement, it is important to remember that pregnancy is associated with a physiologic tachycardia. Heart rate increases throughout pregnancy, reaching a maximum in the third trimester, when it is 15 to 20 beats/min above nonpregnant levels (Schwarz, 1964; Walters et al., 1966). Thus, normal heart rate in late pregnancy is 80 to 95 beats/min. This is true during the sleeping as well as the waking states (Hytten and Lind 1973).

Blood Pressure

In normal pregnancy the systolic and diastolic blood pressures fall 5 to 15 mm Hg during the second trimester, and then rise to nonpregnant levels near term. MacGillivray and co-workers (1969) evaluated serially 226 normal patients throughout pregnancy, and found the following average blood pressures: nonpregnant, 110/70; 16 to 28 weeks, 102/55; 35 to 40 weeks, 108/67. Pressure is usually highest when the patient is seated, intermediate when supine, and lowest when lying on the side. The exception to this is the supine hypotensive syndrome (see above).

Blood pressure greater than that of nonpregnant levels is never normal during pregnancy, and signifies either a possible pregnancy complication (toxemia) or a response to stress (anxiety, trauma).

Venous Pressure

Peripheral venous pressure in the upper extremities is unchanged by pregnancy, but there is progessive rise in venous pressure in the legs secondary to compression of the inferior vena cava by the uterus. At term, femoral venous pressure is 25 cm H_2O (McLennan, 1943), and this elevation in lower extremity venous pressure can cause increased bleeding from leg wounds.

O'Driscoll and McCarthy (1966) found the average central venous pressure in the third trimester to be 8.1 cm H_2O (range, 4 to 12), compared to 3 6 cm H_2O (range, 2 to 5) in nonpregnant controls. If the circulation is full, infusion of 250 ml of fluid into a pregnant woman will raise the central venous pressure 3 to 4 cm H_2O, the same as for the nonpregnant state (Wilson, 1965). In a more recent study of true central venous pressure, Colditz and Josey (1970) reported a progressive fall in central venous pressure during pregnancy. In the third trimester the values were less than half of those of the nonpregnant controls.

Peripheral Blood Flow

Peripheral blood flow in pregnancy is greatly increased due to diminished peripheral vascular resistance. The usual response to stress or noxious stimuli in nonpregnant women is vasoconstriction. However, pregnant women, especially in the first and second trimesters, may react in these situations with peripheral vasodilation. This response is most marked in early pregnancy, and near term the vasoconstrictor response is again predominant (Dolezal and Figor, 1965). Whether this altered vascular reactivity is due to depression of sympathetic activity by estrogen (Lloyd and Pickford, 1961) or secondary to the depressed response to angiotensin seen in pregnant women (Chesley et al., 1963) is not known. Nevertheless, a pregnant woman in shock may not necessarily have cold, clammy skin, especially during the first two trimesters.

Electrocardiographic Changes

Electrocardiograms are frequently necessary in the evaluation of trauma patients, especially those with chest trauma. The normal electrocardiogram during pregnancy is altered because the heart is pushed upward and rotated forward by the elevated diaphragm. The electrical axis deviates to the left about 15 degrees (Hollander and Crawford, 1943), the T waves become flattened or inverted in lead III (Gemzell et al., 1957), and Q waves may appear in leads III and AVF (Burwell and Metcalfe, 1958). Ectopic beats, usually supraventricular, are more frequent during pregnancy.

VOLUME AND COMPOSITION OF BLOOD

Plasma and Erythrocyte Volume

The plasma volume of a pregnant woman begins to increase at about 10 weeks' gestation and thereafter increases rapidly until about 34 weeks, after which the continued increase is somewhat more gradual. The plasma volume increases about 50 per cent from nonpregnant levels of approximately 2600 ml to levels of 3900 to 4000 ml at term (Hytten and Paintin, 1963; Hytten and Leitch, 1971).

There is also a marked rise in erythrocyte volume, although not as great in magnitude as the rise in plasma volume. This increase begins at 10 weeks' gestation and continues progressively to term. Without iron supplementation, the erythrocyte volume of a healthy woman will increase from a nonpregnant level of about 1400 ml to about 1650 ml at term, an increase of 18 per cent (Hytten and Lind, 1973). With iron supplementation the erythrocyte volume will increase an average of 430 ml, or 32 per cent (Pritchard, 1965).

Because the increase in plasma volume is proportionally greater than the increase in erythrocyte volume, the hematocrit falls somewhat during gestation — the so-called "physiologic anemia" of pregnancy. The overall increase in blood volume averages 48 per cent, from 3250 ml in the nonpregnant state to 4820 ml at term. The individual variation in pregancy-induced blood volume increase is quite great, however, ranging from 20 per cent to 100 per cent of nonpregnant blood volume (Pritchard, 1965). It is quite important to remember that small women have smaller blood volumes in both the pregnant and nonpregnant states. Likewise, the patient with pregnancy-induced hypertension (toxemia) has a *contracted* plasma volume, and thus a diminished blood volume despite a normal or elevated hematocrit.

Pregnancy-induced hypervolemia has two important implications for the physician treating pregnant trauma victims. The protective effect of the hypervolemia allows some gravidas to lose 30 to 35 per cent of their blood volume before symptoms such as hypotension develop (Marx, 1965). On the other hand, it may be necessary to replace massive amounts of blood or fluid or both to a pregnant woman in shock before the vital signs return to normal. Monitoring central venous pressure is most helpful in these situations.

Red Blood Cell Indices

As a consequence of the differential rates of increase in plasma and erythrocyte volume (see above), the hematocrit and hemoglobin concentration decline during pregnancy, reaching their lowest values at 32 to 34 weeks, after which they rise somewhat. At 34 weeks, normal mean values for women not supplemented with iron are hematocrit, 32 to 34 per cent. and hemoglobin, 10.5 to 11 gm/dl. For women receiving iron supplementation the mean values for hematocrit and hemoglobin are 36 per cent and 12 gm/dl, respectively (Pitkin, 1977).

Leukocyte Indices

Acute hemorrhage induces a moderate leukocytosis, and after abdominal trauma a marked rise in leukocyte count can suggest rupture of the liver or spleen. Therefore, it is important to remember that pregnancy itself induces a leukocytosis (Table 2–1). This is most marked during the second and third trimesters, when leukocyte counts may range up to 18,000/cu mm, and during labor, when the count may reach 25,000/cu mm (Andrews and Bonsnes, 1951; Efrati et al., 1964; Mitchell et al., 1966). Most of the leukocytosis of pregnancy is

TABLE 2–1   Mean Peripheral Leukocyte Count (per cu mm)

		TRIMESTER		
	NONPREGNANT	*First*	*Second*	*Third*
Andrews and Bonsnes (1951)	7100	9200		10,500
Efrati et al. (1964)*		8700 (6300–15,000)	8730 (6580–21,250)	8500 (4000–18,000)
Mitchell et al. (1966)*	7210 (4750–9600)	9405 (3150–15,300)	10,720 (6300–16,100)	10,350 (5000–16,600)

*Normal range in parentheses.

due to an increased number of neutrophils. The percentage of phagocytic cells increases from 66 per cent in nonpregnant women to 76 per cent in pregnant women (Mitchell, 1966), while the proportion of lymphocytes declines by 10 to 15 per cent during pregnancy (Andrews and Bonsnes, 1951).

Coagulation Factors

Many clotting factors are present in increased amounts in normal pregnancy. Fibrinogen levels rise by 80 to 180 mg/dl, so that at term, levels of 400 to 450 mg/dl are usual (Pechet and Alexander, 1961; Todd et al., 1965; Shaper et al., 1968; Bonnar et al., 1969) (Table 2–2). There are also elevations of Factors VII, VIII, IX, and X, while Factors II and V remain essentially unchanged (Pechet and Alexander, 1961; Todd et al., 1965). Bleeding time, clotting time (Margulis et al., 1954) and prothrombin time (Todd et al., 1965) are unchanged in pregnancy.

Despite the increase in levels of clotting factors and the venous stasis caused by the enlarging uterus, and despite widely held "clinical impressions," it is difficult to demonstrate an increased incidence of spontaneous venous thrombosis during pregnancy. For a pregnant trauma victim requiring prolonged bedrest, pregnancy per se does not create a necessity for prophylactic anticoagulation. However, when it is decided that a pregnant patient should receive anticoagulants, the agent of choice is heparin, which does not cross the placenta. The oral anticoagulants cross the placenta and have been implicated in teratogenesis

TABLE 2–2   Clotting Factors in Term Pregnancy

	TODD ET AL. (1965)		PECHET AND ALEXANDER (1961)		BONNAR ET AL. (1969)	
	Non-pregnant	*Term*	*Non-pregnant*	*Term*	*Non-pregnant*	*Term*
Fibrinogen (mg/dl)	322	419			285	450
Factor VII (% of normal)	100	389	100	130		
Factor VIII (% of normal)	100	126				
Factor IX (% of normal)	100	142				
Factor X (% of normal)	100	259	100	162		
Factor II (units/ml)	294	336		Not increased		
Factor V (% of normal)	100	76		Not increased		

as well as in hemorrhagic problems in the fetus and newborn. The situation post partum is different from that during pregnancy, for during the puerperium there is a definite increase in the incidence of spontaneous thrombosis. If trauma necessitates prolonged bedrest in a patient immediately post partum, serious consideration should be given to the prophylactic use of subclinical doses of heparin.

If trauma leads to abruptio placentae (premature separation of the normally implanted placenta) or amniotic fluid embolism, the patient may develop a rapid, progressive and severe defibrination syndrome, or disseminated intravascular coagulation (DIC). Management of the patient in this situation consists of supportive therapy with fresh whole blood, fresh frozen plasma, or cryoprecipitate, and delivery as efficaciously as possible. The defibrination syndrome resolves promptly once the uterus is emptied. The use of heparin in this type of DIC has not been proved to be beneficial, and is contraindicated (McKay, 1974).

Serum Osmolality and Plasma Proteins

Management of thermal injury during pregnancy requires an understanding of the effects of pregnancy on serum osmolality and colloid-osmotic pressure. For poorly understood reasons, serum osmolality falls about 10 mOsm/L during the first 8 to 10 weeks of pregnancy, and remains at a level of about 280 mOsm/L throughout the remainder of gestation (Robertson, 1968).

Likewise, serum albumin falls by about 1.0 gm/dl during the first trimester, and remains at levels of 2.2 to 2.8 gm/dl until the puerperium (De Alvarez et al., 1961; Reboud et al., 1967). The overall level of serum globulin remains fairly stable throughout gestation, although the alpha-1, alpha-2, and beta fractions increase while the gamma fraction falls (MacGillivray and Tovey, 1957; De Alvarez et al., 1961). The overall fall in total serum protein is about 1.0 gm/dl, and is due almost entirely to the change in albumin concentration. Likewise, the fall in colloid osmotic pressure from nonpregnant levels of 38 cm H_2O to 31 cm H_2O by 24 weeks' gestation (Robertson, 1969) is secondary to and closely parallels the fall in albumin concentration.

Erythrocyte Sedimentation Rate

Due to the increase in serum fibrinogen and alpha and beta globulins, blood from pregnant women sediments very rapidly. For whole blood the mean sedimentation rate is 78 mm/hr, with a range of 44 to 114 mm/hr (Furuhjelm, 1956). Thus the erythrocyte sedimentation rate is of little or no value in the diagnosis of injury or disease during pregnancy.

PULMONARY SYSTEM

Despite the fact that the diaphragm is elevated about 4 cm during late pregnancy (Thomson and Cohen, 1938), the excursion of the diaphragm is increased by 1.0 to 1.5 cm and the tidal volume is increased 40 per cent (Hytten and Lind, 1973). Although the respiratory rate is not changed, the increased tidal volume and decreased residual volume lead to reduced alveolar and arterial pCO_2. Thus normal arterial pCO_2 after the second trimester is about 30 mm Hg (Bouterline-Young and Bouterline-Young, 1956). The sensitivity of the respiratory center is also greatly increased during pregnancy. A rise in arterial pCO_2 of 1 mm Hg in a pregnant woman will cause an increase of 6 L/min in minute ventilation, as compared to a 1.5 L/min increase in nonpregnant women (Prowse and Gaensler, 1965).

GASTROINTESTINAL SYSTEM

Stomach

Gastric motility is reduced in pregnancy, and the emptying time is prolonged. Thirty minutes after a 750 ml watery test meal, the volume remaining in the stomach is 186 ml in the nonpregnant state, 275 ml in the pregnant state, and 393 ml during labor (Davison et al., 1970). Although it is very difficult to quantify experimentally, undoubtedly solid food remains in the stomach for much longer periods during pregnancy. If major anesthesia or surgery is necessary, it should always be assumed that the patient has a full stomach. Therefore, a nasogastric tube is essential prior to any surgery, and if general anesthesia is undertaken, a cuffed endotracheal tube should always be used, with cricoid pressure during intubation to prevent aspiration of gastric contents.

Intestines

Although the motility of the bowel is diminished during pregnancy (Parry et al., 1970), the physiologic changes that occur have little significance in the management of trauma. The anatomic changes in the abdomen, however, are of great significance. The progressive enlargement of the uterus during gestation (Fig. 2–2) compresses the small bowel into an ever smaller volume of the peritoneal cavity. By virtue of its bulk, and by compressing the abdominal viscera into a smaller volume (Fig. 2–3), the uterus may act as a protective shield for the small bowel, especially in cases of penetrating injury (Wright et al., 1954; Beattie and Daly, 1960; Bochner, 1961; Dyer and Barclay, 1962) (see also Chapter 5). However, if penetrating injury to the upper abdomen does occur during pregnancy, multiple loops of bowel may be injured (Buchsbaum, 1968, 1975).

The anatomic changes secondary to pregnancy complicate the diagnosis of abdominal trauma in several ways. The enlargement of the uterus leads to stretching of the abdominal wall and a diminished response to peritoneal irritation. Thus, guarding and rigidity are often diminished or absent after bowel trauma (Buchsbaum, 1968). Because of the rearrangement of the abdominal viscera, pain due to damage of a specific organ may be referred to a different region of the abdomen than that expected in the nonpregnant patient. The displacement of the bowel makes needle paracentesis dangerous and unwarranted during pregnancy.

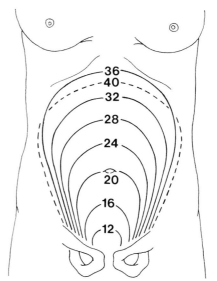

Figure 2-2 The size of the uterus at various weeks of gestation. At 12 weeks the uterus is just palpable behind the symphysis pubis, at 20 weeks it is at the umbilicus, and at 36 weeks it is subcostal.

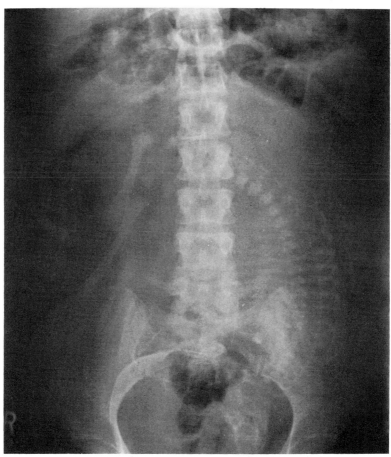

Figure 2-3 Abdominal radiograph at 38 weeks' gestation. The abdominal viscera are compressed into the upper abdomen. Very little bowel gas is seen in the lower three quarters of the peritoneal cavity.

Liver

The human liver is not enlarged during gestation (Combes et al., 1963), and pregnancy does not seem to alter the frequency or outcome of liver injury resulting from trauma.

The serum levels of most "liver enzymes" in pregnancy are unchanged from those found in nonpregnant patients. There is no change during pregnancy in serum levels of glutamic-oxalacetic transaminase (SGOT), glutamic-pyruvic transaminase (SGPT), or lactic dehydrogenase (LDH). This is not true of alkaline phosphatase, however, which increases progressively throughout pregnancy to levels three to four times greater than normal near term. In normal pregnancy at term, alkaline phosphatase activity is 82 ± 35 IU/L (Bodansky method), while in preeclamptic patients, levels of 132 ± 49 IU/L are found (Bagga et al., 1969). This rise is due to alkaline phosphatase of placental origin, and the activity resides in the heat-stable fraction of the enzyme. Sodium sulfo-bromophthalein (BSP) is cleared less rapidly from the circulation during pregnancy — at 45 minutes, the BSP retention is higher than in the nonpregnant state, but it usually is near the upper limits of normal (Tindall and Beazley, 1975).

Pancreas

Traumatic injury to the pancreas results in a clinical picture similar to pancreatitis, including elevations of the enzymes amylase and lipase. Thus, it is important to know that in normal pregnancy, amylase levels are the same as in nonpregnant women (Burt and McAlister, 1966), whereas lipase levels are reduced (mean levels, 15.5 ± 6.2 IU/L during pregnancy, 39.9 ± 4.6 IU/L when nonpregnant) (Hytten and Lind, 1973).

SPLEEN

Since the first reported case in 1803, 69 cases of splenic rupture during pregnancy have been reported. However, there is no good evidence that pregnancy predisposes to splenic rupture. The spleen does not enlarge during gestation (Buchsbaum, 1967), and there is some experimental evidence that, at least in pregnant dogs, the spleen may actually become smaller (Barcroft and Stevens, 1928; Barcroft, 1930). Sparkman (1958) speculates that some cases of "spontaneous" splenic rupture during pregnancy may be secondary to the increased maternal blood volume, which may cause rupture of preexisting splenic parenchymal aneurysms or localized areas of splenic disease.

URINARY SYSTEM

Anatomic Changes

Marked dilatation of the renal pelves and ureters occurs as early as 10 weeks' gestation, and persists until 6 weeks post partum (Fig. 2–4). The right side

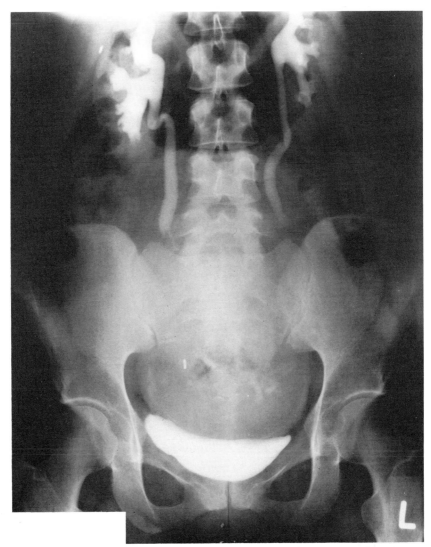

Figure 2-4 Intravenous urogram at 26 weeks' gestation. There is pyeloureteral dilatation above the pelvic brim, more marked on the right.

is usually more dilated than the left, and usually there is no dilatation below the pelvic brim. The best evidence indicates that this dilatation is due primarily to compression of the ureters by the ovarian venous plexuses (Bellina et al., 1970), with a slight contribution from progesterone-induced relaxation of smooth muscle. These anatomic changes must be kept in mind if intravenous urograms become necessary in the evaluation of urinary tract trauma.

The bladder, being attached to the cervix and lower uterine segment, is displaced anteriorly and superiorly as the uterus enlarges, and thus becomes more an abdominal and less a pelvic organ. It therefore becomes more susceptible to injury. Because the bladder, like other pelvic organs, becomes hyperemic during pregnancy, injury to it may be associated with increased blood loss.

Physiologic Changes

Renal plasma flow (RPF) rises early in pregnancy, from nonpregnant levels of about 475 ml/min to about 750 ml/min by 16 weeks' gestation (Sims and Krantz, 1958), and this increase is maintained until delivery. The terminal fall in RPF described in the past is undoubtedly an artefact of studying patients in the supine position. Glomerular filtration rate likewise increases from 16 weeks to term by about 67 per cent, to about 150 ml/min (Sims and Krantz, 1958). As a result of these changes, normal endogenous creatinine clearance in pregnancy rises to about 150 to 200 ml/min (Hytten and Lind, 1973), and serum creatinine and blood urea nitrogen levels fall. Serum creatinine falls from a mean of 0.8 mg/dl in the first trimester to 0.5 mg/dl in late pregnancy (Kuhlback and Widholm, 1966). Normal BUN levels in pregnancy are less than 10 mg/dl. In pregnancies complicated by preeclampsia, creatinine clearance falls and serum creatinine and BUN levels rise.

Despite diminished serum osmolality, the pregnant woman has a greatly enhanced diuretic response to a water load during the first two trimesters. During this time mean maximum urinary flow after a 1 liter water load is 30 ml/min, nearly double the nonpregnant rate of 16 ml/min (Hytten and Klopper, 1963). Nearly 1.5 L may be excreted in the 2 hours following a water load of 1 L (Hytten and Lind, 1973). Thus, the kidneys in early pregnancy are capable of handling the large volumes of fluids that may be necessary to support the circulation of a trauma victim. During the last trimester, the ability of a kidney to excrete a water load falls markedly, to somewhat less than values for nonpregnant women, and this is even more pronounced in patients with preeclampsia (McManus et al., 1934). This, however, is not a reason for withholding large quantities of intravenous fluids when they are needed. In pregnancy, as in the nonpregnant state, the central venous pressure remains one of the best clinical guides to fluid replacement.

Urinalysis

All pregnant patients have an increased amount of glucose in the urine, and nearly half of all nondiabetic pregnant women have glycosuria detectable by usual methods sometime during pregnancy. Amino acid excretions rise markedly during gestation, but unless pregnancy is complicated by renal disease or toxemia, protein excretion is unchanged from nonpregnant levels (Hytten and Lind, 1973). Over 50 per cent of healthy pregnant women have increased leukocyte excretion, and thus the presence of a small number of leukocytes in the urine is not a reliable sign of renal disease or injury during pregnancy (Chadd et al., 1967). The presence of erythrocytes in the urine is not normal during pregnancy, however, and gross or microscopic hematuria is indicative of renal disease or urinary tract injury.

GENITAL SYSTEM

The uterus increases in size during pregnancy from a nearly solid organ 7 cm in length, weighing 70 gm, to a thin-walled muscular sac about 36 cm long, weighing 800 to 1200 gm, with an average volume of 5 L (Pritchard and MacDonald, 1976). By compartmentalizing the peritoneal cavity, this uterine enlargement has a protective effect on many of the abdominal viscera, especially the small bowel (see above), but the increased size makes the uterus and its contents susceptible to injury. Thus, abdominal trauma may lead to many problems peculiar to pregnancy, such as abruptio placentae, uterine rupture, and premature rupture of the membranes (see Chapter 5). Uterine trauma during pregnancy may lead to massive blood loss, for the blood flow through the uterine arteries at term is approximately 500 to 700 ml/min (Pritchard and MacDonald, 1976). Thus, at term, the total circulating blood volume flows through the uterus every 8 to 11 min.

ENDOCRINE SYSTEM

The physiologic changes that occur in the various endocrine organs during gestation are more profound and complex than the changes in any other system. However, the changes with great significance for the trauma victim occur principally in the pituitary and the adrenals.

During pregnancy the pituitary hypertrophies, due to estrogen-induced proliferation of the lactotrophic cells in the anterior pituitary. The pituitary doubles in weight to 1.0 gm, from a nonpregnant average of about 0.5 gm (Daughaday, 1974). The hypertrophic pituitary becomes dependent on a greatly increased blood flow. Hypotension in pregnancy can lead to ischemic necrosis of the anterior pituitary, followed by hemorrhage into the gland when circulation is restored. The resultant destruction of the anterior pituitary, Sheehan's syndrome, is the most common non-neoplastic cause of hypopituitarism. Depending on the magnitude and duration of hypotension, part or all of the function of the anterior pituitary may be lost. The most sensitive hormones, and the first to be lost, are the gonadotropins, followed in order by growth hormone, thyrotropin, ACTH, and prolactin (Daughaday, 1974). Thus, lesser degrees of hypotension may lead to subsequent hypogonadotrophic amenorrhea, while greater degrees may cause panhypopituitarism. Early signs of Sheehan's syndrome in the puerperium are failure of lactation and failure of regrowth of the pubic hair. The prevention of pituitary necrosis is thus a reason for the prevention or rapid treatment of shock in the pregnant woman.

Cortisol metabolism is altered markedly during pregnancy. Plasma glucocorticoid levels rise markedly and progressively (Bayliss et al., 1955; Peterson 1977), and although most of this is bound to transcortin (Katz and Kappas, 1967), the level of which is elevated during pregnancy, there is also a rise in the level of free, and thus active, cortisol (Doe et al., 1960; Burke and Fraser, 1969; O'Connell and Welsh, 1969). Free cortisol levels rise from nonpregnant levels of 1 mcg/dl to levels near 2 mcg/dl at term (Peterson, 1977). The daily secretion rate of cortisol is unchanged during pregnancy, however, and the elevated level of free cortisol is probably secondary to a resetting of the negative feedback set point between unbound cortisol and ACTH (Peterson, 1977). The normal diurnal variation of serum cortisol is maintained during pregnancy. The pregnant woman is as capable of increasing ACTH output and serum cortisol levels in response to stress as is the nonpregnant woman. The fact of pregnancy itself does not necessitate administration of supplemental glucocorticoids to trauma victims.

MUSCULOSKELETAL SYSTEM

During pregnancy, the ligaments of the pubic symphysis and sacroiliac joints loosen, a change which facilitates vaginal delivery by making the rigid pelvis somewhat more flexible. This change is probably secondary to the effects of the hormone relaxin (Hall, 1960), which has been isolated from the blood of many pregnant mammals, including humans (Farrow et al., 1955). Marked widening of the symphysis pubis occurs by the seventh month of gestation (Abramson et al., 1934), when its width has increased by 3 1 to 3 8 mm (Table 2–3). These changes may make the pelvis somewhat less susceptible to fracture during pregnancy by giving it some mobility. However, this mobility of the pelvic joints, coupled with the effects of a protuberant abdomen, leads to unsteadiness of gait. Thus, minor trauma from falls becomes more common during pregnancy than at any other time during adult life (Fort and Harlin, 1970).

In the past, several authors have described cases of delayed healing of fractures during pregnancy (see Buchsbaum, 1968), and osteomalacia with pregnancy has been reported (Felton and Stone, 1966). Buchsbaum (1970) demonstrated that the strength of healing callus in experimental fibula fractures in pregnant rats late in pregnancy was less than that in nonpregnant controls. Certainly there are marked changes in calcium metabolism during pregnancy (Table 2–4). The total calcium concentration in maternal serum falls during pregnancy until 34 to 36 weeks, and then rises slightly so that at term the mean serum calcium concentration is 4.52 (± 0.18) mEq/L, approximately 0.25 mEq/L below nonpregnant levels (Pitkin, 1977; Pitkin and Gebhardt, 1977). However, the fall in total calcium is nearly identical to the fall in serum albumin, and the concentration of ionized calcium remains fairly constant throughout gestation. Maternal parathyroid hormone (PTH) levels rise during pregnancy to about 135 per cent of nonpregnant values (Pitkin, 1977), so that a state of "physiologic hyperparathyroidism" exists during pregnancy. Despite the elevated levels of PTH, and despite previous reports of osteomalacia, the skeleton is well maintained during pregnancy. Studies of bone density reveal no loss in current or past pregnancies (Walker et al., 1972; Christianson et al., 1976). The preservation of the skeleton is probably due to the action of calcitonin

TABLE 2–3   Symphysis Pubis Width (mm)

	Nonpregnant	Pregnant
Males	4.40	—
Nulliparas	4.09	7.90
Multiparas	4.60	7.70

Abramson D, et al.: Surg Gynec Obstet 58:595, 1934

TABLE 2–4   Mean Serum Calcium and Parathyroid Hormone Levels

	IONIZED CALCIUM, mEq/L	TOTAL CALCIUM, mEq/L	PARATHYROID HORMONE, μL-Eq/ML
Nonpregnant	2.30	4.77	
First trimester	2.33	4.80	5.67
Second trimester	2.28	4.56	6.20
Third trimester	2.24	4.46	6.76
Puerperium	2.33	4.50	4.99

Pitkin (1977); Pitkin and Gebhardt (1977).

(CT), which counteracts the effects of PTH on the skeleton while permitting the effects of PTH on the gut (increased absorption of calcium) and kidney (diminished excretion of calcium) to continue. Levels of CT activity during pregnancy are uncertain at present, with one group of investigators reporting a marked increase (Samaan et al., 1973; Samaan et al., 1975), while another (Pitkin, 1977) demonstrates no change or a slight fall.

There is no good clinical evidence, and little experimental evidence, that pregnancy interferes with fracture healing. The rate of bone turnover and remodeling increases throughout pregnancy, so that at term it is twice as great as in nonpregnant individuals (Pitkin, 1977). The rate of turnover in the exchangeable calcium pool increases by 20 per cent. Given a normal calcium intake, the increased metabolic activity of bone during pregnancy could conceivably enhance the healing of fractures.

NERVOUS SYSTEM

Physiologic changes in the nervous system during pregnancy and their significance to trauma victims, though possibly very great, are not known at present. However, complications peculiar to pregnancy may be confused with head trauma with disastrous results, as illustrated by the following case report.

A 28 year old woman at 41 weeks' gestation was found unconscious in a cattle feedlot. It was assumed that she had been attacked by a bull, and she was hospitalized. En route to the hospital she had several grand mal seizures, and on admission was found to have a blood pressure of 170/100 and 3+ proteinuria. On the presumption of head trauma, an extensive neurologic evaluation, including CT scanning was undertaken. Only after this proved negative was it realized that the correct diagnosis was eclampsia. In the interval prior to diagnosis, irreparable damage had been sustained, and both mother and fetus subsequently died.

When seizures begin in the third trimester, the most likely diagnosis is eclampsia. Eclampsia usually, but not invariably, is associated with hypertension and proteinuria. Unless there is incontrovertible evidence of head trauma, a patient with convulsions in late pregnancy should be treated as for eclampsia — with magnesium sulfate infusion and prompt delivery.

WOUND HEALING IN PREGNANCY

Glucocorticoids decrease the rate of collagen biosynthesis, and, as previously noted, during pregnancy the levels of circulating glucocorticoids are markedly increased. Although most of this is bound to transcortin, there is also a small rise in the levels of free, and thus active, cortisol. The clinical significance of these changes is uncertain, however, for normal pregnancy is not a state of hyper-adrenocorticism. There is no evidence that collagen synthesis is decreased during pregnancy. In fact, the activity of proline hydroxylase increases in pregnancy (at least in the uterus), a sign of increased collagen synthesis (Kivirikko and Risteli. 1976).

Graber (1974) states that the incidence of postoperative wound dehiscence is increased in obstetric patients. Most likely in healthy, well-nourished gravidas this increase is slight, and is secondary to (1) an increased incidence of postoperative ileus due to diminished intestinal motility, and (2) difficulty in closing the abdomen if a laparotomy is done for nonobstetric reasons and the uterus is not emptied. In the poorly nourished pregnant woman, both iron and protein deficiency can occur, both of which lead to deficient wound healing. Likewise, dietary zinc deficiency causes poor wound healing (Sandstead. 1973; Burch and Sullivan, 1976), but zinc deficiency does not occur in a well-nourished patient. Thus, the properly nourished gravida probably has only a slightly increased chance of wound dehiscence, but in the undernourished (especially those who exhibit clay or starch pica during pregnancy), this risk is considerably increased. Just as in the nonpregnant patient, however, asepsis, hemostasis, and good surgical technique will minimize the risk.

SUMMARY

During pregnancy the signs, symptoms, and laboratory indices of injury may be changed and the pattern of injury altered. Injury may be complicated by conditions peculiar to pregnancy, and often therapy must be modified to accommodate the anatomic and physiologic changes of gestation. The physician called upon to attend a pregnant trauma victim must remember that he does in fact have *two* patients, and a thorough understanding of the anatomic and physiologic alterations caused by pregnancy is essential if the best interests of both mother and fetus are to be served

REFERENCES

Abramson D, Roberts SM, Wilson PD: Relaxation of the pelvic joints in pregnancy. Surg Gynec Obstet *58*:595, 1934.

Andrews WC, Bonsnes RW: The leucocytes during pregnancy. Am J Obstet Gynecol *61*:1129, 1951.

Bagga OP, Mullick VD, Madan P, Dewan S: Total serum alkaline phosphatase and its isoenzymes in normal and toxemic pregnancies. Am J Obstet Gynecol *104*:850, 1969.

Barcroft J: Alterations in the volume of the normal spleen and their significance. Am J Med Sci *179*:1, 1930.

Barcroft J, Stevens JG: The effect of pregnancy and menstruation on the size of the spleen. J Physiol *66*:32, 1928.

Bayliss RIS, Brown JCM, Pound BP, Steinbeck AW: Plasma-17-hydroxycortico-steroids in pregnancy. Lancet *1*:62, 1955.

Beattie, JF, Daly RF: Gunshot wounds of the pregnant uterus. Am J Obstet Gynecol *80*:772, 1960.

Bellina JA, Dougherty CM, Mickal A: Pyeloureteral dilatation and pregnancy. Am J Obstet Gynecol *108*:356, 1970.

Bochner K: Traumatic perforation of the pregnant uterus. Obstet Gynecol *17*:520, 1961.

Bonnar J, McNicol GP, Douglas AS: Fibrinolytic enzyme system and pregnancy. Br Med J *3*:387, 1969.

Bouterline-Young H, Bouterline-Young E: Alveolar carbon dioxide levels in pregnant, parturient, and lactating subjects. J Obstet Gynaecol Br Emp *63*:509, 1956.

Buchsbaum HJ: Splenic rupture in pregnancy; report of a case and review of the literature. Obstet Gynecol Surv *22*:381, 1967.

Buchsbaum HJ: Accidental injury complicating pregnancy. Am J Obstet Gynecol *102*:752, 1968.

Buchsbaum HJ: Healing of experimental fractures during pregnancy. Obstet Gynecol *35*:613, 1970.

Buchsbaum HJ: Diagnosis and management of abdominal gunshot wounds during pregnancy. J Trauma *15*:425, 1975.

Burch RE, Sullivan JF: Clinical and nutritional aspects of zinc deficiency and excess. Med Clin N Amer *60*:675, 1976.

Burke CW, Fraser JF: Effect of oestrogen treatment and late pregnancy on non-protein-bound cortisol levels and urinary free cortisol excretion. Clin Sci *37*:876, 1969.

Burt CS. McAlister JA: Serum amylase in pregnancy and the puerperium, and in fetal blood. Obstet Gynecol *28*:351, 1966.

Burwell CS, Metcalfe, J: Heart Disease in Pregnancy. London, Churchill, 1958.

Burwell CS, Strayhorn WD, Flickinger D, Corlette MB, Bowerman EP, Kennedy JA: Circulation during pregnancy. Arch Int Med *62*:979, 1938.

Chadd MA, Humphreys DM, Leather HM, Wills SA: Urinary leucocyte excretion in hypertension in pregnancy. Br Med J *4*:655, 1967.

Chesley LC, Wynn RM, Silverman NI: Renal effects of angiotension II infusions in normotensive pregnant women. Circ *13*:232, 1963.

Christianson C, Rodero P, Heinild B: Unchanged total body calcium in normal human pregnancy. Acta Obstet Gynecol Scand *55*:141, 1976.

Colditz RB. Josey WE: Central venous pressure in supine position during normal pregnancy. Obstet Gynecol *36*:769, 1970

Combes B, Shibata H, Adams R, Mitchell BD: Alterations in sulfobromophthalein sodium removal mechanisms from blood during normal pregnancy. J Clin Invest *42*:1431, 1963.

Daughaday WG: The adenohypophysis. *In* Williams RH (ed): Textbook of Endocrinology. 5th Ed Philadelphia, WB Saunders Co 1974.

Davison JS, Davison MC, Hay DM: Gastric emptying time in late pregnancy and labour. J. Obstet Gynaecol Br Commonw *77*:37, 1970.

De Alvarez RR, Alfonso JF, Sherrard DJ: Serum protein fractionation in normal pregnancy. Am J Obstet Gynecol *82*:1096, 1961.

Doe RP, Zinneman HH, Flink EB, Ulstrom RA: Significance of the concentration of non-protein-bound plasma cortisol in normal subjects, Cushing's syndrome, pregnancy, and during estrogen therapy. J Clin Endocr *20*:1484, 1960.

Dolezal A, Figor S: The phenomenon of reactive vasodilatation in pregnancy. Am J Obstet Gynecol *93*:1137, 1965.

Dyer I, Barclay DL: Accidental trauma complicating labor and delivery. Am J Obstet Gynecol *83*:907, 1962.

Efrati P, Presentey B, Margolith M, Rosenszajn L: Leucocytes of normal pregnant women. Obstet Gynecol *23*:429, 1964.

Farrow MX, Holmstrom EG, Salharick HA: The concentration of relaxin in blood serum and other tissues of women during pregnancy. J Clin Endocr *15*:22, 1955.

Felton, DJC, Stone WD: Osteomalacia in Asian immigrants during pregnancy. Br Med J *1*:1521, 1966.

Fort AJ, Harlin RS: Pregnancy outcome after non-catastrophic maternal trauma during pregnancy. Obstet Gynecol *35*:912, 1970.

Furuhjelm U: Maternal and cord blood. A comparative investigation with reference to blood sugar, serum proteins, erythrocyte sedimentation rate and total serum lipids. Ann Paediatr Fenn *2* (Suppl 5): 1, 1956.

Gemzell CA, Robbe H, Ström G: Total amount of haemoglobin and physical working capacity in normal pregnancy and puerperium (with iron medication). Acta Obstet Gynecol Scand *36*:93, 1957.

Graber EA: Management of postpartum and postoperative complications. *In* Barber HRK, Graber EA: Surgical Disease in Pregnancy. Philadelphia, WB Saunders Co, 1974.

Hall K: Relaxin. J Reprod Fertil *1*:368, 1960.

Hollander AG, Crawford JH: Roentgenologic and electrocardiographic changes in the normal heart during pregnancy. Am Heart J *26*:364, 1943.

Howard BK, Goodson JH: Experimental placental abruption. Obstet Gynecol *2*:442, 1953.

Hytten FE, Klopper AI: Response to a water load in pregnancy. J Obstet Gynaecol Br Commonw *70*:811, 1963.

Hytten FE, Leitch I: The Physiology of Human Pregnancy. 2nd Ed. Oxford, Blackwell, 1971.

Hytten FE, Lind T: Diagnostic Indices in Pregnancy. Basle, Ciba-Geigy, Ltd, 1973.

Hytten FE, Paintin DB: Increase in plasma volume during normal pregnancy. J Obstet Gynaecol Br Commonw *70*:402, 1963

Katz FH, Kappas A: The effects of estradiol on plasma levels of cortisol and thyroid hormone-binding globulin and on aldosterone and cortisol secretion rates in man. J Clin Invest *46*:1768, 1967.

Kerr MG, Scott DB, Samuel E: Studies of the inferior vena cava in late pregnancy. Br Med J *1*:532, 1964.

Kivirikko KI, Risteli L: Biosynthesis of collagen and its alterations in pathological states. Medical Biology *54*:159, 1976.

Kuhlback B, Widholm O: Plasma creatinine in normal pregnancy. Scand J Clin Lab Invest *18*:654, 1966.

Lees MM, Scott DB, Kerr, MG, Taylor SH: The circulatory effects of recumbent postural change in late pregnancy. Clin Sci *32*:453, 1967.

Lloyd S, Pickford M: The action of posterior pituitary hormones and oestrogens on the vascular system of the rat. J Physiol (Lond) *155*:161, 1961.

MacGillivray I, Rose GA, Rowe B: Blood pressure survey in pregnancy. Clin Sci *37*:395, 1969.

MacGillivray I, Tovey JE: A study of the serum protein changes in pregnancy and toxaemia, using paper strip electrophoresis. J Obstet Gynaecol Br Emp *61*:361, 1957.

Margulis RR, Luzadre JH, Hodgkinson CP: Fibrinolysis in labor and delivery. Obstet Gynecol *3*:487, 1954.

Marx G: Shock in the obstetric patient. Anesthesiology *26*:423, 1965.

McKay DG: The clinical spectrum and management of acquired coagulopathy in pregnancy. *In* Reid DE. Christian CD (eds): Controversies in Obstetrics and Gynecology II. Philadelphia, WB Saunders Company, 1974.

McLennan CE: Antecubital and femoral venous pressure in normal and toxemic pregnancies. Am J Obstet Gynecol *45*:568, 1943.

McManus MA, Riley, GA, Janney JC: Kidney function in pregnancy. III. Water diuresis in the toxemias of pregnancy. Am J Obstet Gynecol *28*:524, 1934.

Mengert WF, Goodson JH, Campbell RG, Haynes DM: Observations on the pathogenesis of premature separation of the normally implanted placenta. Am J Obstet Gynecol *66*:1104, 1953.

Mitchell, AW, McRipley RJ, Selvarez RJ, Sharra AJ: The role of the phagocyte in host-parasite interactions. IV. The phagocytic activity of leucocytes in pregnancy and its relationship to urinary tract infection. Am J Obstet Gynecol *96*:687, 1966.

O'Connell M, Welsh GW: Unbound plasma cortisol in pregnant and Enovid-E treated women as determined by ultrafiltration. J Clin Endocr *29*:563, 1969.

O'Driscoll K, McCarthy JR: Abruptio placentae and central venous pressure. J Obstet Gynaecol Br Commonw *73*:923, 1966.

Parry E, Shields R, Turnbull AC: Transit time in the small intestine in pregnancy. J Obstet Gynaecol Br Commonw *77*:900, 1970.

Pechet L, Alexander B: Increased clotting factors in pregnancy. N Engl J Med *265*:1093, 1961.

Peterson RE: Cortisol. *In* Fuchs F, Klopper A (eds): Endocrinology of Pregnancy. 2nd Ed. Hagerstown, Md. Harper and Row, 1977.

Pitkin RM: Hematologic indices. *In:* Laboratory Indices of Nutritional Status in Pregnancy. Washington DC, National Academy of Sciences–National Research Council, 1977.

Pitkin RM: Calcium metabolism during pregnancy and its effects on the fetus and newborn. *In* Nirzan M: Pediatric and Adolescent Endocrinology. Basel, S Karger, 1977.

Pitkin RM, Gebhardt MP: Serum calcium concentrations in human pregnancy. Am J Obstet Gynecol *127*:775, 1977.

Pritchard JA: Changes in the blood volume during pregnancy and delivery. Anesthesiology *26*:393, 1965.

Pritchard JA, MacDonald PC: Williams Obstetrics. 15th Ed. New York, Appleton-Century-Crofts, 1976.

Prowse CM, Gaensler E: Respiratory and acid-base changes during pregnancy. Anesthesiology *26*:381, 1965.

Reboud P, Groslambert P, Ollivier M: Protéines et lipides plasmatiques au cours de la gestation normale et du post-partum. Ann Biol Clin 25:383, 1967.

Robertson EG: Increased erythrocyte fragility in association with osmotic changes in pregnancy serum. J Reprod Fertil 16:323, 1968.

Robertson EG: Oedema in normal pregnancy. J Reprod Fertil (Suppl) 9:27, 1969.

Samaan NA, Anderson GD, Adam-Mayne ME: Immunoreactive calcitonin in mother, child and adult. Am J Obstet Gynecol 121:622, 1975

Samaan NA, Hill CS, Beceiro JR, Schultz PN: Immunoreactive calcitonin in medullary carcinoma of the thyroid and in maternal and cord serum. J Lab Clin Med 81:671, 1973.

Sandstead HH: Zinc nutrition in the United States. Am J Clin Nutr 26:1251, 1973.

Schwarz R: Das Verhalten des Kreislaufs in der normalen Schwangerschaft. Archiv Gynak 199:663, 1964.

Shaper AG, Kear J, MacIntosh DM, Kyobe J, Njama D: The platelet count, platelet adhesiveness and aggregation and the mechanism of fibrinolytic inhibition in pregnancy and the puerperium. J Obstet Gynaecol Br Commonw 75:433, 1968.

Sims EAA, Krantz KE: Serial studies of renal function during pregnancy and the puerperium in normal women. J Clin Invest 37:1764, 1958.

Sparkman RS: Rupture of the spleen in pregnancy. Am J Obstet Gynecol 76:587, 1958.

Thomson KJ, Cohen ME: Studies on the circulation in pregnancy. II. Vital capacity observations in normal pregnant women. Surg Gynecol Obstet 66:591, 1938.

Tindall VR, Beazley JM: An assessment of changes in liver function during normal pregnancy using a modified bromsulphthalein test. J Obstet Gynaecol Br Commonw 72:717, 1975

Todd ME, Thompson JH, Bowie EJW, Owens CS: Changes in blood coagulation during pregnancy. Mayo Clin Proc 40:370, 1965.

Trower R, Walters WAW: Brachial artery blood pressure in the lateral recumbent position during pregnancy. Aust NZ J Obstet Gynaecol 8:146, 1968.

Ueland K, Novy MJ, Peterson EN, Metcalfe J: Maternal cardiovascular dynamics. Am J Obstet Gynecol 104:856, 1969.

Walker ARP, Richardson B, Walker F: The influence of numerous pregnancies and lactations on bone dimensions in South African, Bantu, and Caucasian women. Clin Sci 42:189, 1972.

Walters WAW, MacGregor WG, Hills M: Cardiac output at rest during pregnancy and the puerperium. Clin Sci 30:1, 1966.

Wilson JN: Rational approach to management of clinical shock. Arch Surg 91:92, 1965.

Wright CH, Posner AC, Gilchrist J: Penetrating wounds of gravid uterus. Am J Obstet Gynecol 67:1085, 1954.

Chapter 3

DIAGNOSIS AND EARLY MANAGEMENT

Herbert J. Buchsbaum

The early management of the pregnant trauma patient is critical, not only for the mother but also for the outcome of the pregnancy. The physician caring for the injured gravida has two patients, whose sensitivities and responses to trauma differ. Under the stress of trauma, the mother acts to maintain her own homeostasis at the cost of the conceptus. As a result, the uteroplacental circulation is reduced in maternal hemorrhagic shock and in anoxia, with a disproportionately severe effect on the fetus. Resuscitation in maternal hypotension and hypoxia must therefore be instituted early, before irreversible changes take place in the fetus. The immediate, early management of the injured gravida differs little from that of other seriously injured persons.

In the later phases of early management, some modifications are introduced by the pregnancy. The physiologic and anatomic alterations of pregnancy not only alter the type of injury the mother will sustain, and her response to trauma, but also will affect the interpretation of diagnostic studies. A knowledge of these changes is critical in evaluating clinical findings and in interpreting roentgenographic and laboratory results.

Biochemical and Hormonal Alterations

Many subtle biochemical alterations accompany trauma that may affect the conceptus. Some have been assayed, others have not yet been identified. Changes in the endocrine system that help the host respond to trauma have been identified. Among the hormones recognized in the adaptive response are vasopressin, cortisol, aldosterone, and catecholamines. These hormones maintain fluid and electrolyte balance and affect circulation by modifying intravascular volume and blood pressure. Metabolism at the cellular level following trauma is affected by alterations in ACTH, glucocorticoids, growth hormone and glucagon (Jackson, 1973).

Stress elicits an adrenal response with increased epinephrine production. Kaiser and Harris (1950) found that the response of the pregnant uterus to epinephrine depends on its concentration and route of administration. With high exogenous doses it has an oxytocic effect, but these levels are nonphysiologic and elicit severe systemic effects. At lower, more physiologic levels it has an inhibitory effect on the myometrium.

CLINICAL MANAGEMENT

Immediate Measures (Table 3–1)

On her arrival in the emergency room, a quick assessment must be made of the injured gravida to determine the level of consciousness, and cardiovascular and respiratory status. This includes evaluation of breathing and heartbeat, skin temperature and color, and pupillary reaction to light. Vital signs should be taken and recorded. In the absence of a heartbeat and/or breathing, cardiopulmonary resuscitation should be started immediately. This should be done even in the absence of a pupillary response, in preparation for possible postmortem cesarean section (see Chapter 12).

Cardiopulmonary Support

Patency of the airway must be established or maintained; if necessary, endotracheal intubation should be performed. Open chest wounds must be sealed to support respiratory exchange. Oxygen can be administered via a bag, valve, and mask unit until more sophisticated respirators are available. Cardiac activity is monitored with an electrocardiograph. If there is no hearbeat external cardiac compression should be instituted. Pulse, reactivity of pupils, skin color and consciousness should be monitored as parameters of the effectiveness of cardiopulmonary resuscitation.

Intravascular Volume Replacement

A large-bore catheter should be introduced into a peripheral vein and a central vein cannulated for central venous pressure monitoring. When the patient is hypotensive as a result of blood loss, large volumes of lactated Ringer's should be infused until type-specific blood is available. The physiologic hyper-

---

TABLE 3–1   Early Management of the Injured Gravida

1. Determination of ventilatory and cardiovascular status. Institute cardiopulmonary resuscitation as needed Vital signs.
2. Position pregnant patient on her left side.
3. Start intravenous infusions. Insert central and peripheral venous catheters.
4. Draw blood for typing and cross-matching and for laboratory determinations.
5. Insert nasogastric tube; place Foley catheter in bladder.
6. Obtain complete history and perform physical examination.
7. Diagnostic studies—roentgenograms, clinical procedures.
8. Institute tetanus prophylaxis.

volemia of pregnancy (Chapter 2) has a salutary effect in maternal hemorrhage. Clinical signs and symptoms of hypovolemia may not become evident in the pregnant patient until a 30 to 35 per cent reduction in blood volume is reached. Maternal blood pressure therefore is not a satisfactory measure of fetal well-being. Uterine blood flow can be reduced by as much as 10 to 20 per cent following acute hemorrhage, while maternal blood pressure is unchanged (Greiss, 1966).

The treatment of maternal hypovolemia should be directed at restoring both maternal and fetal homeostasis. The most satisfactory response is obtained when both volume and red cell mass are replaced by whole blood. Type-specific blood, if available, should be administered until type-specific cross-matched blood is available. In an acute situation, O negative blood can be used. Whole blood replacement results in restoration of maternal blood pressure and is rapidly followed by return to normal values of uterine blood flow, uterine tissue pO_2. and fetal tissue pO_2.

The use of dextran and lactated Ringer's solution in maternal hemorrhage was studied by Boba and co-workers (1966). They found that both intravenous solutions restored circulating maternal volume and thereby restored maternal arterial blood pressure. Dextran given in a volume equal to the amount of blood removed returns neither fetal arterial oxygenation nor fetal heart rate to normal levels. Lactated Ringer's solution, when used in amounts equal to three times the volume of shed blood, returns the fetal arterial oxygenation to normal levels without increasing fetal heart rate significantly.

Dextran, because of its high oncotic pressure, retains fluid in the intravascular compartment. Lactated Ringer's solution given in large volumes, in contrast, is available to restore the intravascular volume as well as replace the interstitial fluid. The interstitial fluid, which is diminished by the translocation phenomenon following hemorrhage, is necessary for metabolic exchange at the cellular level (Shires et al., 1972). Recent studies suggest that the administration of albumin in patients with hypovolemic shock, while increasing central venous pressure and pulmonary wedge pressure, results in deterioration in pulmonary function (Weaver et al., 1978).

Vasopressors should be avoided in attempts to restore maternal blood pressures in cases of hypovolemia. These drugs, although they restore maternal blood pressure, can cause further decrease in uterine blood flow and result in a worsening of fetal hypoxia (see Chapter 4).

Central Venous Pressure

Clinical measurement of central venous pressure (CVP) is useful in assessing cardiovascular status in trauma patients (Stahl, 1965). In young patients with normal cardiac function the appropriateness of fluid replacement can be assessed by monitoring the CVP. In the trauma patient, intrathoracic pathology can raise central venous pressure. In such patients, the placement of a Swan-Ganz catheter is indicated when central venous pressure readings are inappropriate to the amount of fluid replaced (Swan and Ganz, 1975).

Buchsbaum and White (1973) reported their experience with central venous catheters in obstetrics and gynecology and found monitoring of CVP extremely useful in emergency situations, particularly hemorrhage.

In the pregnant trauma victim, CVP readings must be interpreted with some caution. Colditz and Josey (1970) studied the alterations of central venous pressure during pregnancy. They found a markedly lower basal level in the second and third trimesters than in the first trimester and in the nonpregnant controls. This in no way diminishes the value of central venous pressure monitoring in severely injured gravid patients; the pregnancy alterations must simply be considered in interpreting readings.

Laboratory Studies

Blood should be drawn for typing and cross-matching, and for hematologic studies. Specimens should be sent to the laboratory for SMA 6/60 and 12/60, and for specialized studies as indicated — e.g., serum amylase. A complete blood count, including thrombocyte count, serves as a baseline in patients with suspected internal hemorrhage. An unconscious patient or one with chest wounds should have an arterial blood specimen submitted for pH, pO_2 and pCO_2 determinations.

Although a moderate leukocytosis follows acute hemorrhage, a significant rise suggests a ruptured spleen or liver. Berman and co-workers (1957), studying 338 consecutive patients with abdominal trauma, found an average leukocyte count of 23,890 per cu mm in patients with liver injury, and an average count of 19,050 per cu mm in patients with splenic injury. A count of over 15,000 per cu mm is suggestive of liver or splenic injury.

ALTERATIONS ACCOMPANYING TRAUMA. Attar and colleagues (1969) found changes in blood coagulation — alternating hyper- and hypocoagulability — in severely injured patients. They were unable to identify the precise mechanism leading to this altered coagulation and fibrinolysis, but concluded that a direct relationship existed between the degree of trauma, the alterations in coagulation, and the eventual outcome.

PREGNANCY ALTERATIONS. During pregnancy there is a marked increase in fibrinogen and clotting factors (see Chapter 2). In spite of these changes, maternal bleeding and clotting functions remain unchanged; alterations occur only in pathologic conditions. Abruptio placentae (premature separation of the normally implanted placenta), amniotic fluid embolism, and sepsis can cause a consumptive coagulopathy of pregnancy. A baseline bleeding profile in the injured gravida may be of considerable value. This should include a serum fibrinogen level, fibrin degradation products, platelet count, and examination of a blood smear for schistocytes. Partial thromboplastin time and prothrombin time are slightly prolonged in pregnancy. Since any of the above-mentioned pathologic conditions of pregnancy can accompany severe trauma, it behooves the physician to study the patient's clotting mechanism. A quick method of evaluating clotting and clot retraction is to observe 10 ml of blood in a glass test tube.

In normal pregnancy the leukocyte count can reach 18,000 per cu mm in the last trimester, and can rise to 25,000 per cu mm or more during labor (Efrati et al., 1964). One must therefore interpret a leukocytosis in an injured gravida with caution.

In the presence of clinical clotting disorders of pregnancy secondary to disseminated intravascular coagulation, whole blood replacement, administration of fibrinogen (or preferably cryoprecipitate), and early delivery are the methods of treatment. Disseminated intravascular coagulation can occur secondary to severe trauma but is more common following sepsis. The laboratory findings are those of lowered serum fibrinogen level and an elevated level of fibrin degradation products. A second form of coagulopathy is seen in those patients with massive blood replacement. When large amounts of blood are administered, patients develop a bleeding diathesis. This is characterized by low fibrinogen levels and low platelet counts. This type of coagulopathy is best managed by the administration of fresh whole blood, fresh plasma, and platelet transfusions (Pritchard and Brekken, 1967).

Position of the Patient

Pregnant patients beyond 20 weeks' gestation should not be left on their backs in the supine position while being assessed. The enlarged uterus compresses the vena cava, impeding venous return. Diminished cardiac output results, and the patient becomes hypotensive. This condition has been called the "supine hypotensive syndrome of pregnancy."

Prolonged compression of the vena cava has been shown experimentally to cause abruptio placentae. Reed and co-workers (1970) documented fetal bradycardia electrocardiographically during inferior vena caval obstruction.

The pregnant patient should be placed on her left side, and the position maintained by pillows, folded sheets, or a uterine displacer (Fig. 2–1). This position should be maintained during early assessment, while she is being transported to the Radiology Department or other area, and during surgery as well.

Intestinal Tubes and Bladder Catheter

A nasogastric tube should be placed in the stomach of any patient who sustains serious abdominal trauma, and in any patient who is unconscious. The aspirate is tested for blood. Likewise, a rectal examination should be performed and the stool examined for evidence of blood. In pregnancy there is a decreased motility of the gastrointestinal tract, with prolonged gastric emptying and prolonged intestinal transit. For these reasons the placement of a nasogastric tube is particularly important in the injured gravida.

An indwelling catheter should be placed in the bladder and urine examined for blood. Urine output should be recorded and fluid replacement estimated to maintain an output of 50 ml per hour. Difficulty in inserting the bladder catheter suggests disruption of the urethra secondary to pelvic fracture. Once in place, the Foley catheter should be inflated and can serve for the later performance of a retrograde cystogram to detect rupture of the bladder (Fig. 3–1). The Foley catheter should be left in place and urinary output measured and recorded hourly.

Complete Physical Examination

If the patient is unconscious a complete history should be obtained from relatives or friends. When possible, valuable information can be obtained from the patient's obstetrician.

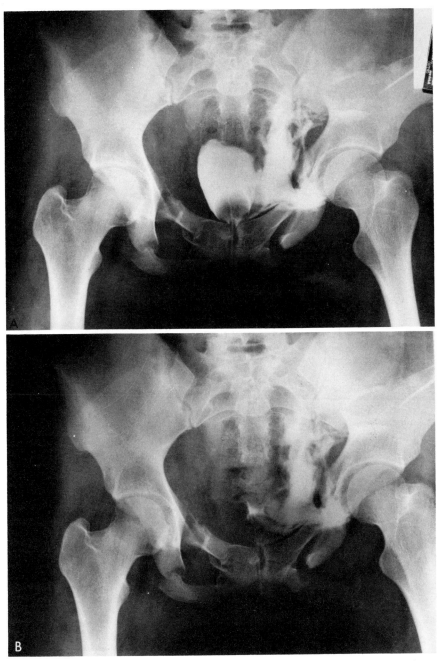

Figure 3–1   Ruptured bladder in female with multiple pelvic fractures. *A*, Retrograde cysto-gram through indwelling Foley catheter showing extravasation of contrast material. *B*, Extra-peritoneal rupture of bladder is demonstrated by contrast material after bladder has been emptied.

A complete physical examination is performed, with particular attention being paid to wounds and areas of ecchymosis. In gunshot wounds, entrance and exit wounds should be identified. A complete neurologic exam should be part of the examination. Fractured ribs on the left should alert the clinician to a possible ruptured spleen; a fractured pelvis, to a ruptured bladder or urethra. Careful examination of the extremities should be carried out and any suspected or documented fractures splinted.

The physical examination should also include a complete obstetric examination. The abdominal portion should include size of the uterus (see Fig. 2–2) for estimations of duration of pregnancy and fetal weight. Auscultation for fetal heart tones and palpation for fetal activity should both be done. Careful attention should be paid to the presence of uterine contractions suggesting early labor. Tetanic contractions accompanied by vaginal bleeding suggest premature rupture of the normally implanted placenta (abruptio placentae).

Any stethoscope will serve for auscultation of fetal heart tones; however, a fetoscope or ultrasonic Doppler cardioscope would help to amplify the sounds. The fetal heart rate and rhythm should be recorded.

A pelvic examination should be performed to determine effacement and dilatation of the cervix. The presentation (vertex, breech, etc.) should be noted, as well as the station of the presenting part. The station is the relationship of the leading pole of the fetus to the ischial spines. One should search carefully for evidence of amniotic fluid in the vagina. If there is any doubt, appropriate tests should be performed. Although no test is completely accurate, the correlation obtained with nitrazin paper is in the range of 97 per cent. The nitrazin test measures the pH of the vagina. The normal pH of the vagina is between 4.5 and 5.5; the pH of amniotic fluid between 7.0 and 7.5.

Laboratory studies are generally of little help in the diagnosis of intrauterine fetal death of short duration. At the earliest biochemical tests and x-ray studies become diagnostic days to weeks after fetal death (Fig. 3–2). The most reliable early finding suggestive of intrauterine fetal death is absence of fetal heart tones. Real-time ultrasound is the most accurate method to detect fetal heart activity, or lack of it (Bang and Holm, 1968; Brown, 1968).

Paracentesis

Diagnostic paracentesis has been widely used in the diagnosis and management of injured patients. The reported accuracy of needle paracentesis varies from 25 per cent to over 90 per cent. A negative tap is inconclusive; a positive tap suggests intraperitoneal hemorrhage.

In late pregnancy the gravid uterus with stretched round and broad ligaments compartmentalizes the peritoneal cavity. The increased anteroposterior diameter of the abdomen, and the compression of the small bowel in the upper abdomen, diminishes the accuracy and increases the hazards of needle paracentesis during pregnancy. For these reasons we have felt that this procedure is unwarranted in pregnancy (Buchsbaum, 1967, 1968).

Four-quadrant taps and culdocentesis have largely been replaced by peritoneal lavage, which appears to be a superior technique. Engrav and associates (1975) report an accuracy of 98.4 per cent with peritoneal lavage in 1465 patients evaluated for blunt abdominal trauma. Rothenberger and colleagues

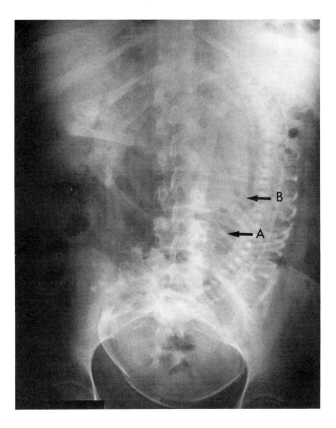

Figure 3–2   Maternal abdominal x-ray with dead fetus in vertex presentation. Roentgen evidence of fetal demise includes overlapping skull bones, air in the heart (*A*) and great vessels (*B*), and hyperflexion of fetal spine.

(1977) used peritoneal lavage in 12 pregnant women following blunt abdominal trauma. They utilized an open technique in which an incision is made into the peritoneum under direct vision, and a peritoneal dialysis catheter is directed toward the pelvis. If over 100 ml of blood is aspirated the test is considered positive; otherwise, one liter of Ringer's lactate is infused through the catheter and later removed by gravity drainage. Their criteria for interpretation of the test are shown in Table 3–2. These authors found peritoneal lavage technically easy to perform and accurate in the evaluation of blunt trauma in pregnant patients. It appears preferable to needle paracentesis.

Antibiotics

The choice of starting antibiotics rests with the surgeon in the management of the injured patient. Although most authorities condemn the use of prophylactic antibiotics, most also agree on the value of "preventive antibiotics." In bowel injury, for example, where peritonitis and abscess formation is likely, most would give antibiotics. The drug can be changed if necessary when cultures are available.

There is evidence that a standard dose of ampicillin administered to a pregnant female results in lower mean plasma levels than in nonpregnant subjects (Phillipson, 1978). To achieve the same antibiotic levels in the pregnant as in the nonpregnant individual it is necessary to double the dose.

TABLE 3–2   Diagnostic Peritoneal Lavage — Criteria for Interpretation*

Positive
1. Aspiration of over 10 ml blood.
2. Grossly bloody lavage fluid.
3. Lavage fluid returned through Foley catheter or chest tube.
4. Red cell count >100,000 per cu mm.
5. White cell count >500 per cu mm.
6. Amylase >175/dl. (Somogyi units)

Indeterminate (Test should be repeated)
1. Red cell count >50,000, <100,000 per cu mm.
2. White blood cell count >100, <500 per cu mm.
3. Amylase >75, <175/dl. (Somogyi units)
4. Dialysis catheter fills with blood.

Negative
1. Red blood cell count <50,000 per cu mm.
2. White blood cell count <100 per cu mm.
3. Amylase <75/dl. (Somogyi units)

---

*From Rothenberger DA, et al.: Am J Obstet Gynecol *129*:479, 1977.

The benefits to the fetus of giving antibiotics to the mother are tenuous. All antibiotics cross the placenta, but fetal serum and tissue levels vary with the agents used. The serum levels achieved in the fetus are approximately half the therapeutic levels in the mother.

Radiographic Studies

The value of x-rays in the diagnosis of fractures and in the management of chest injuries is undisputed; multiple views are useful in localizing a foreign body (Fig. 5–1). Plain films of the abdomen are far less valuable in diagnosing visceral injury. Since there are no pathognomonic roentgenographic signs of visceral injury, changes in and displacement of neighboring structures are suggestive but not diagnostic of organ injury. It is important to coordinate diagnostic studies in the injured patient to save time and unnecessary movement.

Fractures of the lower ribs on the right may be associated with hepatic trauma; fractures of the ninth, tenth and eleventh ribs on the left with splenic rupture. Fractures of the lumbar vertebrae may accompany renal injury. Fractures of the pedicles of the lumbar vertebrae are seen with lacerations of the bowel mesentery, and fractures of the anterior pelvis should arouse suspicion of bladder, urethral, or vascular injury. Free air will be seen below the diaphragm on upright films of the abdomen in 80 to 90 per cent of patients with perforation of the stomach, duodenal bulb, or colon (Love, 1975). Plain abdominal and chest films will identify diaphragmatic injury with herniation. This is a particularly important finding in the pregnant patient (see page 98).

Contrast studies are of great help in diagnosing gastrointestinal or urinary tract injuries. An intravenous pyelogram is helpful in assessing renal or ureteral pathology, and retrograde cystography in determining the integrity of the bladder (Fig. 3–1). When gastrointestinal studies are performed, a water-soluble medium must be used. A fistulogram (in which contrast material is injected into an injury tract) can determine if the peritoneal cavity has been entered (for description, see page 95).

In addition to the traditional roentgen techniques, arteriography, radioisotope scans, and ultrasound have been used to identify visceral injury following abdominal truma. Arteriography is the most widely applied and also the most sensitive, particularly in splenic, hepatic, and vascular injury (Redman, 1977). Nevertheless, it is time-consuming and requires trained personnel and specialized facilities. During pregnancy the dilated pelvic vasculature is particularly susceptible to traumatic injury. When time and conditions permit, pelvic arteriography can be combined with selective embolization to control bleeding (Margolies et al., 1972).

Less well established in the diagnosis of visceral injury is the value of isotope scans and ultrasonography. Technetium (^{99}Tc) scans have been used to identify splenic and hepatic rupture and subcapsular hemorrhage (Kurtzman, 1977). The value of ultrasound in the diagnosis of liver injury needs further evaluation.

While no radiographic study that might aid in the management of maternal injury should be withheld, the value of x-rays must be weighed against the potential risks to the conceptus. Any film of the maternal abdomen represents whole body irradiation to the fetus, with some studies delivering as much as 20 rads. Since negative roentgen findings cannot be accepted as diagnostic, x-rays should be used selectively during pregnancy. The uterus should be shielded during exposure of chest and extremity films. X-ray studies should be coordinated so as to reduce duplication — e.g., KUB (kidney, ureter, and bladder) and plain films of the abdomen. Only films that might dictate changes in the course of management should be taken.

The deleterious effect of ionizing irradiation on the fetus is related to the dose and the period of gestation. While no threshold dose has been established, it is estimated that the fetal tissues are more sensitive to x-rays than are the maternal tissues, particularly during organogenesis (weeks 3 through 12). High doses in very early pregnancy may cause abortion or congenital anomalies; in later pregnancy, the changes may be more subtle — diminished intelligence, genetic damage, or heightened susceptibility to subsequent development of malignancies.

Tetanus Prophylaxis

Most Americans will have received initial immunization against tetanus as infants (DPT), with a reinforcing dose at 18 months and a booster of 0.5 ml at the time they started school. Boosters should be administered at 10 year intervals, but this has not usually been done with women. At the time an injury occurs, 0.5 ml of toxoid should be administered. Ths will elicit adequate antibody levels in an individual previously immunized (Robles et al., 1967). When there is extensive tissue necrosis in conditions favorable to tetanus, human immune globulin (250 to 400 units) should be given intramuscularly with the toxoid booster, but at a different site.

The patient not previously immunized should be given the human immune globulin (200 to 500 units intramuscularly), and the first of three 0.5 ml doses subcutaneously or intramuscularly) of adsorbed toxoid at another site (see Table 3–3).

TABLE 3–3   Prophylactic Treatment of Tetanus*

Type of Wound	Patient Not *Immunized* or Partially *Immunized*	Patient Completely *Immunized* Time Since Last *Booster Dose*		
		1† to 5 years	5 to 10 years	10 years +
Clean minor	Begin or complete immunization per schedule; tetanus toxoid, 0.5 ml	None	Tetanus toxoid, 0.5 ml	Tetanus toxoid, 0.5 ml
Clean major or tetanus prone	In one arm: ‡Human tetanus immune globulin, 250 mg In other arm: ‡Tetanus toxoid, 0.5 ml, complete immunization per schedule	Tetanus toxoid, 0.5 ml	Tetanus toxoid, 0.5 ml	In one arm: ‡Tetanus toxoid, 0.5 ml In other arm: ‡Human tetanus immune globulin, 250 mg
Tetanus prone, delayed or incomplete debridement	In one arm: ‡Human tetanus immune globulin, 500 mg In other arm: ‡Tetanus toxoid, 0.5 ml, complete immunization per schedule thereafter Antibiotic therapy	Tetanus toxoid, 0.5 ml	Tetanus toxoid, 0.5 ml Antibiotic therapy	In one arm: ‡Tetanus toxoid, 0.5 ml In other arm: ‡Human tetanus immune globulin, 500 mg Antibiotic therapy

*From American College of Surgeons: Early Care of the Injured Patient. 2nd Ed. Philadelphia, W.B. Saunders, 1976.

†No prophylactic immunization is required if patient has had a booster within the previous year.

‡Use different syringes, needles and sites.

Note: With different preparations of toxoid, the volume of a single booster dose should be modified as stated on the package label.

REFERENCES

Attar S, Boyd D, Layne E, et al: Alterations in coagulation and fibrinolytic mechanisms in acute trauma. J Trauma 9:939, 1969.

Bang J, Holm HH: Ultrasonics in the demonstration of fetal heart movements. Am J Obstet Gynecol 102:956, 1968.

Berman JK, Habegger ED, Fields DC, et al: Blood studies as an aid in differential diagnosis of abdominal trauma. JAMA 165:1537, 1957.

Boba A, Linkie DM, Plotz EJ: Effects of vasopressor administration and fluid replacement on fetal bradycardia and hypoxia induced by maternal hemorrhage. Obstet Gynecol 27:408, 1966.

Brown RE: Detection of intrauterine death. Am J Obstet Gynecol 102:965, 1968.

Buchsbaum HJ: Splenic rupture in pregnancy. Obstet Gynecol Surv 22:381, 1967.

Buchsbaum HJ: Accidental injury complicating pregnancy. Am J Obstet Gynecol 102:752, 1968.

Buchsbaum HJ, White AJ: The use of subclavian central venous catheters in gynecology and obstetrics. Surg Gynecol Obstet 136:561, 1973.

Colditz RB, Josey WE: Central venous pressure in supine position during normal pregnancy. Obstet Gynecol 36:769, 1970.

Cushing RD: Antibiotics in trauma. Surg Clin North Am 57:165, 1977.

Efrati P, Presently B, Margalith M, et al: Leukocytes of normal pregnant women. Obstet Gynecol 23:429, 1964.

Engrav LH, Benjamin CI, Strate RG, et al: Diagnostic peritoneal lavage in blunt abdominal trauma. J Trauma 15:854, 1975.

Greiss FC: Uterine vascular response to hemorrhage during pregnancy. Obstet Gynecol 27:549, 1966.

Jackson ME: Endocrine aspects of trauma. *In* Bay SB (ed): Trauma. Clinical and Biological Aspects. New York, Plenum Medical Book, 1973.

Kaiser IH, Harris JS: The effect of adrenalin on the pregnant human uterus. Am J Obstet Gynecol 59:775, 1950.

Kurtzman RS: Radiology of blunt abdominal trauma. Surg Clin North Am 57:211, 1977.

Love L: Radiology of abdominal trauma. JAMA 231:1377, 1975.

Margolies MN, King EJ, Waltman AC, et al: Arteriography in the management of hemorrhage from pelvic fractures. N Engl J Med 287:317, 1972.

Phillipson A: Plasma levels of ampicillin in pregnant women following administration of ampicillin and pivampicillin. Am J Obstet Gynecol 130:674, 1978.

Pritchard J, Brekken AL: Clinical and laboratory studies on severe abruptio placentae. Am J Obstet Gynecol 97:681, 1967.

Redman HC: Thoracic, abdominal, and peripheral trauma. Evaluation with angiography. JAMA 237:2415, 1977.

Reed NE Teteris NJ. Essig GF: Inferior vena caval obstruction syndrome with electrocardiographically documented fetal bradycardia. Obstet Gynecol 36:462, 1970.

Robles NL, Walske BR, Personeus G: Delayed recall of tetanus antibodies. Am J Surg 114:627, 1967.

Rothenberger DA, Quattlebaum FW, Zabel J, et al: Diagnostic peritoneal lavage for blunt trauma in pregnant women. Am J Obstet Gynecol 129:479, 1977.

Shires GT, Cunningham JN. Backer CR, et al: Alterations in cellular membrane function during hemorrhagic shock in primates. Ann Surg 176:288, 1972.

Stahl WM: Resuscitation in trauma; the value of central venous pressure monitoring. J Trauma 5:200, 1965.

Swan HJC, Ganz W: Use of balloon flotation catheters in critically ill patients. Surg Clin North Am 55:501, 1975.

Weaver DW, Ledgerwood AM, Lucas CE, et al: Pulmonary effects of albumin resuscitation for severe hypovolemic shock. Arch Surg 113:387, 1978.

Chapter 4

EFFECTS OF HYPOVOLEMIA AND HYPOXIA UPON THE CONCEPTUS

*Charles R. Brinkman, III,
and James R. Woods, Jr.*

Pregnancy represents a state of complete fetal dependence in which the status of the fetus correlates closely with the degree of uteroplacental blood flow and tissue oxygenation. Several years ago an analogy was made between the fetus in utero and the low oxygen conditions existing on Mt. Everest. This concept has since been abandoned (the normal fetus is *not* chronically hypoxic). Nevertheless, the analogy does convey the isolation, dependency and precariousness of the fetus. In this chapter, we will discuss the nature of this dependency and how it is affected by both acute and chronic alterations in maternal circulating blood volume and oxygenation. We will rely heavily on experimental animal data in all sections of our discussion. Following a brief review of the relevant physiologic changes of pregnancy, we will elaborate on the pathophysiology, clinical effects, and treatment modalities of hypovolemia and hypoxia.

NORMAL PHYSIOLOGY

Pregnancy represents a period of dynamic change in the cardiovascular circulation in response to the growing requirements of the developing fetal-placental unit. Estimates of maternal blood volume expansion during gestation

Animal studies reported from the author's (CRB) laboratory have been supported by Grant HL-01755 and Grant HL-13634 from the National Heart and Lung Institute. Dr. Brinkman is the recipient of Career Development Award HL-70237.

The authors express their appreciation to Robert O. Bauer, M. D., and Klaus Staisch, M. D., Departments of Anesthesiology and Obstetrics and Gynecology, UCLA, for their manuscript review and suggestions.

range from 44 to 48 per cent (Pritchard, 1965; Chesley, 1972; Ueland, 1976). Although this increase apparently is progressive throughout pregnancy, the most pronounced increment in blood volume is observed during the second trimester, at a time of rapid placental growth. During the third trimester, reduced placental development is paralleled by a lesser increase in maternal blood volume. The maternal cardiac output also increases to term, peaking at 40 per cent above nonpregnant values. This increase in cardiac output may be partially accounted for by a rise in the heart rate of approximately 10 beats per minute. Although the stroke volume (the second component of the cardiac output) presumably increases to term gestation, this remains to be established.

Significant redistribution of maternal blood volume occurs in response to changes in peripheral vascular resistance and the increasing growth of the uteroplacental mass. Uterine blood flow, which in the nonpregnant state accounts for less than 2 per cent of the cardiac output, may increase to 20 to 30 per cent in late gestation (Lucas et al., 1965). This increase in uteroplacental blood flow may be partially explained on the basis of increased cardiac output and an expanded blood volume, but is primarily due to the low uteroplacental vascular resistance. The fact that the maternal blood pressure does not rise and, in fact, decreases somewhat during the second trimester is further evidence that the placenta offers little resistance to this increase in blood flow.

The regulation of effective circulating volume and the maintenance of vascular tone during pregnancy are quite complex. Rising progesterone levels during normal pregnancy tend to favor vascular smooth muscle relaxation and peripheral pooling. In addition, the increasing mechanical impedance of venous return by the growing uterus and its contents must be taken into account. In response to these hormonal and mechanical factors, the neurogenic tone of the capacitance vessels (venules) increases significantly during pregnancy and contributes to the maintenance of adequate cardiac output and uteroplacental perfusion.

Neurogenic control of uterine blood flow during pregnancy is only partially understood. Alpha adrenergic receptors have been described in the nonpregnant and pregnant uterus (Ladner et al., 1970; Gough and Dyer, 1971; Rosenfeld et al., 1976). Stimulation of these receptors through increased adrenergic tone causes vasoconstriction and reduced blood flow through the involved uterine vessels. Stimulation during pregnancy results in a lesser response than that observed in the nonpregnant patient and presumably reflects the damping effect of the noninnervated placental circulation. A second explanation recently proposed is based upon the depressant effect of the prostaglandin system upon adrenergic receptor activity (Clark et al., 1977).

Beta adrenergic receptors in the uterine vasculature have also been demonstrated but are less well defined than their alpha adrenergic counterparts. Studies of dynamic uterine function, in which neurogenic stimulants and blocking agents were given, suggest that alpha adrenergic receptor activity in the uterine vascular bed predominates over beta receptor activity. Likewise, testing in which uterine blood flow was measured during different perfusion pressures demonstrated no autoregulation. In other words, the uterus, unlike the kidney, brain, myocardium, and skeletal muscle, is incapable of increasing its blood flow in the face of decreasing perfusion pressures (Ladner et al., 1970). The uterine vascular bed late in pregnancy may, therefore, be thought of as a maximally dilated, passive, low resistance system in which uterine blood flow is determined by perfusion pressure (Ladner et al., 1970).

Functional and anatomic changes in the respiratory system result in an increased respiratory minute volume and occur in concert with these important cardiovascular and neurogenic changes. Hyperventilation may then result in a reduced arterial blood and alveolar pCO_2 to 30 mm Hg, without any demonstrable change in the respective oxygen tensions. In addition, there is a lowering of the oxygen capacity, content, and the combined oxygen concentration during pregnancy, reflecting declines in both arterial and venous hemoglobin concentrations. There is less than an 8 per cent decrease in the arteriovenous oxygen content difference during pregnancy when compared with the nonpregnant female. This decrease in tissue oxygen availability is more than adequately compensated for by the increased cardiac output. Indeed, per kilogram of body weight there is no change in the oxygen consumption during pregnancy.

HYPOVOLEMIA

Clinical hypovolemia may be defined in general terms as an acute circulatory insufficiency in which the cardiac output and perfusion pressure are inadequate to provide normal function to major vital organs. Since adequate circulation depends upon the heart, blood volume, and peripheral resistance, insult to any one of these parameters may result in impaired circulatory dynamics. For our purposes, hypovolemia will therefore be subdivided into acute blood loss, nonhemorrhagic volume loss (septic hypovolemia), and loss of effective circulating volume (hypovolemia secondary to conduction anesthesia and the inferior vena cava syndrome). The effects of such changes on the pregnant female are presented first, followed by the effects on the fetus. General principles of management of each type of hypovolemia are reviewed at the end of their respective sections.

Acute Blood Loss

Acute blood loss in the pregnant patient may be related to obstetric (abruptio placentae, placenta previa, postpartum hemorrhage) or nonobstetric nosebleeds, trauma) conditions (Quinlivan et al., 1970). Treatment of acute hypovolemia must take into consideration the nature of the insult and whether delivery of the infant should be part of the treatment regime. It is beyond the scope of this chapter to elaborate on the characteristics of each hemorrhagic condition. It should be emphasized, however, that obstetric and nonobstetric causes of acute blood loss are not mutually exclusive. Although traumatic impact to the pregnant abdomen may be associated with rupture of the liver or spleen, consideration should also be given to the possibility of acute trauma to the uterus or placenta.

The value of delivery by cesarean section at the time of acute hemorrhage hypovolemia depends upon the risk/benefit factors involved and the gestational age of the fetus. Trauma-induced blood loss without evidence of fetoplacental involvement may be managed expectantly. Evidence of placental separation, on the other hand, may dictate cesarean section regardless of gestational age. The points to be emphasized are (1) laparotomy for intraperitoneal bleedings of unknown origin must be done with the full anticipation of both obstetric and nonobstetric causes, and (2) the presence of one source of bleeding should alert one to the possibility of multiple trauma.

The classic responses to acute blood loss are (1) reduced blood volume, cardiac output, and venous return, (2) decreased arterial pressure, (3) reduced baroreceptor activity, (4) vagal inhibition resulting in tachycardia, and (5) stimulation of medullary centers and thoracolumbar sympathetic chains with resultant vasoconstriction and increased systemic vascular resistance (Brinkman et al., 1974). These responses have been described in both unanesthetized and anesthetized animal models. Cerebral and cardiac blood flows are initially maintained at the expense of splanchnic, renal, muscular, and cutaneous vascular beds (Brinkman et al., 1974).

With continued blood loss, a state of reduced cerebral and coronary blood flow is reached, in which even the early neural compensatory mechanisms become impaired. Peripheral vasoconstriction is replaced by venous dilatation and pooling. Impaired venous return and reduced cardiac efficiency further handicap an already low cardiac output. The accumulation of toxic metabolic products from reduced tissue perfusion through capillaries already damaged from intense vasoconstriction leads to capillary congestion with additional loss of plasma volume into the extravascular tissue. It is understandable, then, that all these changes working together lead eventually to a state of "irreversible shock" in which any treatment is unsuccessful and death ensues (Brinkman et al., 1974).

Brinkman and co-workers (1974) studied a group of near-term pregnant sheep in which hemorrhagic hypovolemia was induced by the removal of 50 ml of blood per minute until the arterial pressure had fallen to 50 per cent of the control level. The amount of blood volume removed in order to achieve this end point averaged 20 per cent. There was a progressive decline in the arterial pressure, central venous pressure and uteroplacental blood flow as the hypovolemia was produced. The maternal heart rate initially increased, but with continued blood removal, a progressive heart rate slowing occurred. Figure 4–1 illustrates the maximal maternal cardiovascular changes noted after 15 min of hypovolemia. Values are reported as a per cent change from control. It is important to note that the maximal decrease in uteroplacental blood flow was proportionately greater than the other recorded parameters; this indicates that the uteroplacental vascular resistance increased markedly. The fact that progressive reductions in blood pressure were accompanied by comparable decreases in uterine blood flow is further evidence against autoregulation within the uterine vascular bed. However, once the perfusion pressure fell below 50 mm mean arterial pressure, the uterine blood flow decreased and the uterine vascular resistance increased at a more pronounced rate (Ladner et al., 1970). This suggests that if the perfusing pressure of the uterine arteries drops below a critical level, the extrinsic tissue forces applied to these vessels effect vascular collapse and further impair uterine blood flow. Uterine oxygen transfer ($U\dot{V}O_2$) decreased by 41 per cent in response to the reduction in uterine blood flow. In

MATERNAL RESPONSE TO HEMORRHAGE ± ISE

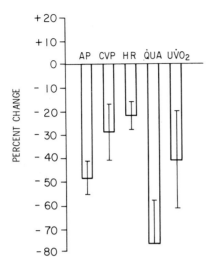

Figure 4-1 Mean percentage change from control, ±1 standard error of the mean (SE) 15 minutes after a 20 per cent reduction in blood volume in a group of near-term pregnant ewes under light pentobarbital anesthesia. AP, Mean arterial pressure; CVP, central venous pressure; HR, heart rate; QUA, uterine blood flow; $U\dot{V}O_2$, uterine oxygen transfer. See text for experimental detail.

contrast, the maternal arterial blood gases and pH changed minimally. Following 20 min of hypovolemic shock, the blood volume was restored by reinfusion of the removed blood, and maternal pressures, heart rate, and uterine blood flow returned to control values.

Other investigators have reported that the uterine perfusion may, in fact, be sacrificed before other vascular beds during acute hemorrhage (Greiss, 1967). In this study, rapid blood removal in the pregnant ewe resulted in a reduction in uterine blood flow before any change in blood pressure was observed. These data provide further evidence that uterine perfusion during acute hemorrhage may be influenced by lower perfusion pressures in addition to vasoconstriction within the uterine vascular bed.

Fetal Effects

The fetal effects of acute maternal blood loss are thought to be primarily a hypoxic response to reduced uteroplacental perfusion. Greiss (1967), studying pregnant sheep, discovered that uterine blood flow could be reduced by 75 per cent for brief periods without producing significant fetal cardiovascular effects. Brinkman and co-workers (1974) studied exteriorized lambs whose mothers had been subjected to a 20 per cent reduction in blood volume by removing 50 ml per min until the maternal arterial pressure had declined by 50 per cent. Figure 4–2 illustrates the changes in fetal arterial pressure (AP), heart rate (HR), blood flow, and umbilical venous oxygen tension resulting from 15 min of maternal hemorrhagic shock. These fetal cardiovascular responses occurred at the same time as the maternal effects illustrated in Figure 4–1. The changes in fetal arterial pressure and heart rate were minimal. There was a progressive increase in ductus arteriosus flow, consistent with increased shunting and increased pulmonary vasoconstriction in response to a declining oxygen transfer across the placenta. Umbilical vein oxygen tension was reduced by 50 per cent. Likewise, umbilical blood flows decreased in spite of an increase in fetal cardiac output (Fig. 4–2). Restoration of maternal blood volume abolished most of the fetal changes, although the fetal cardiac output remained elevated for at least 20 minutes. Fetal oxygen consumption returned to near control levels and a normal acid-base balance was restored.

MANAGEMENT

From the preceding discussion and observations, it is apparent that treatment for acute hemorrhagic hypovolemia must be directed at (1) restoration of circulating blood volume, and (2) prevention of further vasoconstriction in order to correct the maternal insult and to provide maximum clinical benefit to the fetus. Volume replacement with whole blood therefore becomes the first line of approach in hemorrhagic shock. In the event that this choice is not available, volume expansion with plasma, saline or dextrose may be utilized as a temporizing measure.

Various adjunct therapies have been employed and are mentioned here mainly to point out their deficiencies. The administration of oxygen and its transfer to the fetus have been studied in the dog model (Boba et al., 1967). One hundred per cent oxygen administered to the normovolemic mother resulted in an increased pO_2 in the fetal blood. In contrast, 100 per cent oxygen given to a mother during acute hemorrhagic hypovolemia did not change the depressed fetal pO_2 or improve cardiac performance. Thus, with impaired uteroplacental blood flow, improved oxygenation of maternal blood was of little benefit to the endangered fetus. (Oxygen supplementation is discussed further in the sections on hypoxia.) It would follow, then, that appropriate volume expansion, together with oxygen supplementation, during acute hemorrhagic events should be of considerable benefit to fetoplacental oxygen transfer.

Figure 4–2 Mean percentage change from control, ±1 standard error of the mean (SE) in near-term fetal lambs 15 minutes after a 20 per cent reduction in maternal blood volume. AP, Mean arterial pressure; HR, heart rate; QDA, ductus arteriosus blood flow; CO, effective cardiac output; QUV, umbilical blood flow; UVpO₂, umbilical vein oxygen tension. See text and Figure 4–1 for experimental detail and corresponding maternal response. (Effective cardiac output = ascending aortic + ductus arteriosus blood flows.)

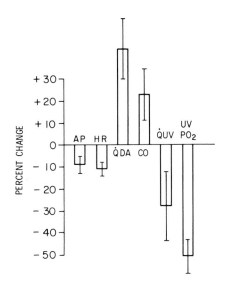

FETAL RESPONSE TO MATERNAL HEMORRHAGE ± 1 SE

The use of vasopressors during acute hemorrhagic hypovolemia is to be avoided except as a last resort for maternal preservation. The anticipated response to vasopressor administration should be a rise in blood pressure in response to drug-induced peripheral vasoconstriction. In hemorrhagic shock studies in the pregnant ewe, administration of phenylephrine (Neosynephrine) during the acute phase resulted in a rise in blood pressure accompanied by a further reduction in uterine blood flow (Greiss and Gobble, 1967). We have discussed the role and activity of the alpha adrenergic system in the uterine vasculature during acute hemorrhagic shock. The administration of a vasopressor under these circumstances would tend to further compromise an already impaired uterine blood flow and with it the status of the fetus.

Septic Hypovolemia

Infection is the leading cause of direct obstetric deaths in many large hospitals in spite of improved culture techniques and antibiotic regimes (Hardy et al., 1974). Septic abortion, pyelonephritis, amnionitis with or without premature rupture of membranes, and postpartum endometritis constitute the major threats. Management must, therefore, be individualized in each case, in terms of both antibiotic coverage and the status of the pregnancy. Pyelonephritis may, on the one hand, be treated with intravenous antibiotics and conservative management of the pregnancy itself. In contrast, amnionitis, in association with premature rupture of the membranes, requires uterine evacuation in addition to appropriate antibiotic coverage for optimal maternal care. Septic abortion may respond to antibiotics and uterine evacuation, but if rapid recovery is not observed, it may require hysterectomy and bilateral salpingo-oophorectomy as a lifesaving effort. Sepsis following major trauma constitutes a unique problem requiring individualized management.

Hypovolemia from overwhelming sepsis is characterized by peripheral pooling of blood volume, and in this sense differs from hemorrhagic hypovolemia, in which blood volume is physically removed from the circulatory system. Endotoxin studies carried out in dog and sheep models have defined three phases or responses leading ultimately to death. Following intravenous bolus injection of *E. coli* endotoxin in pregnant sheep, Bech-Jansen and co-workers (1972) observed a decline in arterial pressure and cardiac output along with an increased systemic vascular resistance. This initial hypotensive phase was followed by a recovery phase in which blood pressure, cardiac output, and regional blood flows returned to or even above control values. This second phase was presumed to be related to an outpouring of catecholamines, primarily from the adrenal gland. The third and terminal phase was characterized by a slowly progressive decrease in arterial pressure, cardiac output, and regional flows and a progressive metabolic acidosis.

FETAL EFFECTS

The ability of the fetus to tolerate such a degree of maternal cardiovascular insult depends largely upon the maintenance of uteroplacental oxygen transfer. Normal maternal oxygenation is of little value to the fetus if uteroplacental oxygen transport is impaired secondary to reduced uterine blood flow. Bech-Jansen and colleagues (1972) found that the fetus appears to tolerate the early stages of maternal septic hypovolemia well. In fact, only in the third and terminal phase of septic hypovolemia were detrimental changes in the fetal cardiovascular system seen.

Many attempts have been made to explain the pathophysiologic changes observed in septic hypovolemia. Although the scope of this chapter does not allow a full discussion of these theories, excellent reviews are available (Speroff, 1966; Cristy, 1971; Kitzmiller, 1971). Nevertheless, increased adrenergic stimulation, systemic hypotension, peripheral vascular pooling, and pulmonary hypertension with reduced cardiac output may all contribute to further impaired uteroplacental blood flow and fetal hypoxia (Bech-Jansen et al., 1972).

MANAGEMENT

Treatment of septic hypovolemia must be directed at (1) volume expansion to compensate for the massive peripheral pooling and loss of fluid into the extravascular space, (2) maintenance of effective cardiac output during volume expansion, and (3) identification of the infectious process, followed by appropriate antibiotic therapy. Bacteriologic studies and antibiotic selection are well defined in standard texts and therefore will not be discussed here. Rapid volume expansion with fresh whole blood accomplishes two purposes: expansion of intravascular volume and correction of red blood cell hemolysis secondary to the infection. Although the value of central venous pressure (CVP) monitoring will be discussed later, suffice it to say that volume expansion with whole blood, saline, or plasma should be undertaken in such a way as to establish an adequate urine output (greater than 30 ml/hour) while maintaining a CVP of less than 10 cm water. The devastating effects of pulmonary edema in the septic patient secondary to volume overload make CVP monitoring during rapid volume expansion essential.

Adequate volume load which is not effectively circulated merely adds to the preexisting peripheral pool. Isoproterenol has become an important adjunct in the management of septic hypovolemia, primarily as a result of its positive inotropic and chronotropic influence upon the heart. When this beta adrenergic drug is administered as an intravenous drip, its effectiveness is reflected in improved mobilization of pooled volume, increased cardiac output, and, as a consequence, stabilization of the blood pressure and uterine blood flow.

The use of steroids in pharmacologic doses during septic shock states has been advocated by numerous investigators. The mechanism by which steroids benefit the patient is controversial, with cited advantages ranging from lysosome stabilization (Weissman, 1965) to decreased peripheral vascular resistance and improved cardiac performance (Sambi, 1965). Nonetheless, improved survival as a result of their administration is well documented. Steroids may be abruptly discontinued at the end of 24 to 48 hours without mishap, once the patient's condition becomes stable.

The use of vasopressors in septic shock has generally been regarded as questionable, if not contraindicated. Metaraminol infusion during septic hypovolemia, while improving the blood pressure, had little effect upon the progressive acidosis and hypoxia accompanying the hemodynamic insult. Likewise, the use of phenoxybenzamine (Dibenzaline), an alpha-receptor blocker, to reduce adrenergic tone and improve tissue perfusion resulted in a faster deterioration than was seen in the untreated group (Bech-Jansen et al., 1972). It is of interest that estrogen administered to pregnant ewes prior to experimental septic hypovolemia markedly reduced the incidence of pulmonary hypertension and systemic hypotension and improved the maternal pO_2 during the septic insult (Crenshaw and Cefalo, 1974). The benefit of estrogen therapy in clinical management remains to be proved.

In addition, recent studies in our laboratory have found dopamine (Intropin) infusion to be a very effective method of maintaining arterial pressure and restoring uterine blood flow in nonpregnant sheep subjected to endotoxic shock. This modality of treatment is likewise in need of further investigation.

Hypovolemia Secondary to Conduction Anesthesia

Conduction anesthesia (spinal, caudal, epidural) has become a well accepted anesthetic tool in obstetrics during the last few years. In the injured pregnant patient, it may be used for cesarean section or for exploratory celiotomy to determine the extent of intraperitoneal injury. The increased usage is understandable when one considers that (1) complete relief of pain may be achieved, (2) the risks of pulmonary aspiration of gastric contents are greatly reduced, (3) continuous therapy (caudal, epidural) may be employed through the labor and delivery period, (4) the risks of maternal or neonatal depression in the absence of other obstetric complications are low, and (5) the same therapy may be used for vaginal delivery or cesarean section with only minor modifications in dosage and timing of drug administration (Bonica, 1972). Further support for this anesthetic modality has come from increased patient interest and participation in labor and delivery. These techniques, in addition, may be used in the pregnant patient for nonobstetric lower abdominal and lower extremity surgical procedures.

The improper use of conduction anesthesia, however, carries with it the risk of hypotension secondary to both blockade of peripheral sympathetic nervous activity and loss of supporting skeletal muscle tone. As was previously mentioned, increased neurogenic tone especially in the capacitance vessels (venules) is characteristically found during pregnancy. Blockade of this elevated neurogenic tone may result in peripheral vasodilatation accompanied by pooling of blood in the venous system, decreased venous return, impaired cardiac output, and systemic hypotension. The degree of peripheral pooling is presumed to correlate with the magnitude of the conduction blockade. It is not surprising, then, that as much as one third of the effective circulating blood volume may be sequestered in the capacitance vessels during the acute hypovolemic episode (Assali, 1972). Little change is seen in the neural activity of the uterine vasculature during this form of hypotension, presumably because of the low resting sympathetic tone in these vessels (Greiss and Gobble, 1967). Impaired cardiac output and marked peripheral vasodilatation in more responsive vascular beds may, therefore, be responsible for shunting blood away from the uteroplacental unit and for reduced oxygen transport to the fetus.

Proper use of conduction anesthesia is based upon patient monitoring and anticipation of related complications. Basic considerations relating to the use of conduction anesthesia include the following: (1) conduction anesthesia should be avoided in patients experiencing hypotension from acute blood loss, sepsis, or supine hypotension; (2) intravenous expansion of the patient's blood volume prior to anesthesia administration has become a common practice and reduces the risk of drug-induced hypotension; (3) close monitoring of the patient's blood pressure allows early detection of blood pressure changes and permits appropriate therapy before marked circulatory changes occur; (4) frequent examination of the level of anesthesia will alert the attending physician to the possibility of too high a level, with its associated respiratory problems.

Once drug-induced hypotension has occurred, however, treatment must be designed primarily to reestablish effective circulating volume and cardiac output. Leg elevation will help reduce peripheral pooling in the lower extremities and improve venous return to the heart. Likewise, volume expansion with normal saline will improve effective circulating volume and with it cardiac output.

VASOPRESSORS

The role of vasopressors in the management of various forms of hypotension has recently been reviewed in depth, and in hypotension secondary to conduction anesthesia they appear to have some limited value (Brinkman et al., 1976). Three groups of vasopressors are currently available (Table 4–1): (1) those with beta-receptor activity, (2) those that stimulate alpha receptors, and (3) those that stimulate both alpha and beta receptors. The cardiovascular properties of the various vasopressors are also shown in Table 4–1. It is clear from our previous discussion that hypotension resulting from conduction anesthesia is based on venous pooling, impaired venous return, and decreased cardiac output. Vasopressors with only alpha stimulating properties (norepinephrine, methoxamine, and phenylephrine) will cause further impairment of peripheral vascular flow through active vasoconstriction. Blood flow to the uteroplacental unit, already impaired by the reduced cardiac output, may be further compromised as a result of the increased adrenergic tone. These drugs are therefore not recommended.

Beta-receptor stimulants (isoproterenol), having both positive inotropic and chronotropic effects upon the heart, would at first glance appear to offer some benefits, primarily through an increase in cardiac output. Vasodilatation in response to isoproterenol administration, however, is accompanied by a 20 per cent decrease in arterial pressure and a 15 per cent decrease in uterine blood flow in the nonpregnant sheep (Ladner et al., 1970). In the pregnant ewe a decline in the blood pressure of only 10 per cent and no change in uterine blood flow have been observed following isoproterenol administration. Although these differences are presumably a result of the maximum dilatation found in the pregnant uterine vasculature, the value of a pure beta-receptor stimulant would seem to be less than optimal.

It is apparent from the preceding discussion that vasopressors with both alpha- and beta-stimulating properties may tend to offset the limitations to their use. Beta stimulation would provide cardiac stimulation to increase the cardiac

TABLE 4–1   Effects of Vasopressors in Pregnancy

	Arterial Pressure		Heart			Vascular Resistance	Uterus	
	Systolic	Diastolic	Rate	Contraction Force	Output		Blood Flow	Contractions
Alpha Stimulating								
Norepinephrine (Levophed)	↑	↑	0	0	0↓	↑	↓↓	↑
Mephentermine (Wyamine)	↑	↑	↑	0	↑	↑	↑	↑
Methoxamine (Vasoxyl)	↑	↑			↓	↑	↓	↑
Phenylephrine (Neosynephrine)	↑	↑	0↑	↓	↓	↑↑	↓	↑
Beta Stimulating								
Isoproterenol (Isuprel)	↓	↓	↑	↑	↑↑	↓	↓	↓
Alpha and Beta Stimulating								
Epinephrine (Adrenalin)	↑	↑	↑	↑	↑	↑	↓↓	↓
Metaraminol (Aramine)	↑	↑		0		↑	↓	0↑
Ephedrine	↑↑	↑	↑		↑	↑	↓	0↓
Dopamine (Intropin)	↑	↑	↑	↑	↑	↑		
Nonadrenergic								
Angiotensin (Hypertensin)	↑↑	↑↑			↓	↑↑	↓	↑

output, while increased alpha adrenergic tone would reduce the risk of peripheral vasodilatation and further peripheral pooling induced by increased beta-receptor activity.

Several studies have shown that metaraminol, administered to sheep made hypotensive by subarachnoid blockade, induces a recovery of the blood pressure and uterine blood flow to control levels (Lucas et al., 1965; Shnider et al., 1970; Assali, 1972). On the other hand, metaraminol administration during a normovolemic, normotensive state results primarily in a pressor response with increased arterial pressure and decreased uterine blood flow (Shnider et al., 1970), From this it would seem that the response to metaraminol may depend upon the status of the cardiovascular system at the time of injection. The fetal response to metaraminol injection during hypotension induced by spinal anesthesia also varies among studies. Lucas and co-workers (1965) found no fetal effects in their study; Shnider and associates (1970), on the other hand, observed a slight improvement in the fetal respiratory gases but no effect upon the progressive fetal metabolic acidosis.

Ephedrine has also been extensively studied during spinal hypotension (Shnider et al., 1968; James et al., 1970; Ralston et al., 1974). Although a predominant pressor response was reported by Ralston and co-workers (1974) in the normotensive pregnant sheep, ephedrine had little effect upon the maternal cardiac output, uterine blood flow, or fetal cardiovascular response. In addition, little or no alteration in the fetal blood respiratory gases was noted. When these studies were repeated in the hypotensive sheep, however, an improvement in the fetal blood respiratory gases was documented (Shnider et al., 1968). Recovery of the uterine blood flow to 90 per cent of control levels was reported by James and colleagues (1970) following ephedrine injection to the hypotensive sheep. The response to mephentermine when studied in the normotensive and hypotensive ewe was similar to that of ephedrine.

The role of dopamine, although inadequately studied at present, may ultimately prove useful in the management of hypotension following conduction anesthesia. When given in low doses, administration of dopamine results in a positive inotropic and chronotropic effect upon the heart, with a resultant increase in cardiac output and reduced systemic vascular resistance (Goldberg, 1972; Rosenblum et al., 1972). Higher doses of dopamine, on the other hand, elicit primarily an alpha adrenergic stimulation, with peripheral vasoconstriction as a consequence. The value of this drug and the dosage schedule necessary to capitalize on the central cardiac response without incurring peripheral vasoconstriction and presumably reduced uterine blood flow are not available at present.

Inferior Vena Cava Syndrome

Women late in gestation, if placed in the supine position, may experience pronounced hypotension and, if this is sufficiently prolonged, impaired uterine blood flow. The response is especially significant in the unconscious trauma patient, who is often left on her back during diagnostic and resuscitative procedures. The major cause of the hypotensive syndrome is compression of the inferior vena cava and major pelvic veins by the heavy gravid uterus. If unrecognized, this form of mechanical pooling may sequester up to 30 per cent of the effective circulating blood volume into the venous system (Assali, 1972). Studies in which pregnant patients late in gestation were moved from the supine to the lateral recumbent position showed a 25 per cent increase in cardiac output (Lees et al., 1968). The uterus may, in addition, compress or partially occlude the abdominal aorta. This unfortunate circumstance will reduce uteroplacental blood flow and may go clinically unrecognized if the fetal heart rate is not monitored. In addition, aortic compression will not be recognized by changes in arterial pressure in the upper extremities.

This form of iatrogenic hypotension is mentioned here because (1) its occurrence is undoubtedly far more frequent than is recognized, and (2) it must be considered each time a pregnant patient is placed in the supine position. It is extremely important that nonobstetric personnel be aware of this problem when caring for the near-term trauma victim. Management is simply directed at removing the mechanical compression (change of position) and mobilizing the pooled venous blood volume through leg elevation. The left lateral recumbent position is the position of choice, although simply pushing the uterus to the left is frequently effective.

Central Venous Pressure (CVP)
Monitoring

No discussion of hypovolemia and its treatment would be complete without emphasizing the value of CVP monitoring. The methods of catheter placement are clearly described elsewhere and so will not be discussed here (Fort, 1969). Several recent studies have appeared in which the use of CVP recordings during hemorrhagic and septic hypotension provided added information regarding the pathologic state of the patient. In every instance the blood pressure alone proved to be a poor index of volume depletion, and only with accurate CVP recording were adequate volume expansion and fluid mobilization accomplished.

The normal central venous pressure ranges from 0 to 5 cm H_2O (O'Driscoll and McCarthy, 1966). In late pregnancy (30 to 42 weeks) these pressures rise to 10 cm H_2O. O'Driscoll and McCarthy (1966) studied 13 patients with hemorrhagic shock in which bolus increments of 250 ml of whole blood were administered in order to raise the CVP to 10 cm H_2O. They found that an average transfusion of 3940 ml volume during the first hour was necessary to achieve these goals. Furthermore, maintenance of renal function was directly related to the aggressiveness with which volume replacement was effected. After volume restoration, the blood pressure in several instances was unchanged from pretreatment values. Only the CVP provided an accurate index of effective circulating blood volume.

Other studies have been equally illuminating. Muldoon (1969) reviewed a two-year experience with hemorrhagic shock. During the first year, patients were treated without the use of CVP, and during the subsequent year, CVP monitoring was employed. The results revealed that CVP monitoring allowed an 80 per cent greater volume replacement, established a more favorable urine output and resulted in no patients with oliguria.

Recently, the development of balloon-directed (Swan-Ganz) cardiac catheters has simplified the placement of catheters in the pulmonary artery and the determination of pulmonary artery and pulmonary wedge pressures. These two parameters give a much more reliable estimate of central intravascular volume and, in addition, provide information on the efficiency of both the right and the left sides of the heart. Placement of a balloon-directed catheter is not a procedure for the inexperienced and in general should be done under fluoroscopy.

In the critically ill or injured pregnant patient, in addition to the usual monitoring of vital signs and functions, an intra-arterial cannula is of great assistance for continuous monitoring of arterial pressure.

HYPOXIA

Hypoxia may be defined as a relative oxygen deficit in which the tissues, for any reason, fail to receive an adequate supply of oxygen. It has been shown that during pregnancy the patient's demands for oxygen become greater as the metabolic demands of breast, uterine, and fetal growth are met. It is not surprising, then, that the pregnant patient is less tolerant of all degrees of hypoxia than the nonpregnant individual. Hypoxia may result from any of several circumstances: (1) decreased delivery of oxygen via the lungs, (2) decreased oxygen-carrying capacity of the blood, (3) decreased tissue perfusion by oxygenated blood, or (4) inability of the tissues to extract or use adequately oxygenated blood. It is important to keep in mind that these hypoxic mechanisms also apply in the patient with acute hypovolemia with reduced cardiac output, reduced blood volume, and constricted vascular beds.

Blood Respiratory Gases and pH During Normal Pregnancy

Kelman and Templeton (1975) studied 12 nonsmoking primigravidas serially at 12, 24. 32, and 38 weeks of gestation. The results of the study are shown in Table 4–2. The progressive decrease observed in the hemoglobin concentration at midgestation is presumed to be a result of hemodilution. Note that there was a progressive decline in the oxygen tension (PaO_2). There was also a slight metabolic acidosis, as calculated by the increased base deficit. As would be expected, the oxygen consumption increased by 43 per cent during pregnancy.

Pathophysiology of Hypoxia

Nonpregnant Patients

It is important in any discussion of the normal pathophysiologic responses to hypoxia to establish the severity of the insult, for this will certainly affect the rate of onset and type of response. It would also appear that the response will vary, depending upon the presence of spontaneous versus artificial respirations. Increasing hypoxia is heralded by dyspnea, tachycardia, and cyanosis, though the latter is not present if hemoglobin concentrations are significantly reduced. With mild hypoxia, or in early, more profound hypoxia, there is a slight elevation of systolic and, to a lesser degree, of diastolic arterial pressures, together with increased cardiac output. As the severity or duration, or both, of the hypoxia increases, the arterial pressure, while decreasing to subnormal values, does not reach shock levels. The changes in cardiac output and cardiac function are less clear in the literature. Downing and co-workers (1966) state that cardiac function was altered only during severe acute hypoxia, when acidosis was present.

TABLE 4–2 **Maternal Hemoglobin, Blood Gases, and Oxygen Consumption During Pregnancy**

Gestational Weeks	12	24	32	38
Hgb (gm/dl)	12.5	11.5	10.8	11.1
PaO_2 (mm Hg)	107.6	104.1	102.5	101.3
$PaCO_2$ (mm Hg)	29.7	28.0	30.2	31.1
$\dot{V}E$ (l/min)	8.4	10.3	10.4	11.1
$\dot{V}O_2$ (ml/min)	160	200	230	280

$\dot{V}E$ = Minute volume.
$\dot{V}O_2$ = Oxygen consumption.

Pregnant Animals

Information regarding the hypoxic response of the dyspneic pregnant organism is limited. Dilts and associates (1969) compared the systemic and uterine hemodynamic responses to mild and severe hypoxia in both pregnant and nonpregnant sheep. Some of these experiments were performed under pentobarbital anesthesia, which is known to blunt the cardiac reflexes. Figure 4–3, redrawn from Dilts and co-workers' data, illustrates the effects of 15 min of severe hypoxia in pregnant and nonpregnant sheep. Maternal respirations were assisted with an intermittent positive pressure breathing respirator driven by a mixture of 6 per cent oxygen and 94 per cent nitrogen. In this group of near-term animals, the cardiac output increased by 11 per cent, whereas the mean arterial pressure fell by about 8 per cent. During this same time-frame, the oxygen tension fell from 99 torr to 32 torr, carbon dioxide tension decreased by 4 mm Hg, and the pH increased slightly. Figure 4–3 also illustrates a group of nonpregnant animals similarly studied for comparison. In the nonpregnant ewe, there were a 40 per cent increase in cardiac output, a 22 per cent decrease in mean arterial pressure and a 43 per cent fall in systemic vascular resistance. Respiratory blood gas changes were similar to those observed in the pregnant animals.

These data very aptly demonstrate the reduced cardiac reserve of the pregnant organism under conditions of severe hypoxia. In addition, the pregnant animal has less of a reduction in arterial pressure and systemic vascular resistance, which probably reflects the high adrenergic tone normally found in pregnancy. At first glance, this adaptation would appear to be a desirable protective mechanism. Unfortunately it does not allow the compensatory vasodilatation which would increase tissue perfusion and enhance tissue oxygen delivery.

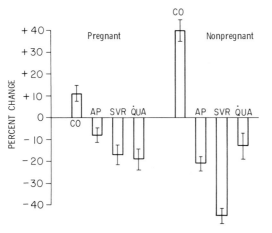

MATERNAL RESPONSE TO HYPOXIA ± ISE

Figure 4–3 Mean percentage change from control, ±1 standard error of the mean (SE) in nonpregnant and near-term pregnant ewes subjected to 15 minutes of severe hypoxia (6 per cent oxygen). CO, Cardiac output; AP, mean arterial pressure; SVR, systemic vascular resistance; $\dot{Q}$UA, uterine blood flow. See text for experimental detail.

Uteroplacental Perfusion

Several studies have examined the influence of hypoxia upon uteroplacental blood flow (Dilts et al., 1969; Greiss et al., 1972; Makowski et al., 1973). Greiss and co-workers (1972) and Makowski and colleagues (1973), each using chronically instrumented pregnant ewes, studied the responses to 10 per cent and 15 per cent oxygen. Greiss and co-workers (1972) reported that reducing the maternal arterial pO_2 to 40 mm Hg decreased placental flow minimally, whereas maternal heart rate increased about 20 beats per min and arterial pressure fell slightly. These observations were constrasted by similar studies carried out in nonpregnant castrated ewes, in which a 25 per cent increase in uterine blood flow was accompanied by tachycardia and a slight decrease in arterial pressure. Makowski and associates (1973), using 15 per cent oxygen for maternal inhalation in a second series of animals, found that this concentration of oxygen resulted in a pO_2 of 44 mm Hg and a minimal decrease in both the arterial pressure and uterine blood flow.

The uteroplacental hemodynamic effects of hypoxia in pregnant sheep have also been studied in our laboratory (Dilts et al., 1969). Near-term pregnant animals were instrumented and studied acutely under spinal anesthesia at 6 per cent (severe hypoxia) and 12 per cent (mild hypoxia) oxygen concentrations. These mixtures produced maternal arterial oxygen tensions of 30 and 55 mm Hg, respectively. Ventilation of the ewe with 6 per cent oxygen resulted in a 22 per cent decrease in uteroplacental blood flow, whereas with 12 per cent oxygen, the blood flow decreased by 17 per cent. In the severely hypoxic animals, the fraction of the cardiac output destined for the pregnant uterus was calculated. Under normal nonstressed conditions, the uterus received between 17 and 20 per cent of the cardiac output. In the severely hypoxic animal, this uterine fraction fell by 30 per cent, or to 12 to 14 per cent of the cardiac output. At a time when the cardiac output was increasing, uteroplacental perfusion was decreasing. Even in the studies by Greiss and Makowski and their colleagues, discussed above, if one assumes that the cardiac output was increasing, a lack of change in the uterine blood flow would mean that the uterine fraction of cardiac output had decreased.

Two possible mechanisms have been postulated for this disproportionate increase in uteroplacental vascular resistance: (1) the decrease in uterine blood flow may be related to an increase in myometrial tone, or (2) hypoxia may elicit a direct vasoconstriction through either increased catecholamine release or sympathetic discharge. Karlsson (1974) studied both these possibilities in pregnant rabbits. Near-term rabbits were acutely subjected to 10 per cent oxygen, and regional blood flows were studied by the microsphere method. The effects were compared with those in animals similarly stressed, but which were subjected to alpha adrenergic receptor blockade with phenoxybenzamine prior to the hypoxic insult. Hypoxia resulted in a consistent and significant decrease in blood flow to the myometrium and an even greater decrease in placental perfusion. Following alpha adrenergic blockade and induction of hypoxia, the decreases were minimal. These findings are in agreement with those of many other investigators regarding the strong dominance of the alpha adrenergic receptors in the uterine circulation.

Placenta and Placental Function
During Hypoxia

We have already established that hypoxia, particularly when severe, reduces uteroplacental blood flow. In addition, when we discuss the fetus in the following section, we shall see that umbilicoplacental blood flow is also reduced. Because blood flow is a very important rate-limiting factor in placental transfer, reductions in flow significantly impair the transfer of substances crossing the placenta by simple diffusion.

Lumley and Wood (1967) studied the response in five women to 10 per cent oxygen during the first stage of labor. The investigators noted that 15 to 30 min after the onset of hypoxia, there was a 35 per cent increase in maternal blood glucose. Simultaneous fetal blood glucose determinations demonstrated a decrease by an average of 5 per cent from maternal levels. To confirm that hypoxia was the important variable, five additional patients breathing room air were given 10 gm of glucose intravenously in order to raise their blood glucose by 35 per cent. In these patients, the fetal blood glucose increased by 33 per cent, demonstrating that maternal hypoxic hyperglycemia causes some impedance to transfer of glucose from the mother to the fetus.

Tominaga and Page (1966) carried out a series of in vitro experiments using both artificially perfused placentas and tissue cultures. They noted that when isolated human placentas were perfused with blood of low oxygen tension, the vascular resistance decreased. This decreased vascular resistance was postulated to be a result of vasodilatation of small tertiary fetal vessels, which would have the effect of increasing the diffusion area of the placenta. Such in vitro studies using an isolated vascular bed are difficult to interpret because in the intact organism, the response of each vascular bed reflects not only its own individual characteristics but also the homeostatic mechanisms of the entire organism. In addition, while there is no evidence that the umbilicoplacental vascular bed is under direct neural control, it is capable of humoral mediated responses.

As a second part of their study, Tominaga and Page (1966) cultured small pieces of human term placentas under oxygen concentrations of 0, 6, 26 and 95 per cent for 24 and 48 hours. At 6 per cent oxygen, they noted that the nuclei of the syncytiotrophoblasts of individual villi tended to cluster together at one pole, resulting in a thinner syncytial layer over the remaining portion of the villi. These changes were detected after 6 hours of hypoxia and were reversible following adequate oxygenation. It was estimated that this change reduced the diffusion distance by 25 per cent and might therefore be a protective mechanism for the fetus.

Oh and co-workers (1975) provided further evidence for the placental vasculature response to hypoxia. Using chronically instrumented near-term pregnant sheep, he determined the distribution of blood between the placenta and the fetus during hypoxia. He found that the placental fraction of the total fetal blood volume decreased progressively during hypoxia, whereas the total placental-fetal blood volume remained unchanged. This study provides further evidence of the increased umbilicoplacental vascular resistance existing during hypoxia and the potential adverse effect it may have upon placental transfer.

No data are available on the effects of hypoxia upon placental and fetoplacental biochemical parameters, such as HPL (human placental lactogen) or estriol. From the data presented, however, it is reasonable to assume that the values would be depressed.

Fetal Response to Maternal Hypoxia

Efforts to assess the effects of hypoxia on maternal and placental physiology have been concentrated largely during late gestation, and comparable information in early pregnancy is sparse. Although one might assume that most of the responses to hypoxia already elucidated occur to some degree at all stages of gestation, additional studies in early pregnancy are desirable.

Rattner and associates (1976) studied the effects of increasing hypoxia upon implantation in mice. On the day following fertilization, the mice were placed in a low oxygen environment for six days and the implantation sites counted on the eighth day. Implantation was not impaired at oxygen concentrations of 21 per cent and 14 per cent, but at 12 per cent and 10 per cent O_2 there was a 50 per cent reduction in implantation sites. At 8 per cent oxygen levels, blastocyte implantation was completely blocked. Unfortunately, the critical duration and timing of hypoxia during the first few days of gestation are unknown.

Additional information regarding the vulnerability of early gestation to hypoxia is derived from the studies of Clemmer and Telford (1966) who exposed pregnant rats to a single 6 hour hypoxic episode between gestational days 9 and 13. Hypoxia was produced by decompression to a simulated altitude of 28,000 feet, a condition comparable to somewhat less than 6 per cent oxygen at sea level. The animals were then sacrificed on the twenty-second day (term) and the fetuses delivered. Ninety-eight per cent of the baby rats survived for 24 hours, after which all were sacrificed and examined for anomalies. The most striking observation was that 28 per cent were found to have cardiac defects, as compared to only 7.5 per cent of fetuses not exposed to hypoxia. In addition, neither the exact timing of hypoxia (ninth day as opposed to thirteenth day) nor the fetal sex seemed to have any effect upon the results. Of the anomalies, 71 per cent were septal defects, the most common being a left ventricular–right atrial opening. The second most common anomaly was an intraventricular defect. Thus, it is apparent that at least in experimental animals, a relatively short duration of severe hypoxia may have a significant effect on the developing fetus.

Hemodynamic and Acid-Base Response of Near-Term Fetus

Hypoxia has long been considered the common denominator of fetal distress and, therefore, has received considerable attention from investigators. Many of the studies were carried out in acute models in which the monitoring equipment and the stress were applied in sequential order. It is important to keep in mind that in such an experimental situation, the preparatory surgery may have influenced the response to induced hypoxia.

Brinkman and co-workers (1970*b*) studied the effects of maternal hypoxia on fetal blood gases, pH, and hemodynamics in pregnant sheep under spinal anesthesia. Figure 4–4 shows the interrelationship of maternal arterial, umbilical

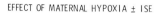

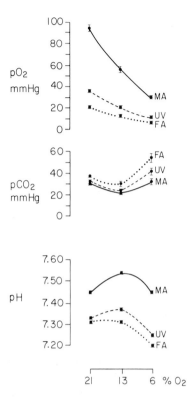

Figure 4–4 Mean values, ±1 standard error of the mean (SE) for blood oxygen (pO_2) and carbon dioxide (pCO_2) tensions and pH during 21 per cent O_2 (room air), 13 per cent O_2 (mild hypoxia) and 6 per cent O_2 (severe hypoxia) respiration by a series of near-term pregnant ewes, and the effects on their fetuses. MA, Maternal arterial blood; UV, fetal umbilical venous blood; FA, fetal arterial blood. (From Brinkman CR III, et al.: Gynecol Invest *1*:115–127, 1970. S. Karger AG, Basel.)

venous, and fetal arterial oxygen, carbon dioxide tension, and pH during exposure to 21 per cent (room air), 13 per cent, and 6 per cent oxygen inhalation by the ewe. Hyperventilation is commonly seen in mild hypoxia (13 per cent) or during the early phases of more severe hypoxia (6 per cent) and results in decreases in both maternal and fetal carbon dioxide tension. This decreased pCO_2 is reflected by an increased maternal pH which, in turn, can be seen in the fetal umbilical vein. Increased metabolic acids in the fetal arterial bed, resulting from tissue hypoxia, may initially balance the maternal respiratory changes. Thus, with continued or severe hypoxia, the maternal organism continues to maintain acid-base stability while the fetus becomes progressively acidotic (Fig. 4–4).

Figure 4–5 illustrates the fetal hemodynamic response to both mild and severe maternal hypoxia (Brinkman et al., 1970*b*). The degree of hypoxia was defined on the basis of the umbilical vein oxygen tension, since there appeared to be two subgroups of umbilical vein pO_2 values when the maternal arterial pO_2 was less than 55 mm Hg. These subgroups were defined as mild hypoxia when the umbilical vein pO_2 was between 14 and 23 mm Hg and severe hypoxia when it was less than 14 mm Hg. Fetal arterial pressure fell slightly and to a comparable degree during both mild and severe hypoxia (Fig. 4–5). In contrast, the outputs of the left and right ventricles, ascending aortic and pulmonary artery flows, respectively, progressively decreased with more severe hypoxia. Furthermore, the ascending aortic flow was proportionally less affected than the pulmonary artery flow. Since the majority of the ascending aortic flow is destined for the head and brain, this observation becomes important when we discuss the effects of hypoxia on regional circulation in the fetus.

Figure 4–5 also illustrates the ability of the ductus arteriosus to shunt blood from nonessential fetal pulmonary circulation to the descending aorta and the systemic circulation. Under conditions of mild fetal hypoxia, blood flow through the ductus arteriosus is maintained or slightly increased. In severe hypoxia, during which a profound decrease in pulmonary artery blood flow occurs, there may be a significant decrease in shunting across the ductus. This decline in ductus arteriosus flow may, in fact, play an important role in the ultimate response of the fetal umbilical circulation to hypoxia. The ductus arteriosus is known to be sensitive to oxygen tension changes. Assali and colleagues (1963) demonstrated that the ductus tends to constrict when the oxygen tension climbs above 50 mm Hg. Indeed, this oxygen sensitivity is important in the transition from a fetal to a neonatal circulation. Whether the ductus arteriosus dilates secondary to a hypoxic stimulus cannot be answered with certainty. It is possible that the maintenance of or increase in ductus shunting during mild hypoxia is primarily the result of a greater increase in pulmonary vascular, rather than systemic vascular, resistance. If so, the altered pressure gradients would favor increased blood flow through the ductus arteriosus.

The fetal response to acute hypoxia is, therefore, similar to that of the adult and is characterized by (1) variable changes in arterial pressure, including both mild increases and decreases, (2) a profound increase in pulmonary vascular resistance, and (3) a reduction in cardiac output. The unique features of the fetal vascular anatomy on the one hand tend to protect the fetal circulation from the effects of hypoxia by shunting blood from the pulmonary to the systemic circulations through the ductus arteriosus. On the other hand, the response of the umbilical circulation to hypoxia does not appear to favor fetal well-being and survival.

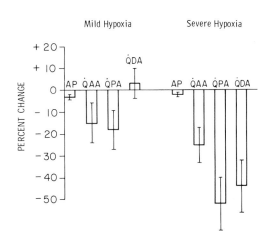

Figure 4–5 Mean percentage change from control, ±1 standard error of the mean (SE) in near-term fetal lambs whose mothers were ventilated with 13 per cent O₂ (mild hypoxia) and 6 per cent O₂ (severe hypoxia) for 15 minutes. AP, Fetal mean arterial pressure; QAA, ascending aortic blood flow; QPA, pulmonary artery blood flow; QDA, ductus arteriosis blood flow. (From Brinkman CR III, et al: Gynecol Invest *1*:115, 1970. S Karger, AG, Basel.)

The maintenance of an adequate umbilico-placental circulation is critical if the fetus is to survive a hypoxic insult. Dilts and associates (1969) found a 40 per cent decrease in umbilical blood flow when the mother was exposed to 15 min of severe 67 per cent oxygen hypoxia. Brinkman and co-workers (1970*a*), using a similar sheep model and the same oxygen concentration, found a 24 per cent decrease in umbilical blood flow. Mann (1970*a*) defined an isoelectric EEG as the end point of hypoxia in the pregnant ewe, and demonstrated a 21 per cent decrease in umbilical flow. Oh and colleagues (1975), using an indicator dilution technique, determined both umbilical blood flow and fetoplacental and placental blood volumes in chronically instrumented (nonanesthetized) sheep. He reported a 20 per cent reduction in umbilical blood flow and a 22 per cent decrease in umbilical blood volume during acute hypoxia.

Cohn and associates (1974) studied a chronic sheep model subjected to 6 per cent oxygen, in which cardiac output and regional blood flows were determined by the labeled microsphere method. The fetal response was studied when the fetal arterial oxygen tension had fallen to 11 to 14 torr, an event which took from 4 to 44 min. In the nonacidemic fetus, arterial pressure increased 14 per cent and the fetal heart rate decreased 25 per cent. Cardiac output decreased by only 5 per cent, whereas umbilical blood flow increased by 12 per cent. The acidemic fetus demonstrated a greater fall in cardiac output (−23 per cent) and only a 5 per cent increase in umbilical blood flow.

Brinkman and co-workers (1970*a*) attempted to isolate the location of the resistance changes in the fetal sheep umbilical circulation. The results of that study (Fig. 4–6) indicate that whereas the placental vascular resistance increased with both mild (13 per cent O_2) and severe (6 per cent O_2) hypoxia, there was a much greater increase in the umbilical sinus vascular resistance in the latter state. The umbilical sinus is the outflow of the umbilical vein through the fetal liver and includes the ductus venosus. Thus, while the fetal placental vessels constrict in the presence of hypoxia, the ductus venosus appears to play a major role in regulating umbilical blood flow in the fetus under hypoxic conditions.

It is apparent from the above discussion that any assessment of the true clinical impact of hypoxia upon mother and fetus is limited by the multiple variables that may occur with such a stress. Although efforts have been made in

PERCENT CHANGE FROM CONTROL
±1 SE

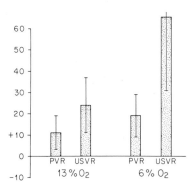

Figure 4–6 Mean percentage change from control, ±1 standard error of the mean (SE) in near-term fetal lambs whose mothers were ventilated with 13% O_2 (mild hypoxia) and 6% O_2 (severe hypoxia). PVR, Placental vascular resistance; USVR, umbilical sinus vascular resistance. (PVR = Umbilical artery − umbilical vein pressure ÷ umbilical blood flow. USVR = Umbilical vein − inferior vena cava pressure ÷ umbilical blood flow.)

some studies to limit the number of variables, in most cases they have been only partially successful. In addition, the duration of gestation may play a role in the outcome of hypoxic testing. It is not surprising, then, that extrapolation of such laboratory studies into the clinical setting may generate some confusion regarding the fetal hemodynamic response to hypoxia. Most investigators agree that fetal exposure to hypoxia is accompanied by bradycardia and a slight to moderate reduction in cardiac output. The response of the umbilical circulation to fetal hypoxia is more controversial. Although the majority of investigators have reported at least a 20 per cent reduction in fetal placental perfusion, further studies are needed.

The influence of hypoxia upon fetal blood flow in selected organ systems has been the subject of several recent reports. Both Cohn and associates (1974) and Mann (1970*b*) demonstrated an increase in cephalic blood flow and a reduction in cerebral vascular resistance in the hypoxic sheep fetus, similar to the response observed in the adult. In other studies, it was shown that the less mature fetus or neonate appears to be less sensitive to the sequelae of hypoxia (Shelley, 1969). From these reports and others, it becomes apparent that severity and duration of hypoxia, in addition to developmental maturity, significantly influence fetal outcome. Support for these observations in the human comes from the fact that survival times are longer following asphyxia in the newborn than after asphyxia occuring at any other time of postnatal life.

Two pathologic lesions of the CNS are typically observed secondary to fetal hypoxia. In the premature infant, cerebral intraventricular hemorrhage with adjacent germinal matrix and white matter infarction are commonly found, whereas in the mature term infant infarction of the cerebral cortex with necrosis and secondary hemorrhage are more frequent. The different sites of reaction to hypoxia between the preterm and term infant are thought to be partly related to the maturation of the central nervous system. Neuronal development begins in the periventricular region, with migration to the cortical areas as term approaches. The reader is referred to the recent excellent reviews of Volpe (1977) and Brann and Sykes (1977) for further information on the effects of hypoxia on the fetal and neonatal central nervous system.

The development of cerebral lesions in the fetus and neonate has been shown to result from metabolic alterations of hypoxia, acidosis, and hypoglycemia. Mann (1970*b*), in his study of cephalic metabolism during hypoxia, found a progressive decrease in the glucose concentration of the carotid arterial blood. Mann (1970*c*) also studied placental gradients of lactate, pyruvate, and glucose in the hypoxic ewe and her fetus. Although no apparent placental transfer of lactate accumulation during hypoxia was found, there was a positive gradient from the fetal to the maternal circulation. A reduction in the umbilical venous-arterial difference of glucose, secondary to an increase in arterial concentrations, and a decrease in umbilical vein glucose concentration were also noted. It is presumed that these two observations relate to increased fetal glycolysis and reduced placental glucose transport. For the reader who is interested in a more complete discussion of the fetal metabolic response and sequelae of hypoxia, the review by Shelley (1969) is recommended.

In addition to the circulatory and metabolic effects of hypoxia, direct and indirect effects upon the centers that control respiration have long been recognized. Dawes (1974) has reported the effects of a variety of stimuli or stresses on fetal sheep breathing activity. He noted that hypercapnea tended to increase the frequency and magnitude of fetal breathing movements, whereas mild degrees of hypoxia greatly reduced or arrested fetal respiratory efforts in the fetal lamb. There is promise that these observations may have some clinical application. Boddy and Robinson (1971) have reported an ultrasound method for recording human fetal chest wall movements.

Clinical Mechanisms of Hypoxia

Up to this point, animal studies have been heavily emphasized as a means for better understanding the mechanisms and sequelae of clinical hypoxia upon both mother and fetus. In addition, a knowledge of the basic pathophysiology of hypoxia is necessary in order to construct proper therapy for such an insult. Clinical conditions predisposing a pregnant patient to hypoxia are limited in number and include chest or airway trauma, airway obstruction, inadequate ventilation (either during anesthesia or due to chronic or acute pulmonary disease), decompression, heart failure or arrest, and epileptic or eclamptic seizure. From this list, it is apparent that the risks to the fetus of hypoxia exceed those of the mother because of fetal dependence on the uterine circulation, on placental transfer, and on its own circulatory system.

Clinical reports describing maternal hypoxia and its sequelae are limited in both number and content. The effects of altitude on arterial oxygen tension and oxygen content and per cent saturation have been studied in unacclimatized human subjects and are available to the interested reader (Luft and Weber, 1974). The chronic response of acclimatized individuals residing at an altitude of 3800 meters (12,000 ft) was reported by Frisancho (1970). Although racial differences in this Peruvian population may have influenced the outcome, lower birth weights, larger placentas and smaller adult stature were the outstanding characteristics of this group of patients. Additional evidence of the relationship of altitude to reduced birth weight was obtained from birth weight statistics for the city of Denver, Colorado (Lichty, 1957).

Acute changes in oxygen tension may occur following cabin pressure decompression during routine commercial airline travel. Modern jet aircraft are pressurized to maintain a cabin altitude of 1524 to 2134 meters (5000 to 7000 ft), a figure well below the level of 3048 meters or 10,000 ft at which symptoms of hypoxia occur. Scholten (1976) recently reviewed the risks of recurrent air travel during pregnancy, particularly as they applied to the cabin attendants. No evidence of increased abortion or perinatal mortality and morbidity was found that could be attributed to mild hypoxia. In his report Scholten did review reasons why pregnant flight attendants should not fly beyond the twentieth week.

Other clinical forms of hypoxia found in association with acute pulmonary insufficiency may occur during induction of anesthesia, shock, aspiration, pulmonary embolization, traumatic pulmonary contusion, respiratory burns, chemical, viral, or bacterial pneumonia, or drug overdosage. Archer and Marx (1974) studied 12 pregnant preoxygenated women who were subjected to 60 seconds of apnea during anesthesia induction. When compared to nonpregnant patients, both groups exhibited a comparable rise in pCO_2, but the pregnant patients had a fall in oxygen tension which was twice as great as that seen in the nonpregnant group. In addition, patients in labor tended to have a lower pO_2 than those not in labor. Marx emphasized the importance of preoxygenation prior to endotracheal intubation and prompt re-oxygenation in parturient women. Futoran and Hill (1975) reported six cases of pulmonary insufficiency in pregnancy from a variety of causes. There were a 66 per cent maternal mortality and a 60 per cent perinatal mortality in the patients studied. Approximately 200 pregnant patients per year may succumb from hypoxia secondary to a damaged lung, based on current estimates. Survival rates may be improved by the use of a volume-controlled respirator delivering 100 per cent oxygen and a positive end-expiratory pressure not to exceed 8 cm H_2O. The use of extracorporeal oxygenation has also been suggested if the arterial oxygen tension cannot be maintained above 50 mm Hg. Obviously one should select patients with a potential for rapid lung recovery before embarking on such a course.

Clinical Effects of Hypoxia on the Human Fetus

Our understanding of the human fetus and its response to hypoxia is limited by the facts that (1) the fetus can suffer the consequences of hypoxia with little or no pathologic change in the mother, and (2) the inaccessibility of the human fetus requires us to rely primarily on fetal heart rate and acid-base changes as indicators of fetal distress. It is of interest that the fetus is able to compensate successfully for chronic hypoxia. Sobrevilla and co-workers (1971) studied fetal scalp blood samples near sea level and at 4200 meters (13,650 ft). Although there was a 33 per cent decrease in the maternal arterial PaO_2 at high altitude, fetal scalp values were comparable at both altitudes. The fetus was observed to compensate or accommodate for the altitude changes by a respiratory alkalosis (decreased pCO_2) and metabolic acidosis (base deficit of 7.4). The scalp pH was similar in the two groups.

The adverse effects of intrapartum fetal hypoxia have been studied by numerous investigators. Low and co-workers (1975a) compared two patient populations on the basis of a decrease in the umbilical arterial buffer base, and utilized a low value as evidence of asphyxia. By using this retrospective parameter, they found that the asphyxic group of fetuses had a lower scalp blood pO_2 and pH at 1 and 2 hours prior to, and at, delivery. There was no difference between the two groups in the maternal venous pH. Low and co-workers (1975b) also noted that if meconium-stained amniotic fluid and fetal bradycardia were used as evidence of fetal hypoxia, only 36 per cent of the group met the metabolic criteria of asphyxia, as established by cord blood sampling. In addition they found that fetuses of mothers with antepartum medical or obstetric complications of labor developed the metabolic abnormalities of hypoxia earlier than the infants of mothers with intrapartum complications.

From the viewpoint of the clinician, a knowledge of the incidence of hypoxia and its early detection is essential for good obstetric management. Low and colleagues (1975b) indicated that 25 per cent of hypertensive pregnancies, 26 per cent of suspected intrauterine growth-retarded pregnancies, and 50 per cent of breech presentations were associated with hypoxic fetuses at delivery. Kubli and associates (1969) concluded that the correlation between baseline fetal heart rate levels and fetal pH was poor. On the other hand, specific heart rate decelerations were statistically associated with pH changes, and a direct relationship between the type and severity of the deceleration and the mean value of the fetal scalp blood pH was shown. Table 4–3 defines the degree of deceleration of the two significant types of fetal heart rate changes, variable decelerations (related to cord compression) and late decelerations (uteroplacental insufficiency). Early decelerations (head compression) are rarely associated with fetal scalp blood pH changes. Figure 4–7 illustrates the relationship between the fetal scalp pH and the types and degree of heart rate deceleration as reported by Kubli and associates.

Khazin and Hon (1971) compared the difference between the maternal arterial and fetal scalp pH in the various types of fetal heart rate decelerations at intervals of 5 to 30 min. In general, severe late decelerations were consistently associated with a pH difference of greater than 0.20. Thirty minutes of mild or moderate late decelerations were also associated with a pH difference of greater than 0.20. Data on severe variable decelerations were lacking except at 5 min, when they were associated with greater than 0.20 pH difference. This study helps to emphasize the importance of the normal pH gradient between mother and fetus. The maternal arterial pH should be higher (more alkaline) than the fetal arterial pH in order for the fetus to eliminate hydrogen ions across the placental barrier. Khazin and Hon (1971) found this difference to be 0.11 of a pH unit in a normal population. A widened gradient in the face of a normal maternal pH probably means fetal hypoxia, whereas a narrowed or reverse gradient may mean primary maternal acid-base pathology. It is apparent from studies such as these that a simultaneous maternal arterial pH may be helpful in evaluating fetal scalp sample results.

TABLE 4–3   Interpretation of Pathologic Fetal Heart Rate Decelerations*

Type		Definition
Late		Rate
1 Mild		decrease <15 beats/min
2 Moderate		decrease 15–45 beats/min
3 Severe		decrease >45 beats/min

Variable	Duration	Rate
1 Mild	<30 sec	>80 beats/min
	or	
	<60 sec	70–80 beats/min
2 Moderate	30–60 sec	<70 beats/min
	or	
	>60 sec	70–80 beats/min
3 Severe	>60 sec	<70 beats/min

*From Kubli FW, et al.: Am J Obstet Gynecol *104*:1190, 1969.

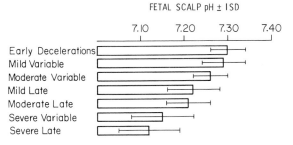

Figure 4-7 Mean pH value ±1 standard deviation (SD) found in fetal scalp blood during various degrees and types of fetal heart decelerations (see Table 4-3). (From Kubli FW. et al: Observations on heart rate and pH in the human fetus during labor. Am J Obstet Gynecol *104*:1190–1206, 1969.)

Neonatal and Childhood Sequelae of Intrauterine Hypoxia

Severe intrauterine hypoxia resulting in birth depression (Apgar score of 3 or less at 1 min) may add additional stress to a newborn infant already at high risk from prematurity, dysmaturity, or sepsis. The organ system most likely to be damaged by hypoxia is the central nervous system. It is not surprising, then, that hypoxia inflicted upon a newborn in an unstable condition may result in permanent sequelae. Subtle signs of CNS dysfunction may occur early in the neonatal period, and seizures are observed in 8 to 22 per cent of low Apgar score infants between 12 and 24 hours of age (Brann and Sykes, 1977). The prognosis for normal development in infants with primary subarachnoid hemorrhage secondary to hypoxia is quite good. In contrast, the developmental prognosis for an infant with seizures secondary to an intraventricular hemorrhage is much worse. Hydrocephalus is a common late sequela of subarachnoid and peri- or intraventricular hemorrhage in the newborn.

Little is known of the long-term consequences of intrauterine hypoxia upon CNS development in the neonate. Dweck and associates (1974) studied 15 hypoxic infants born with 1 min Apgar scores of less than 3, and who required positive pressure O_2 and intravenous buffer for neonatal support. When these babies were compared with 14 nonhypoxic mature infants at 15 to 40 months of age, no differences in IQ scores were found between the two groups. In a much larger study, Niswander and colleagues (1975) reported the results of the Collaborative Study of Cerebral Palsy. Hypoxia was presumed to have occurred in a group of infants whose gestations were complicated by abruptio placentae, placenta previa, or prolapsed umbilical cord. The results of the study revealed comparable values in average motor and mental scores of the surviving infants when comparisons were made with a well-matched control group at eight months and four years of age.

Niswander and co-workers (1975) also reported on a subgroup of low birth weight infants exposed to the same presumed hypoxic stress of abruptio placentae, placenta previa, or prolapsed umbilical cord. Low birth weight infants scored lower on both motor and mental testing at eight months and four years of age than comparable term weight infants, and this difference was true for both the stressed and the control groups. It would seem, then, that long-term CNS sequelae are influenced more by low birth weight than by hypoxia per se. Nonetheless, it is important to keep in mind that the studies conducted by the

Collaborative Study of Cerebral Palsy were carried out prior to routine use of electrophysical and fetal scalp blood monitoring. Current antepartum and intrapartum fetal monitoring might permit a more accurate determination of the presence of fetal hypoxia.

Management

Appropriate management of maternal or fetal hypoxia, or both, during pregnancy is predicated upon (1) prevention, (2) early recognition of predisposing conditions, and (3) aggressive treatment once hypoxia is identified. As has been emphasized in this section, the underlying pathophysiology may be a reflection of an altered maternal environment, respiratory system, placental blood flow or fetal cardiovascular stability. Identification of the appropriate pathophysiologic process is essential before a specific management regime can be developed. It is beyond the scope of this chapter to attempt to review the management of all types of maternal and fetal hypoxia. Therefore, a general scheme of fetal diagnosis and management will be discussed.

Anticipation of specific groups at high risk for hypoxia will help to reduce the size of the population under surveillance. In addition, careful prenatal care and avoidance of unnecessary stress factors will provide a more optimal intrauterine environment for normal fetal development. Antenatal fetal monitoring, using a combination of biophysical methods (such as stress and nonstress fetal heart rate monitoring, and in the future perhaps fetal breathing activity) and biochemical determinations (such as estriol and human placental lactogen), has contributed greatly to our recognition of intrauterine stress and fetal deterioration. Fetuses under stress should be delivered if the potential risks to the neonate are less than the hazards of maintaining the fetus in its intrauterine environment. In those cases in which delivery is elected for fetal or maternal reasons, and where vaginal delivery is not a contraindication, rupture of membranes, placement of internal fetal monitors, fetal scalp blood sampling, and oxytocin administration is an accepted management regimen. It is important to keep in mind that the supine position and also the supine hypotensive syndrome may have an important hemodynamic impact on the potentially hypoxic fetus, as well as on those stressed by maternal hypotension. Therefore, whenever practical or possible, the patient should be placed in the left lateral position.

Many of the stresses of labor should be considered cumulative, and fetal heart rate and scalp blood sampling must be an integral part of any intrapartum monitoring system of high-risk pregnancies. Significant persistent fetal bradycardia patterns that do not respond to change in maternal position and oxygen supplementation should be dealt with. Fetal scalp sampling for acid-base status in this situation may dictate the urgency with which delivery should be effected.

The efficacy of supplemental oxygen administration to the mother in cases of suspected fetal hypoxia is controversial, and data supporting its use are obscured by our limited understanding of the many mechanisms that may impair fetoplacental oxygen transport. In addition, efforts to raise maternal arterial oxygen tension under conditions of impaired uteroplacental blood perfusion may be of minimal benefit to the compromised fetus. On the other hand, there is no question that under normal circumstances raising the maternal oxygen tension will increase slightly but significantly the fetal pO_2. Staisch and co-workers (1976) reported results obtained using a continuous tissue oxygen tension monitor. They demonstrated in pregnant sheep that the fetal arterial oxygen tension responds in a dependent and predictable way to acute changes in maternal pO_2 levels at several concentrations of maternal inspired oxygen. Such continuous methods for oxygen tension or pH monitoring hold promise as an adjunct in the clinical management of the at-risk fetus. We may conclude, then, that supplemental maternal oxygen may be beneficial in some situations. Nevertheless, oxygen supplementation should not be relied upon solely to correct the underlying pathophysiology and instead should be thought of as an adjunct to definitive management.

Maternal oxygen supplementation should be carried out by the use of a leakproof non-rebreathing mask with an attached reservoir (bag),* and an oxygen flow rate of 5 to 6 L/min. A leakproof mask is important so that during inspiration room air is not drawn in; this is best accomplished by a mask with soft, flexible edges. Non-rebreathing allows the pCO_2 to remain in the normal range. A reservoir bag is essential for an adequate oxygen supply during peak inspiration when the instantaneous flow rate may reach 40 L/min. Only with a reservoir bag can this demand be met.

CONCLUSIONS

In this review of the major causes of hypovolemia and hypoxia we have emphasized the pertinent pathophysiology of the mother and fetus. It is only by integrating our knowledge of the effects of and responses to these pathologic processes that a decline in the morbid outcome will be achieved. Our closing admonition to those caring for the critically ill or traumatized pregnant patient is to consider the impact each and every phase of treatment has on both patients — mother and fetus.

REFERENCES

Archer GW Jr, Marx GF: Arterial oxygen tension during apnea in parturient women. Br J Anaesth 46:358, 1974

Assali NS, Bonis JA, Smith RW, Manson WA: Studies on ductus arteriosus circulation. Circ Res 13:478, 1963.

Assali NS: Pathophysiology of Gestation. Vol. I. New York, Academic Press, 1972.

Bech-Jansen P, Brinkman CR III, Johnson GH, Assali NS: Circulatory shock in pregnancy. I. Effects of endotoxin on uteroplacental and fetal umbilical circulation. Am J Obstet Gynecol 112:1084, 1972.

Boba A, Linkie DM, Plotz EJ: Fetal responses to maternal oxygen inhalation during hemorrhagic stress. Am J Obstet Gynecol 97:919, 1967.

Boddy K, Robinson JS: External method for detection of fetal breathing in utero. Lancet 2:1231, 1971.

Bonica JJ: Obstetric Analgesia and Anesthesia. New York, Springer-Verlag, 1972.

Brann AW Jr, Sykes FO: The effects of intrauterine asphyxia on the full-term infant. Clinics in Perinatology 4:149, 1977.

---

*Hudson Oxygen Therapy Sales Co., Temescala, CA, or Wadsworth, OH.

Brinkman CR III, Kirschbaum TH, Assali NS: The role of the umbilical sinus in the regulation of placental vascular resistance. Gynecol Invest *1*:115, 1970*a*.

Brinkman CR III, Weston P, Kirschbaum TH, Assali NS: Effects of maternal hypoxia on fetal cardiovascular hemodynamics. Am J Obstet Gynecol *108*:288, 1970*b*.

Brinkman CR III, Mofid M, Assali NS: Circulatory shock in pregnant sheep. Am J Obstet Gynecol *118*:77, 1974.

Brinkman CR III, Woods JR Jr: Effects of cardiovascular drugs during pregnancy. Cardiovasc Med *1*:231, 1976.

Chesley LC: Plasma and red cell volumes during pregnancy. Am J Obstet Gynecol *112*:440, 1972.

Clemmer TP, Telford IR: Abnormal development of the rat heart during prenatal hypoxic stress. Proc Soc Exp Biol Med *121*:800, 1966.

Clark K, Farley DB, Van Orden DE, Brody MJ: Role of endogenous prostaglandins in regulation of uterine blood flow and adrenergic neurotransmission. Am J Obstet Gynecol *127*:455, 1977.

Cohn HE, Sacks EJ, Heyman MA, Rudolph AM: Cardiovascular responses to hypoxemia and acidemia in fetal lambs. Am J Obstet Gynecol *120*:817, 1974.

Crenshaw C Jr, Cefalo R: Effects of exogenous estrogens on PO_2 and experimental endotoxemia in sheep. Am J Obstet Gynecol *120*:678, 1974.

Cristy JM: Treatment of gram-negative shock. Am J Obstet Gynecol *50*:77, 1971.

Dawes GS: Breathing before birth in animals and man: an essay in developmental medicine. N Engl J Med *290*:557, 1974.

Dilts PV Jr, Brinkman CR III, Kirschbaum TH, Assali NS: Uterine and systemic hemodynamic interrelationships and their response to hypoxia. Am J Obstet Gynecol *103*:138, 1969.

Downing SE, Talner NS, Gardner TH: Influences of hypoxemia and acidemia on left ventricular function. Am J Physiol *210*:1327, 1966.

Dweck HS, Huggins W, Dorman LP, Saron SA, Benton JW, Cassady, G.: Developmental sequelae in infants having suffered severe perinatal asphyxia. Am J Obstet Gynecol *119*:811, 1974.

Fort AT: Hemorrhagic complications of labor and delivery. Obstet Gynecol *34*:717, 1969.

Frisancho AR: Developmental responses to high altitude hypoxia. Am J Phys Anthrop *32*:401, 1970.

Futoran JM, Hill JD: Pulmonary insufficiency associated with pregnancy. Am J Obstet Gynecol *121*:637, 1975.

Goldberg LJ: Cardiovascular and renal actions of dopamine: potential clinical applications. Pharmacol Rev *24*:1, 1972.

Gough ED, Dyer DC: Responses of isolated human uterine arteries to vasoactive drugs. Am J Obstet Gynecol *110*:625, 1971.

Greiss F: A clinical concept of uterine blood flow during pregnancy. Obstet Gynecol *30*:595, 1967.

Greiss F, Gobble FL: The uterine vascular bed: effects of sympathetic nerve stimulation. Am J Obstet Gynecol *97*:962, 1967.

Greiss FC, Anderson SG, King LC: Uterine vascular bed: effects of acute hypoxia. Am J Obstet Gynecol *113*:1057, 1972.

Hardy WE, Freeman MG, Thompson JD: A ten-year review of maternal mortality. Obstet Gynecol *43*:65, 1974.

James FB III, Greiss FC, Kemp RH: An evaluation of vasopressor therapy for maternal hypotension during spinal anesthesia. Anesthesiology *33*:25, 1970.

Karlsson, K.: The influence of hypoxia on uterine and maternal placental blood flow, and the effects of α-adrenergic blockade. J Perinat Med *2*:176, 1974.

Kelman GR, Templeton A: Maternal blood gases during human pregnancy. Physiology *244*:66p, 1975.

Khazin AF, Hon EH: Observations on fetal heart rate and fetal biochemistry. II. Fetal-maternal pH differences. Am J Obstet Gynecol *109*:432, 1971.

Kitzmiller JL: Septic shock: an eclectic view. Obstet Gynecol Surv *26*:105, 1971.

Kubli FW, Hon EH, Khazin AF, Takemura H: Observations on heart rate and pH in the human fetus during labor. Am J Obstet Gynecol *104*:1190, 1969.

Ladner C, Brinkman CR III, Weston P, Assali NS: Dynamics of uterine circulation in pregnant and nonpregnant sheep. Am J Physiol *218*:257, 1970.

Lees MM, Scott DB, Slawson KB, Ken MG: Hemodynamic change during cesarean section. J Obstet Gynaecol Br Commonw *75*:546, 1968.

Lichty JA: Studies of babies born at high altitude. AMA J Dis Child *93*:666, 1957.

Low JA, Pancham SR, Worthington D, Boston RW: The acid-base and biochemical characteristics of intrapartum fetal asphyxia. Am J Obstet Gynecol *121*:446, 1975*a*.

Low JA, Pancham SR, Worthington D, Boston RW.: Clinical characteristics of pregnancies complicated by intrapartum fetal asphyxia. Am J Obstet Gynecol *121*:452, 1975*b*.

Lucas W, Kirschbaum T, Assali NS: Spinal shock and fetal oxygenation. Am J Obstet Gynecol *93*:583, 1965.

Luft UC, Weber KC: Effects of altitude on arterial blood gases: man. Biology Data Book. Vol. III, p. 1890. Bethesda, Md., Federation of American Society for Experimental Biology, 1974.

Lumley JM, Wood C: Influence of hypoxia on glucose transport across the human placenta. Nature *216*:403, 1967.

Makowski EL, Hertz RH, Beschia G: Effects of acute maternal hypoxia and hyperoxia on the blood flow to the pregnant uterus. Am J Obstet Gynecol *115*:624, 1973.

Mann LI, Effects of hypoxia on umbilical circulation and fetal metabolism. Am J Physiol *218*:1453, 1970*a*.

Mann LI: Effect of hypoxia on fetal cephalic blood flow, cephalic metabolism and the electroencephalogram. Exp. Neurol *29*:336, 1970*b*.

Mann LI: Effects in sheep of hypoxia on levels of lactate, pyruvate, and glucose in blood of mothers and fetus. Pediatr Res *4*:46, 1970*c*.

Muldoon MJ: The use of central venous pressure monitoring in abruptio placenta. J Obstet Gynaecol Br Commonw *76*:225, 1969.

Niswander KR, Gordon M, Drage JS: The effect of intrauterine hypoxia on the child surviving to 4 years. Am J Obstet Gynecol *121*:892, 1975.

O'Driscoll K, McCarthy JR: Abruptio placentae and central venous pressure. J Obstet Gynaecol Br Commonw *73*:923, 1966.

Oh W, Omori K, Emmanoulides GC, Phelps DL: Placenta to lamb fetus transfusion in utero during acute hypoxia. Am J Obstet Gynecol *122*:316, 1975.

Pritchard JA: Changes in the blood volume during pregnancy and delivery. Anesthesiology *26*:393, 1965.

Quinlivan WL, Brock TA, Sullivan H: Blood volume changes and blood loss associated with labor. Am J Obstet Gynecol *106*:843, 1970.

Ralston DH, Shnider S, de Lorimier AA: Effects of equipotent ephedrine, metaraminol, mephentermine and methoxamine on uterine blood flow in the pregnant ewe. Anesthesiology *40*:354, 1974.

Rattner BA, Ramm GM, Altland PD: Effects of hypoxic exposure on embryonic implantation in mice. Proc Soc Exp Biol Med *153*:138, 1976.

Rosenblum R, Tai AR, Lawson O: Dopamine in man: cardiorenal hemodynamics in normotensive patients with heart disease. J Pharmacol Exp Ther *163*:256, 1972.

Rosenfeld CR, Barton MD, Meschia G: Effects of epinephrine on distribution of blood flow in pregnant ewes. Am J Obstet Gynecol *124*:618, 1976.

Sambi MP, Weil MH, Udhozi VN: Acute pharmacodynamic effects of glucocorticoids on cardiac output and related hemodynamic changes in normal patients and patients in shock. Circulation *31*:523, 1965.

Scholten P, Pregnant stewardess – should she fly? Aviat Space Environ Med *47*:77, 1976.

Shelley HJ: The metabolic response of the fetus to hypoxia. J Obstet Gynaecol Br Commonw *76*:1, 1969.

Shnider S, de Lorimier AA, Holl JW, Chapler FK, Barishima HO: Vasopressors in obstetrics. I. Correction of fetal acidosis with ephedrine during spinal hypotension. Am J Obstet Gynecol *102*:911, 1968.

Shnider S, de Lorimier AA, Steffenson JL: Vasopressors in obstetrics. III. Fetal effects of metaraminol infusion during obstetric spinal hypotension. Am J Obstet Gynecol *108*:1017, 1970.

Sobrevilla LA, Cassinelli BT, Carcelen A, Malaga JM: Human fetal and maternal oxygen tension and acid-base status during delivery at high altitude. Am J Obstet Gynecol *111*:1111, 1971.

Speroff L: Bacterial shock in obstetrics and gynecology. Am J Obstet Gynecol *95*:139, 1966.

Staisch KJ, Nuwayhid B, Bauer RO, Welsh L, Brinkman CR III: Continuous fetal scalp and carotid artery oxygen tension monitoring in the sheep. Obstet Gynecol *47*:587, 1976.

Tominaga T, Page EW: Accommodation of the human placenta to hypoxia. Am J Obstet Gynecol *94*:679, 1966.

Ueland K: Maternal cardiovascular dynamics. VII. Intrapartum volume changes. Am J Obstet Gynecol *126*:671, 1976.

Volpe JJ: Neonatal intracranial hemorrhage: pathophysiology, neuropathology and clinical features. Clinics in Perinatology *4*:77, 1977.

Weissman G: Lysosomes. N Engl J Med *273*:1143, 1965.

Chapter 5

PENETRATING INJURY OF THE ABDOMEN

Herbert J. Buchsbaum

Penetrating injury of the abdomen during pregnancy has resulted from a great variety of instruments and missiles. Injuries to the gravid uterus have resulted from swords, scythes, sickles, files, wooden stakes, knives, bullets, cannon ball, shrapnel, grenade fragments, and animal horns. A late addition to this extensive list of offending instruments — reflecting the social development of our society — has been maternal and fetal injury resulting from a barbecue fork.

GUNSHOT WOUNDS

The most common type of penetrating injury during pregnancy is the bullet wound. The incidence of gunshot wounds of the abdomen is increasing since Gellhorn's series in 1903. Previously, most cases of gunshot wounds in pregnancy resulted from the accidental discharge of firearms, since military battles were fought away from population centers. The total warfare characteristic of the twentieth century exposed civilians, including pregnant women, to bullet and shrapnel wounds. Even in peacetime the increasing private ownership of guns, civil strife, urban unrest, and terrorist activities have caused an increase in gunshot wounds of the abdomen during pregnancy.

Rushforth and colleagues (1977) documented the dramatic rise in homicides. In both urban and suburban areas, over 80 per cent were committed with firearms. The pregnant woman can be either the intended victim or the wounded bystander.

In addition, reports are appearing of self-inflicted gunshot wounds, attempts at suicide or attempted abortion (Table 5–1). This table lists the recent cases of gunshot wounds of the pregnant uterus reported since the last literature review: nine cases from Viet Nam, two attempted suicides, one attempted abor-

TABLE 5-1 Gunshot Wounds of the Pregnant Uterus

Number	Author/Year	Cause of Injury	Duration of Pregnancy	Associated Maternal Injury	Surgical/Obstetric Management	Fetal Injuries	Outcome Maternal	Outcome Fetal
1	Thonet (1967) (Case 2)	Attempted suicide	8 months	None	Cesarean section	Thorax	Lived	Stillborn, 2150 gm
2	Takki et al. (1969)	Attempted abortion	32 weeks	None	Cesarean section	Head, neck, chest	Lived	Stillborn, 2280 gm
3–11	Din-Van-Tung and Hau-Mac-Suu (1971) (9 cases, including one twin pregnancy)	War wounds	4 months to term	1 of 9	Cesarean section when gestation was over 6 months	Head, 2 neck, 1	9 lived	7 died 3 lived
12	Lins and Schäfer (1972)	Homicide	3rd trimester	Pelvic vessels	Repair, cesarean section	Head, neck, chest	Lived	Stillborn, 2915 gm
13	Devlin (1976)	Accident	37 weeks	None	Cesarean section	Rectal wound	Lived	Lived
14	Zivkovic et al. (1976)	Attempted abortion	8 months	None	Vaginal delivery 4 days later, 2350 gm infant	Colon and forearm	Lived	Lived
15	Gysler et al. (1976)	Accident	8 months	Small bowel	Repair bowel injury; cesarean section	Thorax and anterior mediastinum	Lived	Lived
16	Browns et al. (1977)	Accident	36 weeks	None	Cesarean section	Lung, colon, liver	Lived	Lived

tion, one homicide, and three accidents. Previously reported series of gunshot wounds of the pregnant uterus are listed for comparison in Table 5–2. The true incidence of gunshot wounds in pregnancy probably far exceeds the reported number.

Nonpregnant Persons

The likelihood of an abdominal organ being struck by a bullet is directly related to its size and the space it occupies in the peritoneal cavity; the larger the organ, the more likely it is to be injured. In gunshot wounds of the abdomen the small bowel is the most commonly injured structure, followed by the liver, the colon, and the stomach (Nance et al., 1974; Dawidson et al., 1976).

The mortality and complication rates in gunshot wounds of the abdomen are directly related to the number of organs injured. Dawidson and colleagues (1976), in their series of 277 civilian gunshot wounds of the abdomen, reported serious complications in *all* patients with more than five organs injured, with a mortality of 63 per cent. An average of 2.4 major organs were injured in the 209 survivors, while 4.2 major organs were injured in 28 patients who died.

Pregnant Women

Gunshot wounds of the nonpregnant uterus are a rarity, since the normal sized uterus is sheltered in the bony pelvis (Quast and Jordon, 1964). The gravid uterus transcends the boundaries of the true pelvis in the first trimester, and in late pregnancy is the largest viscus, occupying a considerable portion of the peritoneal cavity.

The gravid uterus acts as a shield for the mother and modifies the type of injury she sustains. This is accomplished by two mechanisms:

1. Because of its size, the uterus is the most likely organ to be injured in penetrating gunshot wounds of the abdomen. It displaces the small intestine into the upper abdomen, compressing it into a smaller space. Since the uterus is not a

TABLE 5–2   Gunshot Wounds of the Pregnant Uterus — Comparison of Series

Author/Year	Number of Cases	Per Cent Associated Maternal Injuries	Per Cent Fetal Injuries	Per Cent Maternal Mortality	Per Cent Perinatal Mortality
Kobak and Hurwitz (1954)	33	24	70	9	70
Martins and Garcia (1964)	45	27	75	6.6	71
Buchsbaum (1968)	16	38	59	0	71
Buchsbaum (1975)	9	33	89	0	66
Present Series	16	19	59	0	41

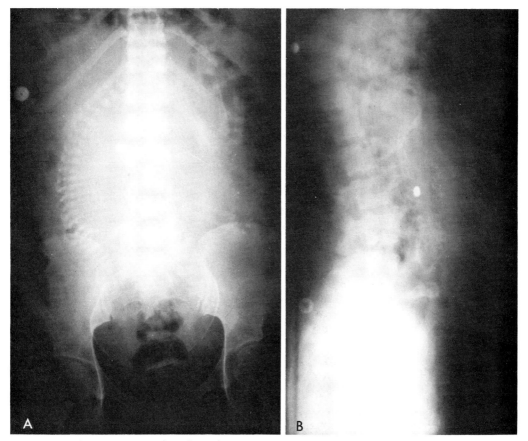

Figure 5–1 Maternal abdominal x-rays (case 1), showing location of the bullet. *A,* Anteroposterior film. *B,* Lateral film. (From Buchsbaum HJ and Caruso PA: Obstet Gynecol *33*:673, 1969.)

vital organ, morbidity is low, and there have been no reported maternal deaths resulting from gunshot wounds of the pregnant uterus since 1912.

2. Any missile, particularly the low velocity bullets producing civilian wounds, that penetrates the abdominal wall and then strikes the uterus, transfers a great proportion of its energy to the relatively dense uterine musculature, which diminishes its velocity. When a bullet enters the uterus, it is likely to come to rest there. This is demonstrated by the following case.

Case 1: The mother was struck in the abdomen by a low velocity, small caliber bullet at 34 to 36 weeks' gestation. X-rays of the maternal abdomen revealed the bullet to be in the uterus, perhaps in the fetal thorax or abdomen (Fig. 5–1*A, B*). At celiotomy, an entrance wound was found on the anterior surface of the uterus; no other organ injury was identified. A cesarean section was performed, with the delivery of a living infant with an Apgar score of 9. Cursory examination of the fetal abdomen and thorax failed to reveal any wounds. The bullet could not be located in the uterine cavity or in the placenta, and there was no exit wound on the posterior aspect of the uterus.

Careful examination of the infant revealed a puncture wound of the right nasolabial fold (Fig. 5–2). There was no injury of the soft or hard palate or tongue,

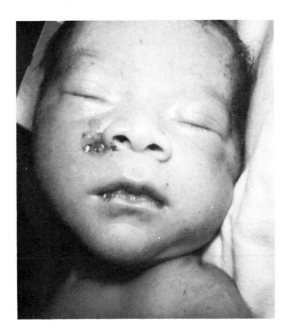

Figure 5-2   Infant in case 1, showing wound at the right nasolabial fold. (From Buchsbaum HJ and Caruso PA: Obstet Gynecol *33*:673, 1969.)

and the bullet was not in the infant's mouth. A whole body x-ray of the newborn revealed the location of the errant bullet (Fig. 5–3).

After penetrating the cheek, the bullet came to rest in the infant's mouth. The infant subsequently swallowed the bullet in utero. The missile was retrieved 110 hours later when the infant passed it per rectum (Buchsbaum and Caruso, 1969).

The diminished velocity of the bullet and the shielding effect of the gravid uterus is further manifested by the low incidence of associated maternal injury. Only 19 per cent of women who sustain gunshot wounds of the gravid uterus have associated visceral injuries (Tables 5–1 and 5–2). As a result of improvements in firearms the velocity of bullets is increasing, yet associated injury occurred in only 19 per cent of the most recently reported cases.

The frequency with whch gunshot wounds of the abdomen in pregnancy miss striking the uterus is unknown. Dyer and Barclay (1962) noted: "We are aware of no report of a penetrating wound of the abdomen during pregnancy not involving the uterus." There are such cases in the recent literature (Thonet, 1967; Buchsbaum, 1968; Din-Van-Tung and Hau-Mac-Suu, 1971), and the incidence is probably far higher than the reported cases would indicate, since a bullet wound of the small bowel, without the drama of uterine injury, is hardly a reportable condition. Din-Van-Tung and Hau-Mac-Suu (1971), reporting battlefield wounds sustained by civilians, cited nine women with bullet wounds of the pregnant uterus and noted in passing that seven other pregnant women were seen during the same time period in whom the bullet did not injure the uterus.

Unfortunately, the same mechanism that spares the small bowel from injury in penetrating wounds (compression of the intestine in the upper abdomen) can also place it at greater jeopardy. When a bullet enters the upper abdomen, the shielding effect of the gravid uterus is lost and the mother is likely to sustain more entry and exit wounds of the small intestine, in addition to other visceral injury.

Fetal Wounds

Fetuses have sustained wounds in utero that vary from trivial to fatal. Fetal injuries occurred in 59 per cent of the recent cases of gunshot wounds of the gravid uterus. In previous series, this varied from 59 to 89 per cent (Table 5–2). The conceptus has fared far worse than the mother, with perinatal mortality ranging from 41 to 71 per cent.

In addition to direct injuries that can cause fetal death in utero, the pregnancy can be compromised by injury to the membranes, the cord, and the placenta. Isolated injuries to these structures have occurred as a result of gunshot wounds (Eckerling and Teaff, 1950; Dyer and Barclay, 1962; Martins and Garcia, 1964; Buchsbaum, 1968; Wray and Burnett, 1971).

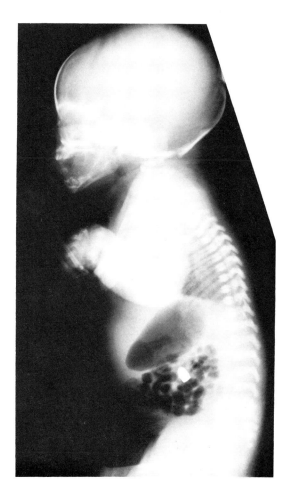

Figure 5–3 Postpartum x-ray of infant (case 1), showing bullet in abdomen. (From Buchsbaum HJ and Caruso PA: Obstet Gynecol 33:673, 1969.)

Management of Abdominal Gunshot Wounds

The early management of patients with gunshot wounds of the abdomen is listed in Table 3–1. Part of the initial physical examination should be a search for entry and exit wounds. Entry wounds are generally smaller, exit wounds larger, because the bullet, deflected by abdominal structures, starts to tumble, increasing the size of the exit wound. It is usually impossible to predict the course of a bullet after it has entered the body. It can be deflected and even embolized in the gastrointestinal or genitourinary tract, veins, or arteries (Ledgerwood, 1967). It is therefore important to search for pulmonary or cardiac wounds resulting from bullets that enter the upper abdomen and penetrate the diaphragm.

When vital signs are stable, appropriate x-ray studies of the abdomen should be taken to localize the bullet if it has not exited. At least two views are needed. In recognition of the risks of x-rays to the conceptus and their limited value, x-ray films should be taken judiciously. When the bullet appears to be in the uterus, both the likelihood of and the extent of fetal injury are impossible to determine radiographically. The size of the gravid uterus should carefully be determined and the presence or absence of fetal heart tones documented.

Although there is increasing interest in expectant therapy of penetrating wounds, even gunshot wounds of the abdomen, this is not practical for the gravid patient. Most authorities agree that peritoneal irritation with tenderness, guarding, or rigidity is the most important sign identifying patients who need celiotomy. Shaftan's criteria (1960) have been widely applied and the validity of conservative management has now been documented. The passive and active stretching of the abdominal wall in pregnancy alters its response to intraperitoneal stimuli. During pregnancy tenderness may appear later than in the nonpregnant state; guarding and rigidity are often absent or diminished. Alterations of vital signs, increasing pulse rate, and falling blood pressure, the usual criteria for early celiotomy, are not valid parameters in the injured gravida. The physiologic hypervolemia of pregnancy appears to have a salutary effect in maternal hemorrhage. A clinically measurable fall in blood pressure or a rise in pulse may not develop in the gravid patient until a reduction of 30 to 35 per cent in blood volume has occurred (Romney et al., 1963; Marx, 1965). The mother maintains her own homeostasis at the expense of the fetus by reducing uteroplacental blood flow.

We feel that early exploration should be performed in pregnant patients with penetrating gunshot wounds of the abdomen. The infant can well tolerate the stress of surgery and anesthesia, and may even benefit by delivery and early surgery when it has sustained intrauterine injury.

EXPLORATION

A vertical paramedian incision should be utilized which can be extended cranially into the epigastrium for adequate exploration and repair, and caudally for performing cesarean section if necessary. Upon opening the peritoneal cavity, the surgeon should look carefully for the presence of amniotic fluid. A systematic examination of the peritoneal viscera should be performed if no obvious bleeding sites are identified. In the upper abdomen, the liver should be palpated and examined visually, the spleen observed for perforation and bleeding, and the stomach, small bowel, and colon examined carefully. Undiagnosed duodenal injury can cause serious morbidity and mortality. All injuries should be treated by appropriate surgical techniques. As long as the mother's vital signs remain stable and the size and location of the gravid uterus do not interfere with adequate exploration and repair of injuries, the uterus should not be emptied. When the missile passes through the colon, surgical management should include aggressive debridement of the missile tract, with irrigation of the wound and removal of accessible missiles. Such patients also benefit from adjuvant antibiotic therapy (Flint et al., 1978).

When repair of visceral injuries has been completed and no uterine wounds are found, the abdomen should be closed and the pregnancy left undisturbed. *Celiotomy should not be a license for cesarean section.* Saunders and Milton (1973) reported that the risks of precipitating labor by diagnostic celiotomy are "negligible, provided no unnecessary surgical measures are undertaken." Thonet (1967, Case 1) reported a pregnancy undisturbed following the repair of a gastric wound and a nephrectomy necessitated by a gunshot wound during early pregnancy.

The fetus can tolerate the stress of surgery and anesthesia (Schnider and Webster, 1965; Slater, 1970). Alterations in maternal homeostasis — hypoxia and hypovolemia — have a far greater effect on the course of pregnancy. Labor and delivery of a live or dead infant in the postoperative period has no deleterious effect on the mother.

As already stated, when a bullet strikes the uterus it often comes to rest in that structure. Nevertheless, at the time of celiotomy the surgeon should perform a careful examination of the structures of the upper abdomen, since the bullet may have entered the uterus after striking other peritoneal viscera, or may have injured these organs after passing through the uterus. The enlarged veins of the broad ligament and pelvis are particularly susceptible to injury.

In the case of penetrating wounds of the uterus, the surgeon is faced with the problem of whether to do a cesarean section or leave the pregnancy undisturbed. When a bullet has penetrated the uterus, there is a great likelihood that the fetus has sustained injury. If the fetus is dead and uterine bleeding can be controlled with ligatures, cesarean section need not be performed.

As noted above, x-rays of the maternal abdomen can rarely be of help in determining the severity of fetal injury. This can be appreciated by comparing the anteroposterior and lateral maternal abdominal roentgenograms shown in Figures 5–1, 5–4 (*A, B*), and 5–6 (*A, B*). In these cases the mother sustained an abdominal gunshot wound during the third trimester and the bullet came to rest in the uterus. The infant shown in Figure 5–1 (Case 1) sustained a minor wound of the cheek and swallowed the bullet, whereas the infant in Figure 5–4 was delivered with a pneumothorax and a bullet lodged in the spine and died 75 hours post partum (Fig. 5–5*A, B*).

If there is extensive uterine injury with bleeding or injury to the parametria or uterine vessels, cesarean hysterectomy should be performed.

If the infant is alive and near term, the surgeon must weigh the potential benefits of surgical repair of intrauterine-sustained injuries against the risks of

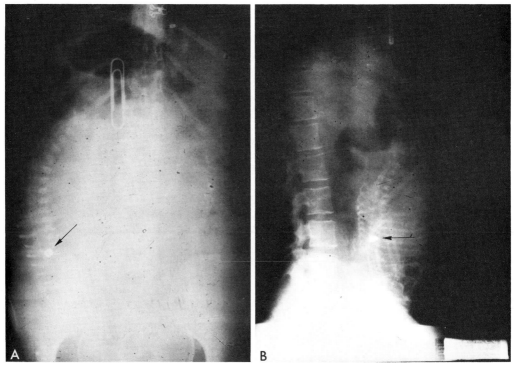

Figure 5–4   Abdominal films of gravida who sustained gunshot wound of the abdomen in the third trimester. Bullet can be seen overlying maternal spinal column (arrow). *A*, Anteroposterior view. *B*, Lateral view.

prematurity. In Buchsbaum's series (1968), the disparity between fetal injury in utero (59 per cent) and perinatal mortality (71 per cent) was explained by the high number of fetal deaths resulting from complications of prematurity in noninjured infants delivered by incidental cesarean section.

With increasing sophistication in the care of premature infants, and with the availability of pediatric surgeons, the indications for cesarean section have increased. Remarkable results in repair of fetal injuries, with resultant fetal survival, have been achieved when personnel and facilities are available, as shown in the case reported by Browns and colleagues (1977).

> *Case 2:*   A 23 year old multiparous patient was shot in the mid-portion of the abdomen at 36 weeks' gestation with a low velocity 0.38 caliber bullet. X-rays of the maternal abdomen showed the bullet in the uterus, evidently lodged in the arm of the fetus (Fig. 5–6 *A, B*). Celiotomy and cesarean section were performed, with the delivery of a living 1700 gm infant. The mother had sustained no associated injuries.
>
> The infant had an entrance wound posteriorly in the right flank and an exit wound in the right anterior chest wall. The bullet came to rest in the upper right arm (Fig. 5–7). The infant's right tension pneumothorax was managed with a thoracostomy tube and respirations assisted via a nasotracheal tube. At 12 hours of age, meconium was noted oozing from the entrance wound in the flank.
>
> The infant was explored, and wounds of the kidney, colon, liver, and diaphragm were appropriately repaired. The infant was discharged from the hospital on day 34 in satisfactory condition.

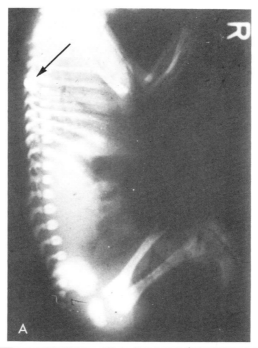

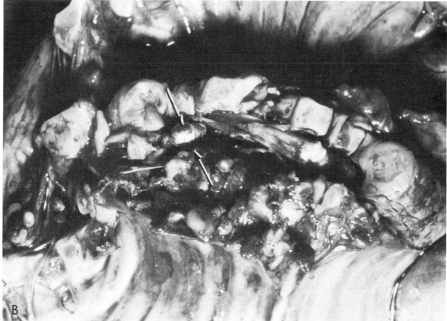

Figure 5-5 *A*, Postpartum x-ray of infant born to the woman in Figure 5–4. Arrow marks bullet lodged in the thoracic spine. *B*, Autopsy preparation showing bullet (arrows) at the level of T4–T5.

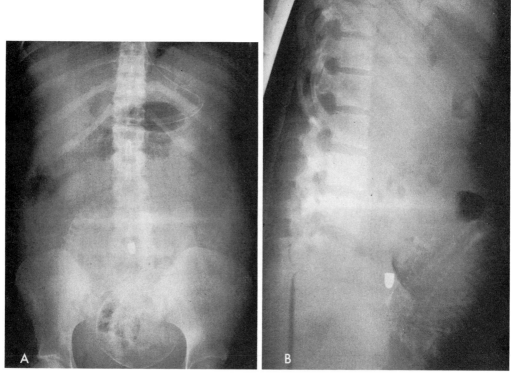

Figure 5-6   Maternal abdominal x-rays (case 2). *A*, Anteroposterior film showing bullet over-lying maternal spine. Fetal head in pelvis, fetal spine on the right. *B*, Lateral view. Bullet is seen anterior to maternal spinal column, suggesting intrauterine location. (From Browns K, et al: JAMA 237:2409, 1977. Copyright 1977 by the American Medical Association.)

This case demonstrates the value of cesarean section in severely injured fetuses, though one must remember that infants have been delivered alive vaginally after having sustained intrauterine injury. The perinatal mortality in the current series is the lowest reported to date (Table 5–2). The perinatal mortality was 41 per cent, whereas 59 per cent of the infants sustained intrauterine injury. Four infants clearly benefited from cesarean section followed by early surgical intervention, contributing to the lower perinatal mortality.

In the event that the fetus is dead, delivery will generally occur within 48 hours. If the uterus does not empty itself spontaneously, intrauterine saline or prostaglandins can be used to induce labor for delivery of the dead fetus.

FETAL INDICATIONS FOR CESAREAN SECTION.   There are three rare and difficult-to-diagnose fetal indications for cesarean section: (1) hemorrhage; (2) interference with fetal/maternal exchange; and (3) infection. It is unlikely that the mother could be prepared and cesarean section performed in time to control fetal hemorrhage and save the infant. The same could be said about injury to the cord or placenta, since the infant's buffers against hypoxia and hypovolemia are very limited. It is unclear how frequently amnionitis would occur in gunshot wounds of the pregnant uterus. The bullet is contaminated from the time it leaves the barrel of the gun, and in addition carries with it pieces of clothing and skin. This has not proved to be a problem in cases of perforation of the uterus when the pregnancy was allowed to progress. The uterus has a unique resistance to infection, an immunologic factor that progressively increases during the third trimester (Larsen et al., 1974; Schlievert et al., 1975).

STAB WOUNDS

Stab wounds of the abdomen during pregnancy have resulted from common household instruments like the knife, file, and barbecue fork; from farm tools like the scythe and sickle; and from farm posts and wooden pegs. Historically, invading armies put civilians to death, particularly women "big with child," with sword, saber and bayonet. Goring by animal horns represents an uncommon form of penetrating injury.

Animal Horns

Injury to the pregnant abdomen resulting from goring by animal horns was known in the time of Moses, and still occurs. The horns of oxen, bulls, cows, water buffalo, and bison have all been implicated (Harris, 1878). Although a rare occurrence now, animal goring of the pregnant uterus still occurs on farms, particularly in developing countries.

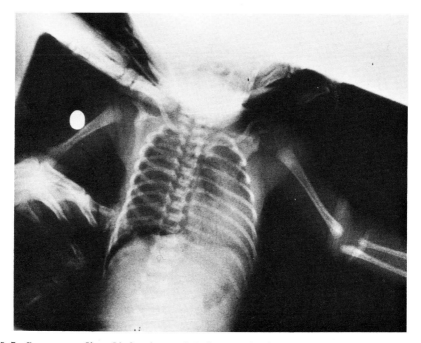

Figure 5–7 Postpartum film of infant in case 2. Infant sustained abdominal and chest wounds in utero, with bullet lodged in the right upper arm. (From Browns K, et al: JAMA *237*:2409, 1977. Copyright 1977 by the American Medical Association.)

The outcome of such cases can be quite varied. Harris, in 1878, reported the survival of six of nine mothers and the live birth of five children following maternal goring. As recently as 1973, Tanga and Kawathekar reported a gravida, charged by a bull, who sustained a transverse wound in the lower abdomen. The laceration extended from flank to flank, through the full thickness of the abdominal wall. The uterine was also lacerated, with placenta extruding. The mother survived, and was delivered of a 2500 gm stillborn infant.

MANAGEMENT

This type of injury represents a unique situation with considerable tissue destruction and wound contamination. The management of such injuries must be individualized. Wide debridement of the wound is necessary, and tetanus prophylaxis (page 49) should be started early. Since animals charge with their heads down, the standing gravida usually sustains injury of the lower abdomen, the vulva and vagina, and the lower extremities. If the peritoneum is penetrated, uterine injury usually results; viscera in the upper abdomen are usually spared. Particular attention should be paid to identifying any bladder injury; catheterization with an indwelling catheter and retrograde cystography should be performed. Careful observation of vital signs is necessary to identify pelvic vessel injury.

It is best for such patients to undergo exploration. If only a puncture wound of the uterus is present and the bleeding can be controlled by sutures, the pregnancy is best left undisturbed. If the placenta or cord is injured, or fetal injury has occurred, cesarean section cannot generally be performed in time to save the conceptus. If fetal death has occurred, the patient will go into labor spontaneously and deliver vaginally. In the presence of major myometrial or vascular wounds, cesarean hysterectomy should be performed.

Knife Wounds

Stab wounds of the abdomen are less common than bullet wounds and the prognosis is far better. In gunshot wounds, injury to the abdominal wall and viscera is increased by the shock waves and temporary cavitation; all organs in the path of a bullet are injured. The likelihood of visceral injury in stab wounds is far less than in gunshot wounds; an organ can slide away from the advancing blade, so that about half of patients with stab wounds of the abdomen sustain an injury requiring surgical repair (Smithwick et al., 1968; Bull and Mathewson, 1968; Carter and Sawyers, 1969; Nance and Cohn, 1969). Since the prognosis in penetrating injuries is related to the number of organs injured, mortality in stab wounds is far lower than in gunshot wounds. Nance and colleagues (1974) reported deaths in 1.4 per cent of 1180 stab wounds and in 12.5 per cent of 1032 civilian gunshot wounds.

In the nonpregnant victim the structures most commonly injured in stab wounds of the abdomen are the liver, small bowel, colon, and spleen. As already noted, an injury to the nonpregnant uterus is extremely rare. In late pregnancy, any stab wound of the lower abdomen is likely to injure the uterus, and other organs are spared by its shielding effect. This effect is lost in stab wounds of the upper abdomen, and indeed the small bowel may be placed in greater jeopardy as the result of compression into the upper abdomen.

The frequency with which stab wounds occur during pregnancy is difficult to assess. Bochner (1961) reviewed stab wounds of the pregnant uterus and reported four cases, including one of his own. Buchsbaum reviewed the subject again in 1968 and was able to cite six additional reports. Since that last report, four cases have appeared (Knapp and Drucker, 1972; McNabney and Smith, 1973; Malinovski, 1974; Amine, 1976).

MANAGEMENT

As in the management of all other injuries in pregnancy, the physician is faced with two patients whose sensitivities to the trauma vary and both of whose needs must be addressed. In the last 20 years there has been a shift in the management of stab wounds of the abdomen. Previously, all penetrating wounds of the abdomen were explored. But since there is no penetration of the peritoneum in more than 30 per cent of cases, and in an additional 15 to 20 per cent of patients there is no injury that requires repair, methods were sought to reduce the morbidity of nonproductive celiotomy. Shaftan (1960) proposed the selective conservative management of penetrating wounds of the abdomen. As a result of this technique, clinics have reduced the number of explorations significantly. Printen and colleagues (1968) reduced the number of patients explored to 47.1 per cent, McNabney and McCause (1967) reduced theirs from 63 to 32 per cent, and Nance and Cohn (1969) reduced the nonproductive celiotomies from 61 to 13 per cent. These results were achieved utilizing Shaftan's strict criteria. Since the pregnant patient's abdominal wall may not respond to intraperitoneal stimuli as quickly or to the same degree as in the nonpregnant state, additional techniques to identify those patients with peritoneal penetration and intraperitoneal injury are of value.

One such technique is the fistulogram (Cornell et al., 1965). The wound site is appropriately cleansed and a #16 or #18 French catheter is passed into the tract and fixed to the abdominal wall with a purse-string suture. A syringe is attached to the catheter and 75 ml of Hypaque (sodium diatrizoate) is injected rapidly. The catheter is then clamped and the patient's position changed, and anteroposterior and lateral abdominal x-rays are taken. The x-rays must be examined carefully to determine if the contrast material has entered the peritoneal cavity. In wounds that have not penetrated the peritoneum, the contrast material is restricted to the layers of the abdominal wall. With peritoneal perforation, the contrast material spills into the peritoneal cavity, outlining loops of bowel and pooling under the diaphragm and in the pelvis.

This study can be performed in the emergency room and does not require special equipment or highly trained personnel. It can help to identify those patients without peritoneal penetration who can be managed conservatively.

The management of the pregnant patient with a stab wound entering the peritoneal cavity must be individualized. As noted above, the clinical criteria based on abdominal findings first suggested by Shaftan and then supported by others may not be appropriate for the gravid patient. The mechanism of visceral injuries varies as a result of the large gravid uterus. Since over two thirds of stab wounds of the anterior abdominal wall (comprising approximately 90 per cent of all wounds) are in the upper abdomen (above the umbilicus), an area where the small bowel is compressed into a smaller than normal area, the small bowel is placed at greater risk. The stab wounds of the abdomen can conveniently be divided into those of the lower and those of the upper abdomen for purposes of management.

WOUNDS OF THE LOWER ABDOMEN.   In later pregnancy a stab wound of the lower abdomen that enters the peritoneum with a great enough force and a long enough instrument will generally injure the uterus. If penetration is suspected, the physician is faced with the problem of whether to explore the abdomen or not. Peritoneal lavage (p. 46) can be used to determine if uterine bleeding is severe enough to justify surgical intervention. Since the major uterine vessels are on the lateral aspect of the uterus, they may be removed enough from the entry wound to escape injury from a small blade. A Foley catheter and retrograde cystogram can rule out urinary bladder injury. Close monitoring of vital signs, and a negative peritoneal lavage, can generally rule out pelvic vessel injury and would suggest that the patient could be followed by careful observation. Amniocentesis can be performed to see if there is bleeding into the amniotic cavity. A negative amniocentesis does not rule out concealed hemorrhage. The amniotic fluid can be further studied to assess fetal maturity and fetal well-being.

Fetal Wounds.   If the knife penetrates both the abdomen and the uterine wall the fetus is likely to sustain injury. The severity of the injury can vary from superficial soft tissue wounds to severe, life-threatening ones. If celiotomy is undertaken, the physician must decide whether to perform a cesarean section or leave the pregnancy undisturbed. Since it is impossible to determine the severity of the wound, the physician must weigh the potential benefits of corrective surgery in an injured infant delivered by cesarean section against the risks of premature delivery. Cases have been reported in which uterine wounds have been repaired and the pregnancy continued. These infants have been born alive with stab wounds sustained in utero. The fetal wounds heal, albeit slowly.

Hammar and Carter (1960) reported a maternal stab wound of the abdomen at 32 weeks' gestation. At celiotomy a stab wound of the anterior uterine wall was found, which was repaired, and the pregnancy continued undisturbed. Six weeks later the patient was delivered of a mature infant weighing 2838 gm, with a gaping wound of the thigh.

Wright and colleagues (1954) reported a similar experience, in which amniotic fluid was found in the peritoneal cavity at the time of exploration. The uterine-myometrial wound was repaired and the abdomen closed. Following the procedure, amniotic fluid was noted in the vagina for several days. The leaking stopped and the patient was delivered of a term, living infant nearly 4 months later. The infant had a healing soft tissue wound.

Although a penetrating wound of the uterus is likely to affect the conceptus, the severity of the wound is difficult to predict. In a recently reported case, a pregnancy continued for 1 week after a maternal stab wound of the abdomen with a barbecue fork at 8 months' gestation (Amine, 1976). The patient was managed conservatively and delivered 1 week later. The infant had two healing puncture wounds on the back at the level of T6–T7. On examination the infant was found to have flaccid legs, later determined to be a result of scarring of the spinal cord and the arachnoid membrane secondary to the trauma.

In all three of these cases the myometrial wound was repaired and the pregnancy continued. These cases give clinical support to the research evidence that membranes can seal by regeneration (Wynn et al., 1967). But the membranes are not the only fetal appendages that can sustain injury. Dyer and Barclay (1962) reported the delivery of a stillborn infant following maternal stab wound where the umbilical cord had been partially severed.

Although we feel that conservative management of the pregnancy is in order in penetrating wounds of the abdomen, others have elected to perform cesarean section when uterine stab wounds are found at exploration. Knapp and Drucker (1972) performed a cesarean section on a woman with seven self-inflicted stab wounds of the abdomen at term. The uterus had four wounds on its anterior surface. A live, 2835 gm infant was delivered that had only two superficial lacerations, one on the back, the other on the flank. McNabney and Smith (1973) performed cesarean section in one case of stab wound of the abdomen with uterine perforation. The mother sustained no other viscus injuries, but amniotic fluid and blood were found in the peritoneal cavity. A 2500 gm infant with an Apgar score of 8 was delivered with a 1 cm stab wound in the right lower quadrant. The infant was explored after delivery and was found to have no wounds requiring intervention.

Under no circumstances should consideration of maintaining the pregnancy compromise management of the maternal wounds. If the gravid uterus limits exploration or repair of injury, the uterus should be emptied regardless of duration of gestation. Malinovski (1974) reported a case of stab wound of the left lower quadrant at 37 weeks' gestation. The mother sustained a through-and-through wound of the sigmoid and its mesentery, and there was a wound of the uterus through which amniotic fluid was leaking and through which placenta was visible. Cesarean section was performed, with the delivery of a 3200 gm infant without injury that later developed normally. In this case the duration of gestation, the uterine injury, and the associated injuries all directed that cesarean section be performed.

The hardiness of the conceptus and its ability to withstand the trauma of vaginal delivery is demonstrated by a case reported by Steele (1941). The mother sustained a penetrating wound of the lower abdomen. She was subsequently delivered vaginally of a live infant with a laceration of the abdominal wall and evisceration of bowel. The infant's wound was treated surgically in the early neonatal period with successful outcome.

If the surgeon, at the time of exploration, undertakes delivery by cesarean section of either a mature or a premature infant, every effort should be made to have a neonatologist and a pediatric surgeon available. Unless severe injury has occurred, the uterine wounds can generally be repaired and the patient's reproductive capacity maintained. Patients have conceived after repair of extensive uterine wounds (Aguero and Kizer, 1968). If, on the other hand, the uterine injury is severe or the organ limits access to repair of maternal injury, cesarean hysterectomy should be performed.

WOUNDS IN THE UPPER ABDOMEN. In wounds of the upper abdomen, constituting 60 per cent of stab wounds in the nonpregnant population, the same conditions apply as in gunshot wounds. The difficulty in assessing the abdominal wall response to peritoneal irritation, the less satisfactory results with peritoneal lavage, and increased likelihood of viscus injury suggest that pregnant patients should be explored.

Of particular interest in stab wounds of the upper abdomen (i.e., those above the umbilicus) are lacerations of the diaphragm. While not a frequent occurrence — 13 of 4000 cases (Kessler and Stein, 1976) — an unsuspected diaphragmatic laceration presents great risk in pregnancy. The pathophysiology of diaphragmatic hernia is not completely understood, particularly whether herniation occurs immediately following injury or whether it requires an increase in intraperitoneal pressure. Kessler and Stein (1976) suggested three phases in the clinical course of diaphragmatic hernias: (1) The initial phase of injury; (2) the interval phase, during which there may be no symptoms or only vague symptoms; and (3) the acute or obstructive phase with obstruction or strangulation of the hernia contents.

Unlike congenital and acquired abdominal hernias, posttraumatic diaphragmatic hernias have no peritoneal sac. Right sided diaphragmatic wounds are generally sealed by the liver. The colon is the most commonly herniated organ; stomach, small bowel, or liver can also be displaced into the thoracic cavity. The seriousness of this condition is demonstrated by a mortality of 16 to 20 per cent, which rises to 25 to 66 per cent when strangulation is present. Kessler and Stein (1976) report a mortality of 23 per cent in their series, documenting the importance of early diagnosis and appropriate management. A diaphragmatic hernia following trauma may remain asymptomatic for a long period of time. Conditions which increase the intraperitoneal pressure, like the growing uterus, the nausea and vomiting of pregnancy, and the stress of labor, are likely to cause herniation of viscera.

Shortness of breath, epigastric discomfort, nausea, and vomiting are the common symptoms. The diagnosis can usually be established by chest x-rays or by contrast studies of the bowel.

Osborne and Foster (1953) reported a maternal death resulting from a posttraumatic diaphragmatic hernia in pregnancy. Stomach and transverse colon herniated into the chest through a 6 cm defect. The stomach had ruptured after acute dilatation. The maternal mortality in reported cases, including his own, was 58.3 per cent (7 of 12). Additional cases have been reported since Osborne and Foster's review, suggesting that this is not a rare entity (Kasim and Podelets, 1967; Morosini and Manfredi, 1973; Stevenson, 1974; Kessler and Stein, 1976). In these four recently reported cases there were one maternal death and three fetal deaths.

Appropriate surgical management should be undertaken as soon as the diagnosis of diaphragmatic hernia in pregnancy is established. Following repair, delivery should be accomplished by cesarean section in order to avoid the stress of labor and the Valsalva maneuver.

REFERENCES

Aguero O, Kizer S: Obstetric prognosis of the repair of uterine rupture. Surg Gynecol Obstet *127*:528, 1968.

Amine ARC: Spinal cord injury in a fetus. Surg Neurol *6*:369, 1976.

Bochner K: Traumatic perforation of the pregnant uterus. Report of two cases. Obstet Gynecol *17*:520, 1961.

Browns K, Bhat R, Jonasson O, Vidyasagar D: Thoracoabdominal gunshot wound with survival of a 36-week fetus. JAMA *237*:2409, 1977.

Buchsbaum HJ: Accidental injury complicating pregnancy. Am J Obstet Gynecol *102*:752, 1968.

Buchsbaum HJ: Diagnosis and management of abdominal gunshot wounds during pregnancy. J Trauma *15*:425, 1975.

Buchsbaum HJ, Caruso PA: Gunshot wound of the pregnant uterus. Case report of fetal injury, deglutition of missile, and survival. Obstet Gynecol *33*:673, 1969.

Bull JC Jr, Mathewson C Jr: Exploratory laparotomy in patients with penetrating wounds of the abdomen. Am J Surg *116*:223, 1968.

Carter JW, Sawyers JL: Pitfalls in diagnosis of abdominal stab wounds by contrast media injection. Am Surg *35*:107, 1969.

Cornell WP, Ebert PA, Zuidema GD: X-ray diagnosis of penetrating wounds of the abdomen. J Surg Res *5*:142, 1965.

Dawidson I, Miller E, Litwin MS: Gunshot wounds of the abdomen. A review of 277 cases. Arch Surg *111*:862, 1976.

Devlin A: Nursing care study: Innocent victim — shot before birth. Nurs Mirror *143*:45, 1976.

Din-Van-Tung, Hau-Mac-Suu: Les plaies de guerre de l'appariel génital féminin. Gyn Obst (Paris) 70:179, 1971.

Dyer I, Barclay DL: Accidental trauma complicating pregnancy and delivery. Am J Obstet Gynecol *83*:907, 1962.

Eckerling B, Teaff R: Obstetrical approach to abdominal war wounds in late pregnancy. J Obstet Gynaecol Br Emp *57*:747, 1950.

Flint LM Jr, Voyles CR, Richardson D, et al: Missile tract infections after transcolonic gunshot wounds. Arch Surg *113*:727, 1978.

Gellhorn G: Schusswunden des Schwangern Uterus. Zbl Gynaek *27*:781, 1903.

Gysler R, Haller R, Morger R: Intrauterine gunshot wound. J Pediatr Surg *11*:589, 1976.

Hammar B, Carter TD: Intrauterine stab wound of foetus. Cent Afr J Med *6*:362, 1960.

Harris RP: Horn goring in pregnancy. Am J Med Sci *75*:338, 1878.

Kasim IM, Podelets VF: Combination of traumatic right-sided diaphragmatic hernia with pregnancy. Vestn Khir *98*:117, 1967.

Kessler E, Stein A: Diaphragmatic hernia as a long-term complication of stab wounds of the chest. Am J Surg *132*:34, 1972.

Knapp RC, Drucker DH: Self-inflicted stab wounds to pregnant uterus and fetus at term. NY State J Med *72*:391, 1972.

Kobak AJ, Hurwitz CH: Gunshot wounds of the pregnant uterus. Review of the literature and 2 case reports. Obstet Gynecol *4*:383, 1954.

Larsen B, Galask RP, Snyder IS: Nuramidase and peroxidase activity of human amniotic fluid. Obstet Gynecol *44*:219, 1974.

Ledgerwood AM: The wandering bullet. Surg Clin North Am *57*:97, 1977.

Lins G, Schäfer A: Forensische Probleme bei Abtreibung durch Schuss. Zeitsch Rechtsmed *71*:108, 1972.

Malinovski I: Penetrating abdominal wound with injury of the pregnant uterus. Vestn Khir *113*:62, 1974.

Martins CP, Garcia OM: Ferimentos do utero gravido por arma de fogo. An Brasil Ginec *58*:229, 1964.

Marx GF: Shock in the obstetric patient. Anesth *26*:423, 1965.

McNabney WK, McCause A: Management of abdominal stab wounds. Am J Surg *114*:726, 1967.

McNabney WK, Smith EI: Penetrating wounds of the gravid uterus. J. Trauma *12*:1024, 1973.

Morosini S, Manfredi A: Ernia traumatica del diaframma in gravidanza. Atteneo Parmense Acta Biomed *44*:199, 1973.

Nance FC, Cohn I Jr: Surgical judgment in the management of stab wounds: A retrospective and prospective analysis based on a study of 600 stab wounds. Ann Surg *170*:569, 1969.

Nance FC, Wennar MH, Johson LW, et al: Surgical judgment in the management of penetrating wounds of the abdomen: Experience with 2212 patients. Ann Surg *179*:639, 1974.

Osborne WW, Foster CD: Diaphragmatic hernia complicating pregnancy. Am J Obstet Gynecol *66*:682, 1953.

Printen KJ, Freeark RJ, Shoemaker WC: Conservative management of penetrating abdominal stab wounds. Arch Surg *96*:899, 1968.

Quast DC, Jordan GL Jr: Traumatic wounds of the female reproductive organs. J Trauma *4*:839, 1964.

Romney SL, Gabel PV, Takeda Y: Experimental hemorrhage in pregnancy. Am J Obstet Gynecol *87*:636, 1963.

Rushforth NB, Ford AB, Hirsch CS, et al: Violent death in a metropolitan county. Changing patterns in homicide (1958–74). N Engl J Med *297*:531, 1977.

Saunders P, Milton PJD: Laparotomy during pregnancy: An assessment of diagnostic accuracy and fetal wastage. Br Med J 3:165, 1973.

Schlievert P, Larsen B, Johnson W, et al: Bacterial growth inhibition by amniotic fluid. III. Demonstration of the variability of bacterial growth inhibition by amniotic fluid with a new plate-count technique. Am J Obstet Gynecol 122:809, 1975.

Schnider SM, Webster GM: Maternal and fetal hazards of surgery during pregnancy. Am J Obstet Gynecol 92:891, 1965.

Shaftan GW: Indications for operation in abdominal trauma. Ann Surg 99:657, 1960.

Slater BL: Multiple anaesthetics during pregnancy. A case report. Br J Anaesth 42:1131, 1970.

Smithwick W III, Gertner HR Jr, Zuidema GD: Injection of Hypaque (sodium diatrizoate) in the management of abdominal stab wounds. Surg Gynecol Obstet 127:1215, 1968.

Steele: *In* Flamrich E: Schussverletzung des Schwangeren Uterus. Zbl Gynaek 65:25, 1941.

Stevenson HM: Diaphragmatic injuries. Proc R Soc Med 67:1, 1974.

Takki S, Pollanen L, Ertama P, Lehtonen T: Criminal abortion by gunshot. A case report. Ann Chir Gynaecol Fenn 58:122, 1969.

Tanga MR, Kawathekar P: Injury due to bull goring. Int Surg 58:635, 1973.

Thonet C: Suicidio frustrado durante el embarazo. Rev Chil Obstet Ginecol 32:166, 1967.

Wray RC Jr, Burnett WF: Gunshot wound of the intestine, pregnant uterus, and placenta with maternal and fetal survival. Am Surg 37:308, 1971.

Wright CH, Posner AC, Gilchrist J: Penetrating wounds of the gravid uterus. Am J Obstet Gynecol 67:1085, 1954.

Wynn RM, Sever PS, Hellman LM: Morphologic studies of the ruptured amnion. Am J Obstet Gynecol 99:359, 1967.

Zivkovic S, Milosevic V, Stanivukovic V: Prenatal gunshot perforation of the colon. J Pediatr Surg 11:591, 1976.

Chapter 6

AUTOMOBILE INJURIES AND BLUNT ABDOMINAL TRAUMA

Warren M. Crosby

Introduction

The automobile epitomizes the American way of life. Collisions between automobiles are common occurrences in the United States, and nearly 50,000 persons lose their lives annually from this cause. Automobile-induced trauma is the most common cause of death in the 15 to 24 year age group—in males more frequently than in females—and ranks third after heart disease and cancer for all age groups. It is not known if pregnancy alters women's or their husbands' driving habits; it is presumed that pregnant women have essentially the same risk of being in an automobile collision as nonpregnant women. Barno and colleagues (1962) reported that trauma was the leading nonobstetric cause of death among pregnant women in Minnesota in the decade preceding 1960, and that half of these deaths were due to automobile collisions. More recently, Jimerson and Crosby (1977) found that 0.9 per cent of all maternal deaths in Oklahoma were caused by the automobile.

Although the deaths in the Jimerson and Crosby study were considered "accidental" almost by definition (the term "automobile accident" is firmly ingrained in the language and applies to all automobile collisions, whether the collision was willful or accidental), many were actually preventable. For instance, death of one pregnant woman was the result of a combination of alcohol, poor road conditions and nonuse of available restraint systems. The pregnant victim was in the passenger seat of a relatively new car outfitted with lap belts and shoulder harnesses, but these were not in use. Her husband was driving at a legal rate of speed on a four-lane road at night. An inebriated driver coming from the opposite direction crossed the median strip and hit them head-on. The maneuver must have been fairly sudden, because neither car made any evasive or braking action. The combined rate of speed at the moment of collision was estimated to be around 50 to 60 mph; the woman was killed. An "accidental" death, yes, but clearly preventable. The collision would probably have not occurred at all had the driver of the opposing car not had an elevated blood alcohol level. Modern road construction with separation of the two opposing lanes of traffic is very successful in avoiding head-on collisions and in preventing deaths therefrom. Failure of the pregnant victim to use available restraint systems certainly reduced her chances for surviving the collision. It is, of course, beyond the scope of this chapter to discuss possibilities for road improvement or control of drunken driving. Emphasis should be given, however, to the nature of the automobile accident; the tragedy is all the greater when a little thought could have prevented it. The purposes of this chapter are:

1. To derive general conclusions about crash injury patterns seen in pregnant automobile victims;

2. To derive general guidelines for treatment of pregnant accident victims; and

3. To discuss presently available and future restraint systems and to comment upon their use by pregnant passengers.

Principles of Automotive Injury

Every automobile collision is a unique event. Indeed, the forces involved in an experimental impact are difficult to estimate even when collisions are reproduced under laboratory conditions. But specific types of automobile collisions do tend to produce similar injuries. Whatever the type of collision, being thrown out of the car is very hazardous. If restraint systems did nothing else but prevent ejection, the mortality rate would decline with their use (Huelke and Gikas, 1968).

Unrestrained Passengers

The basic features of the impact sequence are necessarily complicated. When the occupant is unrestrained, virtually any part of the body may be injured. In head-on collisions, the driver's chest becomes impacted against the steering wheel and his knees against the dashboard. The collapsible steering column and improvements in the design of steering wheels and dashboards have reduced injuries from these factors. Right front seat passengers do not have the restraining advantage of the steering wheel, and are propelled directly into the windshield, the A pillar, or the roof header. Their injuries are likely to be more serious than those of the driver or rear seat passengers, and they more often involve the head rather than the chest. Head injury is the most frequent cause of death from automotive crashes, and head injury alone accounts for the higher mortality rate for nondriver accident victims (Huelke and Gikas, 1968). Back seat passengers are less often fatally injured, largely because of the restraining influence of the front seat.

In side impacts, lateral motion causes more injuries to the occupants on the side impacted. Rear-end collisions also injure front seat passengers more severely than rear passengers, perhaps because the heads of the front seat occupants initially are propelled backwards into the forward moving seat and then rebound forward, with the angular momentum of the head increasing with the velocity of the impacting vehicle; the head then may strike the dashboard, steering wheel, A pillar, or roof header in a secondary collision. Again, drivers fare somewhat better than other front seat riders because of the protecting steering wheel. Rear seat passengers have a relative advantage because the rear deck absorbs some of the momentum of the passenger's head impacting against it; this reduces the velocity of forward rebound and may diminish head and neck injury. Roll-over accidents are more complicated; head and neck injuries still predominate, but multiple extremity fractures are often produced by the tumbling action of the occupant's body within the vehicle (Huelke and Gikas, 1968). The roof often collapses, crushing the occupants with serious head and torso injuries.

Ejection from the vehicle is especially dangerous, again because of secondary and tertiary impacts of the body with the road bed, surrounding trees, road signs or oncoming cars, or crushing by the vehicle itself. Improvements in design to reduce ejection have reduced fatal injuries considerably. Laminated windshields that shatter but maintain their resistance to penetration have decreased the incidence of ejection via this route. Door latches are now much less likely to give way, thus reducing ejection through doors. These improvements followed suggestions in the initial studies of impact injuries by Tourin and Garrett (1960) and Huelke and Gikas (1968).

Restrained Passengers

Restrained victims fare considerably better in all collisions (Table 6–1). The fear that the victim will be trapped in a burning vehicle is almost completely unwarranted (Modern Medicine, 1968). It is true that occasionally a freak situation may occur in which being ejected from a vehicle may prove beneficial for the occupant; a low-velocity roll-over accident involving passengers in a convertible may be such a situation. But this is so rare that it is statistically negligible.

The first widely available automobile restraint system was the lap belt. This device, if properly applied across the upper thighs and pelvis, restrains the body by fixing the pelvis to the seat. During the impact sequence, the

TABLE 6–1 Maternal Injuries in Severe Collisions

	NUMBER	DEATHS (PER CENT)	INJURED (PER CENT)	TOTAL MORTALITY (PER CENT)
Lap belt restraint	24	1 (3.6)	2 (7.4)	3 (10.7)
No restraint	180	14 (7.8)	24 (14.4)	38 (21.1)

lower part of the body remains more or less stationary (Fig. 6–1). The lower legs below the knee are free to rotate laterally or forward, and ankle and foot injuries may occur. The pelvis absorbs the restraining force of the lap belt and forces the body to decelerate with the car seat and the car. The upper body, however, is free to rotate on the lower spine. In head-on collisions, the body jack-knifes forward with the head impinging on the dashboard. With side collisions, the upper body again flexes forward and laterally, impacting against the A pillar, the seat, or the door. Injury is prevented largely by preventing ejection through the door or windshield. Survival in rear-end collisions is not affected as much by lap belt restraint; however, it is effective in reducing injury by preventing secondary and tertiary impact within the car (Huelke and Gikas, 1968). Roll-over collisions invariably produce secondary and tertiary impacts within the rolling vehicle, and lap belt restraint reduces the number and severity of these impacts. Above all, prevention of ejection results in considerable reduction in the injury incidence and severity in roll-over collisions.

BLUNT ABDOMINAL TRAUMA IN NONPREGNANT AND PREGNANT VICTIMS

The automobile is responsible for nearly half of nonpenetrating abdominal injuries (Griswold and Collier, 1961). Blunt traumatic injury is frequently multiple, with injuries to the head, the chest, and the extremities accompanying damage to the viscera. The fact that head injury may cause coma, or chest injury require immediate life-saving attention, or extremity fractures catch the attention of the attendants, should not eliminate the trauma physician's vigilance in searching for nonpenetrating injury to the major organs of the abdomen. Rupture of the bladder or bowel is a life-threatening injury, but the signs and symptoms of these injuries take time to develop and thus an accurate diagnosis cannot be made immediately. Rupture of solid organs, such as the liver or spleen, causes hemorrhage. The hemorrhage may be self-limited or continuous and may be relatively minimal or massive. Either way, the passage of a certain amount of time is also required before the diagnosis can be made. Frequently shock in a person with a head or chest injury is treated without recognition that the cause of the shock was rupture of an abdominal organ rather than the more obvious injury to the head, chest, or extremities.

According to Griswold and Collier (1961), trauma to the spleen or to one or both kidneys accounts for half of the injuries to the abdominal viscera. Intestinal injury and hepatic rupture account for one third, and the remaining injuries involve trauma to the abdominal wall, the mesentery, the diaphragm, the pancreas, and retroperitoneal hemorrhage (Griswold and Collier, 1961).

General Mechanism of Injury

The mechanism of blunt abdominal injury is only speculative, and very little work has been done to determine the factors responsible for variations

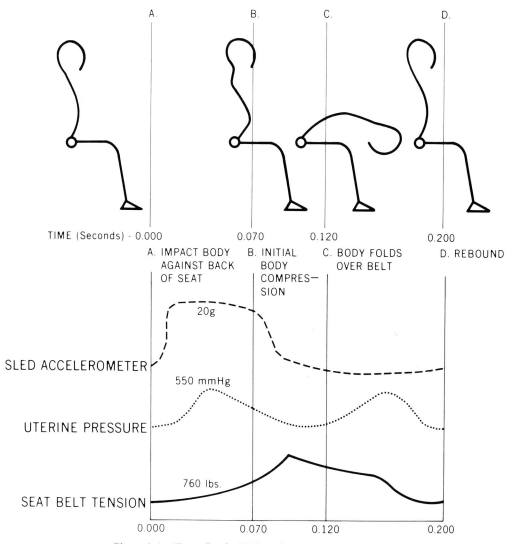

Figure 6-1 (From Crosby WM. et al.: Am J Obstet Gynecol *101*:108, 1968).

in organ involvement. It would appear that most of the abdominal viscera have some degree of mobility, and thus force applied to the abdomen over a relatively long period of time will be less damaging than a short, sharp blow. The spleen or liver may be ruptured by relatively minor forces that are applied abruptly, but the bowel is unlikely to be ruptured except by forces of great magnitude. Inward compression of the abdominal wall produces crushing of the bowel wall itself, between the blunt object and some other unyielding portion of the abdomen. Sudden entrapment of gas in a closed loop with increasing pressure may rupture the bowel. Similar deformation of the abdominal cavity may also cause shearing of the bowel from its vascular attachments, or it may rupture the diaphragm or the anterior abdominal wall itself.

The pancreas and other extraperitoneal organs are not injured as often because they are solid organs and protected by the strong muscles of the back and the ribs. These organs are relatively delicate, however, and the fact that the kidneys are injured nearly as often as apparently more vulnerable organs such as the spleen or liver indicates that the protection offered by the muscles of the back and the rib cage is not as effective as it might seem. This is probably because force can be transmitted through the protective structures directly to the capsule of the kidney, which is torn rather easily. Similarly, rapid flexion or extension of the body may disrupt the continuity of the pancreas, without any force being applied directly to the abdomen.

MECHANISM IN PREGNANCY. In Crosby and Costiloe's (1971) series, 5 of 14 fatally injured pregnant victims of automobile collisions died from blunt abdominal trauma. In two, major abdominal blood vessels were ruptured; in two others the liver or the spleen, or both, was ruptured, and in one the uterus was ruptured. In each case the mother died of exsanguination. Sparkman (1958) reviewed 44 patients who had splenic rupture during pregnancy. Sixteen ruptures were attributed to trauma, although in 10 the trauma was apparently trivial in nature. In a later study by Buchsbaum (1967), trauma was the etiologic factor in 6 of 21 splenic ruptures occurring during pregnancy. Because of this relatively minor amount of trauma associated with splenic rupture, Sparkman concluded that pregnancy itself predisposes the woman to splenic rupture. In comparison with the frequency of spontaneous rupture of the spleen in various diseases, he judged that pregnancy was second only to malaria in the frequency of reported cases.

In contrast, it has been observed that the bowel is injured somewhat less frequently when the victim is pregnant. This is apparently because the bulk of the fluid-filled pregnant uterus protects the bowel from direct force applied to the anterior abdominal wall (Buchsbaum, 1968; Crosby, 1974). In pregnant women after the first trimester, the dissipation of the traumatic force may occur within the uterus itself, because of its size. Uterine rupture or, more frequently, separation of the placenta may then result.

Retroperitoneal Hemorrhage

During pregnancy, blunt abdominal trauma is more likely to produce hemorrhage than in the nonpregnant state. Elliott (1966) reported 39 pregnant women seriously injured in automobile collisions in Australia. Eight died and each had multiple injuries. The primary cause of death in each was uncontrollable hemorrhage. In five of the eight the hemorrhage was confined to the retroperitoneal space. This potential space offers very little resistance to bleeding; it has been estimated that it can hold as much as 4 liters of blood at the pressure normally present in pelvic veins (Gomcyekow, 1962). Retroperitoneal hemorrhage is enhanced by the increased vascularity surrounding the pregnant uterus; the hemorrhage originates from small, thin-walled vessels in the broad ligament that are engorged with blood draining the uterus. In the Elliott study, intraperitoneal bleeding caused the death of three patients, owing to rupture of the liver or the spleen or to disruption of the mesentery from its vascular attachments.

Biomechanics

The biomechanics of impact when the victim is pregnant have been studied using the pregnant baboon as the test subject (Crosby et al., 1968). Controlled and reproducible impacts were utilized. The animals were prepared for both physical and physiologic measurements (intrauterine and intraperitoneal pressure, vehicular deceleration forces, lap belt and shoulder harness tension, fetal and maternal heart rate by electrocardiogram and maternal blood pressure). Impacts with an unrestrained subject were felt to be impractical and thus were not performed.

Head-on impacts of 20 G were carried out repeatedly, and each animal underwent essentially the same impact sequence. In each case, following impact into the brake, the body of the animal continued forward, following the dictates of inertia. As depicted in Figure 6–1, the lower torso was restrained by the lap belt, the tension of which rose to very high values. The legs of the animal rotated upward until they were completely extended. The upper torso continued forward, but because the pelvis was restrained by the lap belt, it underwent rotation through the arc required by the spine fixed at the pelvis. The head followed the arc along with the extended arms until the arms struck the floor of the sled and the chest impinged upon the seat pan. The body then rebounded back to the normal upright position and came to a stop. The lower abdominal organs were compressed between the lap belt and the maternal spine. Thus, the pressure within the large pregnant uterus rose to levels 10 times that observed during labor. This intrauterine pressure was partially offset by a concomitant rise in intraperitoneal pressure, but these levels were generally less than half the intraperitoneal pressure. The maternal heart rate slowed briefly and a similar reduction in fetal heart rate occurred, but it lasted considerably longer than the maternal bradycardia.

Uterus

The pregnant uterus varies in shape, size, and vulnerability with advancing pregnancy. During the first trimester, it is well protected, being contained entirely within the bony pelvis. One of the fatally injured patients reported by Crosby and Costiloe was in her third month of gestation when the car in which she was a passenger ran off the road at a high rate of speed and hit several tree stumps. All four occupants were killed. The pregnant victim suffered extensive injuries, including rupture of the left renal artery, pulmonary artery, and left hemidiaphragm, but the uterus, placenta, and fetus were unharmed (Crosby and Costiloe, 1971). This finding suggests that in the first trimester, the uterus is not subject to direct trauma, unless the pelvic ring collapses inwardly or an external structure (such as the steering column or a glass or metal object) is thrust into the pelvic cavity through the abdominal wall or the perineum. Penetration injuries are more often associated with falls than with automobile collisions. Three months' gestation is the earliest time that the uterus has been reported to have been ruptured in an automobile collision (McCarty and Risely, 1956).

Beyond the first trimester, the uterus extends out of the pelvis, and becomes more vulnerable to direct injury. The pregnant uterus is a fluid-filled sac, surrounded by a variety of cushioning materials. The bowel, bladder and anterior abdominal wall tend to cushion blows from the front, and the strong back muscles and spine shield the pregnant uterus from injury from the back. Thus protected, the uterus, fetus, and placenta are usually uninjured, even at term. This is illustrated by another California automobile collision. This victim was at term and was ejected when the vehicle in which she was riding was hit from the rear by another car. Autopsy revealed the cause of death to be subarachnoid hemorrhage. The fetus and uterus were intact in spite of what must have been severe compression of the extensively bruised lower abdomen (Crosby and Costiloe, 1971).

During a collision, the uterus follows the laws of inertia, as does the rest of the woman's body: it continues in the direction the body was going until the body decelerates. The uterus then elongates and flattens itself against the anterior abdominal wall. The amount of deformation of the uterus depends upon the velocity of deceleration and the elasticity of the uterus. Abrupt deceleration may rupture the uterus directly without external penetration, but this is quite unusual. If the uterus remains intact, the elastic recoil of the uterine walls produces a wave-like motion in the amniotic fluid. This causes a reversal of the sequence and the uterus flattens in the opposite plane and becomes shorter. The concomitant rise in uterine pressure may be extreme, as depicted in Figure 6–1. With pressures 10 times that observed in labor, it is apparent that the fetus may be squeezed considerably by the amniotic fluid pressure and cessation of flow through the umbilical cord may very well occur. However, these extreme pressures are of short duration and it is unlikely that the fetus would be killed by compression alone in such a short period of time.

Placenta

The violent motions are more likely to cause a disruption of placental attachments than they are to disrupt the uterine wall or crush the fetus. The placenta does not contain elastic tissue, and cannot stretch or contract to adjust to sudden increases or decreases in the area of its attachment to the uterine wall. Placental tearing or rupture is quite unusual; separation from the uterine wall is much more common. The anchoring villi may be sheared off during these violent motions and the result is the same as when the placenta is separated for any other reason. Blood escapes from the intervillous space, dissects through the decidua and may cause shock and uterine contractions, whether there is external bleeding or not.

Because the uterus must decelerate in every collision, no matter how minor, and because of the extreme variability of the forces involved, the possibility of placental separation is ever-present, yet it was clinically apparent in only about 4 per cent of collisions reported by Crosby and Costiloe (1971). Subclinical placental separation can occur, with the bleeding being confined to the decidua. Under these circumstances the uterus is usually irritable for a period of a few hours, and there may even be a minor amount of vaginal bleeding. The subsequent hematoma, if it remains limited, may become organized in the usual way and ultimately present as an infarct of the placenta. The incidence of subclinical placental separation and infarction following automobile collisions is unknown, but minor separations appear to be of little clinical significance (Crosby, 1974). Based on data from collected cases, Crosby estimates that if labor does not ensue within a week following the collision, the hematoma will be self-limited and will not cause subsequent premature labor or fetal demise.

The larger the decidual hematoma, the greater will be the clinical effect. Involvement of 10 to 25 per cent of the placental surface regularly initiates labor, but there will usually be no untoward effect to the mother or the fetus, because such small abruptions are usually self-limited (Page et al., 1954). Of course, if the baby is born prematurely under these circumstances, the after-effects may be devastating. When 25 to 50 per cent of the placental surface is involved, fetal distress is usually seen and intrapartum death may occur if there is delay in delivery. Involvement of more than half of the placental surface in the separation almost invariably is associated with fetal demise (Page et al., 1954). Placental separation may be also accompanied by maternal shock, uterine tetany and hypofibrinogenemia. According to the authors of this clinical classification of abruptio placentae, the perinatal mortality associated with Grade I abruption (10 to 25 per cent involved) was 30 per cent; Grade II abruption (25 to 50 per cent involved) was 80 per cent, and for greater than 50 per cent (Grade III) it was 100 per cent (Page et al., 1954).

Fetal Injury

Injury to the fetus caused by blunt abdominal trauma is unusual. The fetus is protected by the cushioning effect of the amniotic fluid and the elasticity of the uterus; even the effects of inertial forces are damped by the fluid medium. However, flexion of the mother's body over a lap belt with the buckle or the belt itself crushing the fetal skull has been reported by Crosby (1974). The fetus may be directly injured by objects penetrating the uterus, and such injuries are usually fatal for both mother and fetus.

Parkinson (1964) reported a fetal skull fracture that occurred during a head-on collision in which the mother drove into a utility pole. Apparently the fracture was brought about by the bilateral fractures of her superior ischial rami. Parkinson refers to seven other, similar cases with either fetal intracranial bleeding or fetal skull fracture. He believes that at the time of the publication of the article the eight cases were the only reported instances of traumatic direct fetal injury without uterine rupture. In a discussion of that article, McNeil estimated the incidence of direct fetal injury due to external trauma to be less than 1 per 10,000 births. For the most part, fetal skull injury is due to maternal pelvic fracture in which the dislocation of the pelvic bones during the fracture process crushes the entrapped fetal skull. Three baboon fetuses involved in experimental impacts suffered head injury; one had compression of the skull between the lap belt and the maternal spine, and two fetuses in breech position sustained head injuries, presumably when the upper part of the uterus was compressed between the seat pan and the maternal spine (Crosby et al., 1968).

Incidence and Severity of Injuries During Pregnancy (Tables 6–1 and 6–2)

The many variables that influence the pattern and severity of injury include the type of collision (head-on, rear-end, side and roll-over are the generally used categories), the seating position and posture of the victim at the moment of impact, the size and velocity of the automobile, its compressibility, the occupant restraint system and how it was used at the moment of impact, and the resistance of the passenger shell to collapse from external force. Yet among these and other complicated factors, general patterns do exist. It is well established, for instance, that rear-end collisions are much more likely to injure the neck than the body of a front seat victim. Similarly, head-on collisions cause head and knee injury more often than do rear-end or broadside collisions, and injuries to the chest occur more often among drivers than among passengers (Huelke and Gikas, 1968).

As noted earlier, the only prospective study of pregnant victims of automobile collisions was conducted by Crosby and Costiloe (1971), using automobile collisions investigated by the California Highway Patrol. In each accident investigated, the patrolman asked all female occupants if they were pregnant, so that the study would not be biased to include only victims in late pregnancy who were obviously pregnant. The authors contacted the victim and her physicians and the hospitals that cared for her. Data were complete for 406 pregnant victims. Severity of passenger injury closely paralleled the severity of physical damage to the vehicle. Each car was classified according to standards of damage by the investigating officer. The categories of damage were minor or no damage, moderate, and severe or total damage.

TABLE 6–2 Fetal Injuries in Severe Collisions

	Number	Died with Mother	Abruptio Placentae	Maternal Shock	Unknown Cause	RDS	Total (Per Cent)
Lap belt restraint	24	1 (4.2)	1	0	2	3	4 (16.7)
No restraint	166	13 (7.8)	5	3	2	11	24 (14.4)

Minor and Moderate Collisions

The minor and moderate categories were combined because the incidence of injuries was very small in each. Among 233 pregnant victims of minor to moderate collisions, only three mothers were injured. Two had rib fractures and one sustained a fracture of the radius. Although six of the mothers ultimately lost their babies, in only three was there evidence that the fetal loss was directly related to the collision. In each of these three, the fetus was said to have stopped moving soon after the collision, and a macerated stillborn was delivered within 3 or 4 days of the impact. Neurogenic shock is a reaction to stressful situations that often results in a hypotensive state, characterized by syncope, slow pulse rate, peripheral vasoconstriction and central vasodilatation and essentially uniform recovery. Pregnancy seems to be accompanied by an increase in susceptibility to neurogenic shock. We hypothesize that the uterine arteries undergo vasoconstriction during the sequence of neurogenic shock (Crosby and Costiloe, 1971). The fetus "faints" along with the mother, but because of its initially lower pO_2 and the continued inadequacy of uterine artery flow, fails to recover as often as the mother does. Since none of the belted mothers or fetuses were directly injured, it may be concluded that lap belts usually are not harmful to the conceptus in minor to moderate collisions.

Severe Collisions

In this study, there were 204 pregnant victims of automobile collisions that caused major or total damage to the car (Table 6–1) One hundred eighty victims were not restrained and 14 of them died (7.8 per cent). Death was most often caused by head injury. However, internal injuries tended to be multiple, and death commonly resulted from exsanguination: three patients had rupture of major blood vessels, such as the aorta, pulmonary artery, and renal artery, along with rupture of the spleen or liver, placental separation, or multiple fractures of ribs or extremities. Three died of intra- or extraperitoneal bleeding following pelvic fractures, and in two of these victims the uterine wall was also ruptured. One patient died of burns but was otherwise uninjured. Only one of 28 belted victims was fatally injured (3.6 per cent), and that was the result of a ruptured spleen and diaphragm. Since two nonbelted victims, but none of the belted victims, had uterine rupture, it seems that the lap belt does not have any special propensity for contributing to this type of abdominal compression injury.

Among 166 unrestrained survivors, there were 24 victims with significant injuries (Table 6–1). Three separate injury patterns emerged from this group:

1. *Severe and life-threatening injuries:* Four victims had internal abdominal injuries (ruptured spleen, liver, bladder), and three of these had associated multiple fractures. Only one of the babies survived; two fetuses died of placental separation and one of maternal shock. One victim survived a severe head injury and was still in coma a year later; her fetus also died of placental separation. None of these victims were ejected from the car.

2. *Moderate severity (not life-threatening)*: Five victims had multiple fractures without internal injury. Three had pelvic fractures and one had three frac-

tured vertebrae. Three fetuses succumbed to placental separation. None of these victims were ejected from the vehicle.

3. *Mild severity:* There were 14 victims with fractures of patella, ribs, clavicles, arms, wrists, or jaw. Only one fetus was lost from this group. In this case the mother sustained only a rib fracture in a roll-over collision. She was near term and the fetus was macerated when delivered two days following the impact. The fetus apparently died of maternal shock, since there was no evidence of trauma or placental separation. From these injury patterns the following generalizations are warranted:

1. Severe, life-threatening injuries are usually multiple.

2. Internal injuries are usually accompanied by intraperitoneal bleeding and shock.

3. Victims with multiple injuries are likely to lose the fetus, usually from placental separation or maternal shock or both.

4. The likelihood of fetal loss is usually proportional to the severity of maternal injury, and the most frequent cause of fetal death is death of the mother.

5. The high incidence of pelvic fracture and the likelihood of placental separation in association with pelvic fracture make it imperative to obtain x-rays of the pelvis in pregnant victims of severe collisions.

The number of belted victims in this study was considerably smaller, and the conclusions drawn are necessarily tentative. Only one of the 27 belted *survivors* suffered any significant injury — several fractured ribs which produced a pneumothorax. Following prompt treatment, mother and baby did well.

However, the fetus fared less well among this small group of restrained passengers than among those that were unrestrained (Table 6–2). The overall perinatal mortality resulting from collision in belted victims was 13 per cent among survivors as opposed to 7.2 per cent for unrestrained surviving mothers. However, since these differences were not statistically significant, and because the maternal plus fetal death rate was almost exactly equal among the two groups (12.9 per cent versus 13.0 per cent), we felt that there was no evidence that lap belt restraint was harmful for the mother or the fetus and suggested that lap belts be worn (Crosby and Costiloe, 1971).

Data on additional 19 belted victims had been gathered by correspondence and from the literature (Rubovitz, 1964; Theurer and Kaiser, 1963). In many of these, the injuries were spectacular, which probably accounted for their having been brought to my attention. The patterns of injury in this group differ somewhat from the unrestrained group:

1. There was almost a total absence of fatal head injuries, indicating perhaps that death from head injury may be reduced by wearing lap belts. This has been noted by others (Huelke and Gikas, 1968), and occurs because there is less opportunity for the head to strike solid objects when the victim is restrained by a belt. This is true because the victim is prevented from being ejected from the vehicle, under which circumstance many fatal head injuries are incurred.

2. Several victims had uterine ruptures and several more had placental

separation, implying that lap belt restraint may increase the risk of these uterine catastrophes by focusing much of the decelerative force on the lower abdomen. This question may never be satisfactorily answered because cars are now equipped with three-point restraint systems rather than single lap belts. It is my assumption that women who usually use their restraint system will have less reluctance to use the three-point system than the lap belt alone when they become pregnant.

DIAGNOSIS AND TREATMENT OF AUTOMOTIVE INJURIES

At the Scene: Triage

The emergency medical technician at the scene of an accident and the physician in the hospital emergency ward have essentially the same goal in treating the victims of automobile collisions. First they must assess who is dead and who is beyond help, who has sustained minor injury and can be left untreated for the time being, and who needs help immediately. The chances for the seriously injured victim depend greatly on the personnel's degree of experience in triage. Unfortunately, few emergency technicians or physicians have much training in trauma of pregnant victims.

Several texts dealing with the total care of injured patients (e.g., Nahum, 1966; Shires, 1966; American College of Surgeons, 1976) are available. These provide excellent guidelines for initial and for more prolonged care of the injured patient. It is interesting to note, however, that of a random sampling of available books on the care of the injured patient in medical school libraries, not one mentioned the condition of pregnancy or the unique problems associated with pregnant trauma victims.

Initial emergency treatment of the seriously injured pregnant victim of an automobile collision will not differ significantly from that of a nonpregnant woman. The primary aim is to reconstitute or preserve vital functions: the airway must be kept open by an oral or nasal tube or opened by tracheostomy if obstructed; visible hemorrhage must be attended to, and concealed hemorrhage sought out and vigorously treated. Blood volume replacement, of course, is mandatory for acute blood loss and shock, but if the source of the hemorrhage is not controlled, blood replacement will be ineffective and will help only temporarily. Surgical exploration for the source of concealed hemorrhage is often life-saving. Most authorities suggest passage of a nasogastric tube and a bladder catheter on arrival in the emergency room. Intravenous fluids are begun through the needle from which blood was obtained for typing and cross matching and other baseline and diagnostic blood studies. A brief perusal for major fractures is made; if any are found, they should be splinted. X-rays of such fractures and their definitive therapy should wait, however, until more important head and internal injuries are ruled out and the patient's condition stabilizes.

Shock

BLOOD LOSS.   The pregnant trauma victim may have hypotension and shock from several mechanisms. At times it is difficult to tell which of these might be the major cause, and not infrequently several factors combine to produce shock. In most severe injuries, hypovolemic shock will predominate, and the immediate administration of lactated Ringer's solution followed as soon as possible by type-specific and (later) cross-matched blood is the most appropriate treatment. Regardless of the apparent origin of shock, however, a large bore intravenous line needs to be established. Since blood volume is increased during pregnancy, blood replacement should be more generous than usual. By the end of the first trimester, blood volume has risen 15 to 30 per cent above the normal nonpregnant level, and rises slowly from there to term (Chapter 2). Blood replacement should thus achieve a final blood volume at least 25 per cent above the calculated norm for a woman of the patient's height and nonpregnant weight. Healthy young women, particularly when pregnant, often do not develop clinically recognizable signs and symptoms of blood loss until it is almost too late to treat it. As much as 30 to 35 per cent of total blood volume can be lost in the pregnant victim before tachycardia, hypotension, pallor, weak pulse — the generally recognized signs of shock — become clinically apparent (Romney et al., 1963).

NEUROGENIC SHOCK.   If the shock-like state is clearly neurogenic and there is no evidence of internal bleeding, and particularly if volume replacement has not elevated the blood pressure to an acceptable level, vasopressors may be helpful. But the uterine artery and its branches are unusually sensitive to vasoconstrictors during pregnancy (Greiss, 1963). Because of this, the 15 to 20 per cent of cardiac output devoted to uteroplacental blood flow is immediately available for more vital maternal functions during times of stress. In hemorrhagic or neurogenic shock, epinephrine levels are immediately increased in the blood; blood flow is directed away from the uterus to the mother's heart and brain. Nature has recognized that the fetus is a parasite, and attempts to preserve fetal life at the expense of the mother result in death of both, whereas if the mother's life were salvaged, the mother could live on to reproduce again. While the fetus represents a very successful parasite under ordinary circumstances, under conditions of competition between mother and fetus in life-threatening situations, the mother usually wins. With maternal hypotension, therefore, volume replacement offers maternal as well as fetal relief, while the combination of vasoconstrictors and hypotension may so reduce uteroplacental blood flow that the fetus may die unnecessarily.

If vasopressors must be used when volume replacement fails, it is best to choose ephedrine, given in doses of 12.5 to 25 mg intravenously. Ephedrine appears to be the vasopressor of choice during pregnancy because it has very little alpha adrenergic stimulation; its effect lies mainly in increasing cardiac output and not in vasoconstriction. This drug has been used successfully to treat the "neurogenic" variety of shock from spinal anesthesia during pregnancy with little apparent effect on fetal well-being. The same cannot be said of the more potent alpha adrenergic stimulating drugs, such as Neosynephrine (phenylephrine), Vasoxyl (methoxamine), or Levophed (levarterenol).

SEPTIC SHOCK.   Septic shock is more common during and following termination of pregnancy, presumably because bacterial contamination of the urinary tract and uterus is more likely during pregnancy and the puerperium than any other time. Consequently, fecally contaminated wounds and post-abortal trauma victims should be treated expectantly for septic shock with central venous pressure monitoring and massive antibiotic therapy. Should septic shock develop, Isuprel (isoproterenol) still seems to offer the best pharmacologic support, even when the victim is pregnant.

SUPINE HYPOTENSIVE SYNDROME (see also Chapter 2).   Approximately 10 per cent of women in the latter half of pregnancy will demonstrate hypotension when lying supine (Howard et al., 1953). This "supine hypotensive syndrome" is caused by uterine compression of the vena cava in the supine position. If the position of the patient is not changed within a few minutes, cardiac output will decline and hypotension may occur. While clinically apparent hypotension is not seen in every pregnant woman in the supine position, vena caval compression to a greater or lesser degree will occur in each. Such compression can only contribute to the unstable state of the injured trauma victim. Thus, pregnant accident victims should be transported in the lateral position, preferably lying on their left side — from the initial aid at the scene through the emergency room, in the x-ray department, to and from the operating suite, and finally in their rooms. Even during surgery, the pregnant patient should have a wedge-shaped bolster under the right hip and flank so that the uterus will not compress the vena cava as much as if she were lying flat on her back. Recovery room and ward nurses should be instructed to keep the patient lying on her side.

Internal Abdominal Injuries: Diagnosis

The diagnosis of closed abdominal injury is more difficult to establish in late pregnancy than earlier. Absent bowel sounds, rebound tenderness, and leukocytosis are the signs of closed abdominal injury, which is often accompanied by internal hemorrhage. When these signs are accompanied by hypotension, tachycardia, and a falling hematocrit, a search for internal bleeding must be made promptly. Four quadrant needle aspiration not only is nonproductive during pregnancy but is contraindicated in the presence of the enlarged uterus. Culdocentesis, on the other hand, is clearly superior to the abdominal approach during pregnancy. The finding of nonclotting blood in the cul de sac is a clear indication of internal hemorrhage and requires immediate surgical exploration regardless of fetal status or the presence of fractures or other less important injuries. Most authorities also agree that should blood be found on nasogastric suction in quantities large enough to suggest intragastric hemorrhage, abdominal exploration must be carried out.

Farrell (1959) classified closed abdominal injuries as causing (1) hemorrhage, (2) peritonitis, or (3) disruption of the abdominal wall, mesentery or diaphragm, without hemorrhage or peritonitis. Virtually all patients with closed abdominal injuries will show some degree of shock and abdominal pain, unless they have head injuries or have been given narcotics to mask such symptoms. The intoxicated victim may also have her pain threshold obtunded by elevated blood alcohol concentrations. Physical findings of blunt abdominal injury include abdominal rigidity, absent bowel sounds, rebound tenderness, dullness to percussion in the flanks (indicative of fluid accumulation), and frequently what appear to be minor contusions to the anterior abdominal wall giving indications of the direction from which the injury occurred. Pain referred to the shoulder may be mistaken for orthopedic injury to that region. Referred pain to the shoulder may indicate intra-abdominal blood, air, or bowel fluid under the diaphragm. Painful shoulders, particularly when exaggerated by deep breathing, should be considered an indication of intraperitoneal injury.

Laboratory Studies

Laboratory studies may be of help in diagnosing intra-abdominal injuries, but usually these are helpful only when repeated over a period of several hours. Leukocytosis is a common concomitant of concealed hemorrhage, as is a falling hemoglobin or hematocrit. Liver function tests are not of much value in the diagnosis of an acutely injured liver. X-rays are often taken in trauma victims and may occasionally be diagnostic of an otherwise unsuspected, ruptured abdominal viscus, when free air appears under the diaphragm. In those rare cases of ruptured hemidiaphragm, the appearance of bowel loops in the chest is also diagnostic. Obliteration of the psoas muscle shadow is indicative of fluid in the extraperitoneal space. Displacement of the stomach either upwards or downwards indicates the presence of intra-abdominal injury, usually that related to an upper abdominal hemorrhage.

The increased vascularity of the pelvic region and increased blood volume and cardiac output make retroperitoneal as well as intraperitoneal hemorrhage a very real threat during pregnancy. Retroperitoneal hemorrhage may involve the pancreas as well as the uterine parametria, and serum amylase determinations should be made during the recovery period of seriously injured trauma victims to rule out pancreatic injury.

Management

Although the welfare of two people must be considered when the accident victim is pregnant, for the most part the interests of the fetus coincide with those of the mother. The mother's vital signs are to be maintained or corrected, which gives the fetus a better chance of surviving as well. At operation, however, the well-being of the fetus may have to be compromised by surgical necessity. The uterus may have to be emptied in order to control bleeding and repair retroperitoneal lacerations or bowel injury. Indeed, the uterus may have to be removed if it is lacerated or avulsed. In the latter instance, however, the fetus is invariably dead. Bowel and other injuries should be repaired whenever possible without violating the pregnant uterus. If one suspects that the patient is in labor, vaginal delivery, even within a few hours of laparotomy, is entirely feasible. Cesarean section, even if the fetus is known to be dead prior to emergency laparotomy, would not offer any particular advantage to either the mother or the fetus, and would require the mother to have another cesarean section should she again become pregnant.

PELVIC FRACTURES.   The management of fractures in pregnancy is covered in Chapter 8. Pelvic fractures will be discussed here because they are commonly seen and often cause hemorrhage and disability in pregnant automotive crash victims. Bleeding from pelvic fractures is generally concealed in the retroperitoneal space, but when the fracture involves the bladder and urethra, blood may be present in the urine. If a catheter cannot be passed into the bladder, it is usually because there has been disruption of the continuity of the urethra. Surgical reconstitution will be necessary along with suprapubic bladder drainage.

Displaced pelvic fractures are fairly obvious in the trauma room. The impression of pelvic fracture can be corroborated by grating crepitation when the pelvis is moved by the examiner's hands. This should not be done any more than is absolutely required for the diagnosis, however, because the retroperitoneal hemorrhage from pelvic fractures will be increased by movement at the fracture site. Fracture of the pelvis, even when displaced, does not ordinarily interfere with vaginal delivery. When healing takes place, the displaced fracture may have a large callus and the distortion of the pelvis may obstruct labor progress, but this occurs in fewer than 10 per cent of cases (Eastman, 1958). Certainly in premature labor there is no need to perform a cesarean section when there is only a minor degree of dislocation. Dyer and Barclay (1962) observed that labor and vaginal delivery through a fractured pelvis are well tolerated.

ANESTHESIA.   Anesthesia techniques should not vary when the trauma victim happens to be pregnant. The aims of anesthesia in such victims are to achieve the maximum amount of oxygenation along with maximum cardiovascular support; therefore, major conduction anesthetics that contribute to hypotension are contraindicated, whether or not the trauma victim is pregnant. Cyclopropane is well tolerated by pregnant victims and has the advantage of high oxygenation with a minimum of uterine relaxation. Halothane and other chlorinated hydrocarbons have the disadvantage of causing uterine relaxation, which may contribute to hemorrhage, should the uterus be lacerated or emptied by cesarean section. On the other hand, this effect may be an advantage when the trauma victim is undergoing surgery and has uterine contractions of premature labor. The halogenated hydrocarbons may prevent labor from becoming progressive, at least during the time of the operation, and may be beneficial in preventing labor following the operation.

ABRUPTIO PLACENTAE.   Abruptio placentae is a common concomitant of serious injury in automobile collisions. In Crosby and Costiloe's study (1971), 4 per cent of seriously injured trauma victims sustained a clinically apparent placental separation. Aside from death of the mother, premature separation of the placenta was the most common cause of fetal death. The pregnant trauma victim should be observed for uterine tetany, uterine tenderness, and vaginal bleeding — the clinical manifestations of abruptio placentae. Near term, an immediate cesarean section may salvage the fetus, whereas if the placental separation is ignored and injuries of lesser importance are treated, the fetus may die unnecessarily and the mother's condition be complicated by the hypotension and shock that accompanies severe abruptio placentae. Furthermore, the more severe grades of placental separation may be accompanied by depletion of serum fibrinogen, and the resultant hemorrhagic state may be overlooked while trying to treat other injuries. When an injured patient in the third trimester of pregnancy has vaginal bleeding, repeated clot observation tests or, preferably, serum fibrinogen levels should be obtained periodically during the course of management. It should go without saying that all trauma victims have a potential for hemorrhage. Thus, the treatment for hypofibrinogenemia should be fibrinogen replacement.

URINARY INJURIES. Blunt abdominal trauma can lead to perirenal hemorrhage due to avulsion or laceration of the kidney. Accident victims with otherwise unexplained flank pain, particularly when there is blood in the urine, should have intravenous pyelography, which may help establish the integrity of the renal collecting system and that of the ureters and bladder. However, one author states that 20 per cent of patients who ultimately prove to have renal injuries have normal urinalysis findings on admission (Peters, 1968). Repeated urinalysis is more likely to produce abnormal results if the kidney is injured. Renal injury is often masked, and because of this fact, when the surgeon is exploring the abdomen of the trauma victim he should make certain that the kidneys are both intact and uninjured. During the stabilization period in severely injured patients with suspected intra-abdominal injuries, intravenous pyelography should be accomplished when other x-rays are being taken (Peters, 1968). The ureter is rarely involved with survivable automobile injuries, particularly in pregnant women; but the bladder and urethra may be severely damaged by pelvic fracture. As noted earlier, passage of a bladder catheter should be accomplished in all seriously injured trauma victims; the inability to pass the catheter indicates disruption of the urethra and base of the bladder.

Assessment of Fetal Status

The fetus is frequently ignored during the immediate management of the mother's injuries. This is appropriate when life-saving measures are being taken, because the fetus's life is totally dependent upon the integrity of the mother's vital functions. However, in less severe injuries, in which the mother's vital organs continue to function reasonably well, and particularly when the fetus is large enough to survive outside the mother, fetal monitoring should be accomplished so that the fetus will not die unnecessarily from an unrecognized and unlooked for complication. Premature separation of the placenta, premature rupture of the membranes and uterine rupture all can occur and compromise the fetus without having been apparent to the emergency room physician. In the less severely injured pregnant victim or in the stabilization phase of the severely injured victim in which the acute resuscitative measures have been successful, fetal monitoring should be begun with a standard fetal monitor, which may be borrowed from the obstetrical unit. Figure 6–2 depicts a typical fetal monitor record from a fetus in distress.

Occasionally, it may become necessary to assess the maturity of the fetus in order to determine future care. An example of such a situation might be a seriously injured mother whose condition is now stable, but whose intracranial

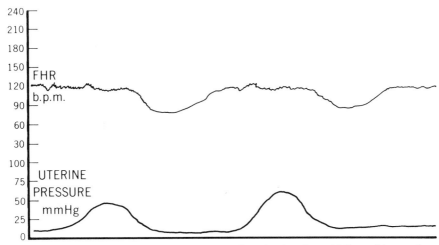

Figure 6-2 Fetal monitor tracing showing severe late deceleration with loss of beat-to-beat variability, indicative of severe fetal distress.

or chest injuries are so serious that she is not expected to live. The physician must then decide whether to perform a cesarean section on the dying or dead mother (Chapter 12).

PREVENTION OF AUTOMOTIVE INJURIES

Restraint Systems

The increases in automobile usage have been accompanied by an increased toll of injuries and deaths. The public for the most part has considered this an unavoidable concomitant of driving: since the numbers were fairly small, there was little interest in trying to reduce the toll. Automobile crash research began with racing drivers and among the first restraint systems designed for use to reduce crash injury were the lap belts Barney Oldfield installed in his racing car in 1922 (Snyder, 1968). As the road toll approached 50 thousand deaths per year in the 1950's, various private and governmental agencies began to develop programs for crash injury research. The initial studies identified the most lethal factors in crash injury deaths. Ejection through doors and windshields prompted design changes that have been effective as has been the collapsible steering column, but restraint systems still offer the most promise of reducing death and injury from automotive collisions. Snyder, one of the more prolific writers on crash injury research, states that "It is possible that no single device has contributed as effectively to the protection and survival of vehicle occupants involved in crash impacts as has the occupant restraint system" (Snyder, 1968). Several studies have compared the injury and death rates from automobile impacts for belted and nonbelted victims (Tourin and Garrett, 1960; Huelke and Gikas, 1968; Crosby and Costiloe, 1971; Van Kampen and Edelman, 1975). In every report the lap belt has been found to be effective in reducing injuries. It is also true that the lap belt may focus decelerative force on those parts of the body that are being restrained.

Seat Belt Injuries

The change in injury pattern brought about by using restraint systems has been called seat belt injury. While this term seems to imply that the seat belt somehow caused the injury, in most situations the impact involved would have proved more serious without the belt. Huelke and Gikas (1968) showed that upper torso restraint, by preventing jackknifing of the body over the lap belt, would have provided more protection than the lap belt alone. However, the major decrease in death rate was attributable to the lap belt alone, and only a few more victims would have been salvaged by the addition of a diagonal belt. Indeed, in one recent study of nonpregnant occupants, the lap belt was found to be as effective as three point restraint (Van Kampen and Edelman, 1975). A major study from Sweden, however, points out the exceptional injury prevention effectiveness of modern automobile engineering in conjunction with the three point restraint system. In this study, Bohlin (1967) reported on 28,780 automobile collisions involving 42,813 occupants, a study of exceptional size. He believes the data to be unusually complete, because the manufacturer of the automobile guaranteed every car for accident repair costs in excess of $80. Each owner was required to fill out an extensive questionnaire in order to have his car repaired. Most of the cars had three point restraint systems installed, but only about 25 per cent of drivers and 30 per cent of front seat passengers used them. Bohlin showed that not only were the belted victims injured both less often and less severely, but not one properly restrained victim with a three point harness was killed in an impact of under 60 mph! In comparison, unrestrained victims were killed in collisions occurring over the entire range of velocities, including one at 12 mph.

Seat Belt Usage in Pregnancy

However, should the pregnant traveler use a restraint system? Should she run the risk of focusing impact forces on the abdomen and pelvis? Would the fetus be killed in a low velocity impact when the mother was belted when it might have survived if she had not had the belt on? Many pregnant women have intuitively felt that the lap belt would cause more harm than good, and some of those few women who were accustomed to fastening their seat belts would avoid doing so if they became pregnant. Their fear was that in a collision, the presence of the lap belt would increase fetal loss more than it would reduce maternal injury; none of the women wanted to sacrifice her baby to save herself. This attitude was reinforced by isolated case reports of "seat belt injuries" to pregnant victims (Theurer and Kaiser, 1963; Rubovitz, 1964). Anecdotal reports such as these, however, do not give a realistic picture of the actual incidence of such injuries, and cannot provide usable data on which to make recommendations for lap belt use by pregnant travelers. Crosby and Costiloe's prospective studies (1971) of pregnant victims of automobile collisions do provide such data. Their study showed that the leading cause of fetal death was death of the mother. Lap belt restraint, which clearly is effective in reducing fatal injuries, is also effective in reducing death of both the fetus and the mother. Pepperell and co-workers (1977) reported a series of 27 pregnant women injured in automobile accidents. Five mothers died; none wore seat belts. The three point belt appears to increase the likelihood of fetal injury, but it prevented maternal deaths. Careful analysis of Crosby and Costiloe's study (1971) did show some possible detrimental effects of lap belt restraint alone. The incidence of fetal death among belted survivors of severe collisions was somewhat higher than among unbelted survivors. While this difference was not statistically significant, it does show that the benefits of lap belt restraint are not realized as much by the fetus as they are by the mother. This effect is probably due to the forward flexion of the mother's body over the lap belt in most impact situations. Prevention of forward flexion would thus be expected to reduce fetal loss. Experimental studies performed on pregnant baboons clearly showed this assumption to be true.

In this study, pregnant baboons were impacted at 20 G in an impact configuration that previously had resulted in a 50 per cent death rate for fetuses whose mothers were restrained by a lap belt alone (Crosby, 1968). Lap belt or three point restraint was chosen randomly. With the lap belts alone, five of 10 fetuses succumbed, while only one of 12 fetuses whose mothers were restrained by three point system lost its life. The difference in fetal death rate is statistically significant; apart from bruises, none of the mothers were injured with either type of restraint (Crosby et al., 1972). Prevention of forward flexion is thus helpful in preventing both maternal and fetal injuries.

Since three point restraint systems have become mandatory in United States cars, such restraint is available for nearly everyone. To purposefully avoid such effective restraint is folly; traveling unrestrained in an automobile or an aircraft invites personal disaster. Why fewer than 30 per cent of vehicle occupants avail themselves of such superb protection is difficult to explain. Restraint system usage has not changed appreciably over the past decade, despite several federally mandated devices installed in cars. Warning lights and buzzers were looked upon as a nuisance. The interlock system, which prevented ignition unless the restraint system was buckled in place, was rejected so violently by the public that Congress overrode the regulation that required them. Those concerned with automotive safety have apparently decided it is impossible to change the habits and personalities of the traveling (and voting!) public, and have begun to focus their attention on alternative methods of increasing occupant protection.

As a result of what has been called "the Australian experience" in automotive safety circles, occupant restraint has become nearly universal on that continent. This was brought about by a series of state laws which prescribed a modest fine if an occupant of a moving vehicle were observed without the restraint system in use. According to Australian authorities, the laws were objected to at first, but the public soon adjusted to them. Increased auto safety became an accepted goal. Almost daily newspaper reminders of the decrease in auto fatalities helped reinforce acceptance. Now, apparently only the most "devil may care" adventurers avoid using restraint systems. Whether or not such an approach would be accepted in the United States is another question. Public reaction to the interlock system would seem to militate against such a law's ever being passed. But it is also possible that the public was reacting more against the incessant nagging of their cars than the restraint system itself. If that impression is even partly true, it may be that a fine for nonuse of restraint systems might have a beneficial effect; the "nagging" would be less frequent and less irritating and the fine would result from ignoring the dictates of the law rather than those of the car. Except for voter reaction, the cost of such a law would be infinitely smaller than the cost of the interlock system or the more advanced "passive" restraint systems now in development under mandates from the U.S. Department of Transportation.

Airbags

Of the various forms of passive restraint systems, the airbag seems to offer the most promise; it is the most tested device and has had the greatest amount of federal support. The airbag system does not require any participation by the occupant of the car. Essentially, airbags are inflatable plastic pillows installed in the dashboard and the steering wheel that inflate extremely rapidly on impact. The occupants of the car, as they are propelled forward, impact against the inflating airbag instead of against the dashboard or the steering wheel. In order to avoid the harmful effect of multiple impacts, rebounding back and forth between the bag and the seat, airbags are vented so that they deflate as the occupant impacts against them. The effect is one of cushioning rather than bouncing, much as would occur in falling against a large downfilled pillow.

The airbag passive restraint system has been tested in both experimental and "real world" situations. We have subjected pregnant and nonpregnant baboons to experimental impacts using the airbag system. We felt that they inflated properly and on time (if they had not the baboon would have suffered severe injuries). There is little question that a baboon, restrained actively by a lap belt and passively at impact by an airbag, can withstand forces considerably greater than those tolerated with lap belt restraint alone. A 50 G forward impact was tolerated by one nonpregnant baboon with nothing more than momentary dazing (Snyder, 1970). Such observations are directly applicable to human impact situations in head-on collisions, and there is little doubt that under similar impact situations with lap belt and airbag restraints, humans also would enjoy a reduction in fatal injuries. Insurance companies, impressed by the injury reduction potential of such systems, have supported installation of airbag systems in American automobiles. They are urging the federal government to make the airbag system mandatory, so that the public will have to pay for its own protection. This of course would benefit the insurance companies as well as the public, provided that the airbag system lives up to its claim.

Several fleets of cars have been equipped with airbags, and they have been made commercially available in some cars. In general, the bags did not inflate inadvertently and did work under conditions in which they were designed to work. However, these facts do not satisfactorily answer all of the objections to the mandatory requirement of installing the system in all production model cars. In lateral impacts for instance, the bags will not protect against occupant impacts against the doors or pillars along the side of the car, unless the cars are equipped with airbags installed in the doors as well; door airbags are planned as a part of the system at present. Rear seat passengers are also being ignored by present airbag planners. No airbag system as yet has been tested over a large enough segment of the population or a long enough period of time to know how well it will work 5 to 10 years after its installation. Bags inflating due to equipment failure rather than impact could increase crash injuries by causing inadvertent loss of control of the car. There is mounting evidence that proper use of the lap belt is also necessary to receive the full benefit of airbag deployment (Snyder, 1968). Without the lap belt, occupants tend to "submarine" below the inflated bag. Since only 20 to 30 per cent of occupants bother to use any restraint system now, it is difficult to see how the use of airbags will improve matters much, unless occupant seating is remodeled in such a way that the position in the car seat accomplishes the same effect as fastening the lap belt now does for passengers seated on the typical "bench seat" found in most United States cars. Bucket seats, particularly if they are more deeply cushioned and wrap around the sides of the occupants, might accomplish such an effect (Snyder, 1968). Other objections to the airbag system involve the high cost (several hundred dollars if installed in production models), or (unproved) charges that their deployment might rupture ear drums. Department of Transportation Secretary William T. Coleman in 1976 effected a compromise between these factions by holding off instituting regulations requiring airbag installation in all production model cars, and at the same time authorizing continuation of field testing of the system.

What the future of this or other passive restraint systems will be is unclear. What is evident, however, is that the public will have to make one of three choices: using no restraint and thus having no protection; using restraint systems that require a positive action on the part of the vehicle occupant to become operational; or using restraint systems that require no active role on the part of the occupant. Whether the public will leave the choice to individuals or will ask their governments to settle the issue for them remains to be seen. Whatever choice is made will affect pregnant as well as nonpregnant travelers.

APPENDIX

BIOMECHANICS OF AUTOMOTIVE INJURY

Kinetics

All moving bodies have kinetic energy which must be dissipated before they can come to a stop. In the moving automobile, kinetic energy is imparted by the engine and dissipated by the friction of the tires on the road and the brake linings on the brake drum. The occupants are slowed along with the car because of their friction against the seats. The energy involved is arithmetically related to the mass of the vehicle and its occupants, but is geometrically related to their velocity and the stopping time. The formulas dictating these features are as follows:

1. The kinetic energy of a moving body equals mass times acceleration ($e = mA$).

2. Deceleration is equal to the square of the velocity divided by twice the stopping distance ($A = \dfrac{V^2}{2S}$).

3. Stopping distance is equal to half the rate of decleration times the square of the time ($S = \frac{1}{2} AT^2$).

4. At the earth's surface, gravity causes an acceleration of 32 feet per second in a freely falling body. Thus, a 1 G force may be defined as that force which will produce a similar acceleration or deceleration in a freely moving body (Schilling, 1968).

These formulas for mass and velocity also apply to the occupant of the vehicle. If the occupant becomes decelerated uniformly and slowly enough, nothing happens: by bracing his feet and hands, the occupant is able to keep from hitting the interior of the car and thus avoid injury. But at higher rates of deceleration, bracing oneself becomes totally ineffective. For instance, a "30 G" stop means that the body undergoing deceleration is subjected to forces equaling 30 times that of gravity. Thus a 200 pound man would in effect weigh 6000 pounds during deceleration, and no one can control such a weight by bracing himself. Using the above formulas, a car going 60 mph at the moment of impact into a solid bridge abutment can be expected to decelerate in a distance of, let us say, 4 feet. Under these circumstances the force of deceleration on the occupants of the car is 30 G. Thus, the bodies of the occupants, each weighing about 3 tons, will continue forward and impact against parts of the car.

Tolerance Limits

The force formula is even more devastating when one considers parts of the body impacting against relatively unyielding parts of the car. In the case of the head of the occupant traveling at 60 mph hitting the A pillar supporting the windshield and the roof, the distance over which it comes to a stop is about 1 inch. The forces applied to the head would be 300 G! One inch stopping distance is approximately the "crumpling distance of the skull" (Schilling, 1968). Tolerance of the human body to the force of acceleration or deceleration is dependent upon many variables. The amount of force is obviously important, but the time over which it is applied to the body is equally, if not more, important. The initial studies of whole body tolerance to deceleration were begun by deHaven and carried on by Snyder and others (deHaven, 1942; Synder, 1963).

The relationship between time and decelerative force is depicted in Figure 6–3. It can be seen that fairly low decelerative force (5 to 10 G) can cause disability if applied to the body over a full second. The harmful effect is largely due to the hydraulic effect of blood. Applying the force of deceleration to the blood in the vascular system will overcome the normal blood pressure and force the blood in the direction of deceleration. If applied over 0.3 second or less, blood has little time to flow over much distance; normal flow is resumed when the force stops. If the force is applied for 0.4 to 0.9 second, however, blood may flow for a considerable distance away from organs that need it most, principally the heart and brain. Under these conditions the

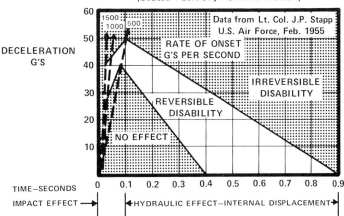

Figure 6-3 Relationship of decelerative force and time of impact with injury produced. (From Kulowski J: Crash Injuries, 1960. Courtesy of Charles C Thomas, Publisher, Springfield, Illinois.)

usual reaction is syncope. Over a longer period of time, the hydraulic effect of blood itself may rupture blood vessels and cause irreversible damage from hemorrhage into tissues. While there are marked individual differences between persons due to age, sex, and physical conditions (Snyder, 1970), maximum human tolerance to decelerative force is about 50 G over a stopping time interval of 0.2 second. Figure 6–3 was derived from experiments performed by Stapp and are confined to a well restrained subject facing forward. The limits to tolerance described would only apply to adequately restrained occupants of automobiles in head-on collisions. The body can apparently tolerate considerably greater G forces applied in the backward facing positions under similar experimental conditions. Stapp estimated that with adequate restraint and cushioning of the seat back the human can tolerate a 90 G stop facing backward, with 200 G being required to inflict fatal injury (Kulowski, 1960). More remarkable tolerance to impact has been described by Snyder, and his studies point out the importance of the length of time over which the deceleration occurs. He studied suicides, homicides, and accident victims that had fallen from heights, impacting on concrete and other incompressible surfaces. He showed that if the impact was sufficiently abrupt, humans could survive very high G forces. At decelerations that lasted less than 0.0006 second, these study subjects had survived impact velocities of up to 116 ft/sec (79 mph)! Under these conditions, calculation of G forces actually becomes meaningless. Such extremely abrupt impacts are not seen in automotive collisions, but Snyder's study does point out that the human body can tolerate extreme impact forces if they are applied over an extremely short period of time (Snyder, 1963). The results in Figure 6–2 apply to the whole body, however, and rest on the assumption that it is decelerated evenly.

Injury then is due mostly to organ displacement and hemorrhage. Individual organs and tissues have widely varying tolerances to impact, and, since function of some organs is more important than function of others, the effect of a given impact will depend largely upon the organs injured rather than the G forces applied to the entire body. It is here that the vagaries and inconsistencies of crash injuries arise: some unfortunate victims die from what appears to be a relatively minor collision, but in which large forces came to bear on susceptible and vital organs. An example would be a relatively low velocity collision in which the driver's aorta was ruptured by the lower part of the steering wheel. Conversely, an occupant lying down asleep in the back seat might survive without a scratch a rear-end collision that completely demolishes the car. Tolerances of individual organs and structures are difficult to derive because the protection of each varies with its position in the body. The liver, kidneys, and spleen are friable and poorly supported, but are surrounded by the ribcage anteriorly and laterally and the back muscles and vertebrae posteriorly. As a result, these organs are usually damaged only in severe collisions. Similarly, the heart, lungs and great vessels are usually left intact unless the collision is severe enough to crush the chest. Because the majority of collisions involve forward moving cars, there is continued forward motion of the body after impact. The head most frequently impacts against something in the car. In one study, 81 per cent of injured victims sustained head injuries. Arms and legs are free to rotate as they will, and are injured in nearly as many victims (78 per cent). The injuries received in automobile collisions involve the chest in 25 per cent and the pelvic and abdominal contents in 12 per cent (Modern Medicine, 1968). Another study of fatal collisions showed that being ejected from the vehicle was the leading cause of death, and again, the immediate cause of death was head injury (Huelke and Gikas, 1968). This study involved 139 automobile collisions in which 177 occupants died. After ejection, the most frequent instruments that caused death included (in this order) the front door, steering assembly, instrument panel, rear door, roof header, and A pillar, with the windshield ranking at the bottom of the list. The authors estimated that 38 of the 48 ejected victims would have survived the collision had they been restrained by a lap belt alone, and three others would have survived if they had used the three point system now available (Huelke and Gikas, 1968).

REFERENCES

American College of Surgeons, Committee on Trauma: Early Care of the Injured Patient. 2nd ed. Philadelphia, WB Saunders 1976.
Barno A, Freeman DW, and Baker MP, Jr: Minnesota mortality study. Minn Med 45:847, 947, 1962.
Bohlin NI: A statistical analysis of 28,000 accident cases with emphasis on occupant restraint value. Proceeding 11th Stapp Car Crash Conference, October, 1967.
Buchsbaum HJ: Splenic rupture in pregnancy. Obstet Gynecol Surv 22:381, 1967.
Buchsbaum HJ: Accidental injury complicating pregnancy. Am J Obstet Gynecol 102:752, 1968.
Crosby WM, Synder RG, Snow CC, et al: Impact injuries in pregnancy. I. Experimental studies. Am J Obstet Gynecol 101:108, 1968.
Crosby WM, Costiloe JP: Safety of lap belt restraint for pregnant victims of automobile collisions. N Engl J Med 284:632, 1971.
Crosby WM, King AI, Stout CC: Fetal survival following impact: improvement with shoulder harness restraint. Am J Obstet Gynecol 112:1101, 1972.
Crosby WM: Trauma during pregnancy: maternal and fetal injury. Obstet Gynecol Surv 29:683, 1974.

deHaven H: Mechanical analysis of survival in falls from heights of fifty to one-hundred and fifty feet. War Med 2:586, 1942.

Delaney, JJ: Obstetrical and gynecological injuries. *In* Barnes AC, Holzman GB, Rutherford RB, Zuidema GD (eds): The Management of Trauma. 2nd ed. Philadelphia, WB Saunders, 1968.

Dyer I, Barclay DL: Accidental trauma complicating pregnancy and delivery. Am J Obstet Gynecol 83:907, 1962.

Eastman NJ: Editorial comment. Obstet Gynecol Surv 13:69, 1958.

Elliott M: Vehicular accidents and pregnancy. Aust NZ J Obstet Gynaecol 6:279, 1966.

Farrell JJ: Non-penetrating abdominal trauma. J Fla Med Assoc 43:1104, 1959.

Gomcyekow GE: *In* Baylis SM, et al: Traumatic retroperitoneal hematoma. Am J Surg 103:477, 1962.

Griess FC: The uterine vascular bed: the effect of adrenergic stimulation. Obstet Gynecol 21:295, 1963.

Griswold RA, Collier HS: Blunt abdominal trauma. Int Abstr Surg 112:309, 1961.

Howard BK, Goodson JH, Mengert, WF: Supine hypotensive syndrome in late pregnancy. Obstet Gynecol 1:371, 1953.

Huelke DF, Gikas PW: Causes of deaths in automobile accidents. JAMA 203:1100, 1968.

Jimerson S, Crosby WM: Unpublished data, 1977.

Kulowski, J.: Crash Injuries. Springfield, Ill, Charles C Thomas, 1960.

McCarty V, Risely DR: Traumatic rupture of the uterus in early pregnancy. J Int Coll Surg 26:228, 1956.

McNeil JP Jr: *In* Parkinson EB: Prenatal loss due to external trauma to the uterus. Am J Obstet Gynecol 90:30, 1964.

Modern Medicine: p. 68, Jan 15, 1968.

Nahum AM: Early Management of Acute Trauma. St Louis, CV Mosby, 1966.

Page EW, King EB, Merrill JA: Abruptio placentae: dangers of delay in delivery. Obstet Gynecol 3:385, 1954.

Parkinson EB: Perinatal loss due to external trauma to the uterus. Am J Obstet Gynecol 90:30, 1964.

Pepperell RJ, Rubinstein E, MacIsaac IA: Motor-car accidents during pregnancy. Med J Aust. 1:203, 1977.

Peters PC: Trauma to the genitourinary system. *In* Shires GT: Care of the Trauma Patient. New York, McGraw-Hill, 1968.

Romney SL, Gabel PV, Takada Y: Experimental hemorrhage in late pregnancy. Am J Obstet Gynecol 87:636, 1963.

Rubovitz FE: Traumatic rupture of the pregnant uterus from "seat belt" injury. Am J Obstet Gynecol 90:828, 1964.

Schilling JA: Trauma. Okla State Med Assoc J 61:499, 1968.

Shires GT: Care of the Trauma Patient. New York, McGraw-Hill, 1966.

Snyder RG: Occupant restraint systems of automotive, aircraft, and manned space vehicles. *In* Proceedings of Impact Injury and Crash Protection Bioengineering Symposium. Detroit, Wayne State University Press, 1968.

Snyder RG: Human impact tolerances. International Automobile Safety Conference Compendium. New York, Society for Automobile Engineering, 1970.

Snyder RG: Human tolerance to extreme impacts in true fall. Aerosp Med 34:695, 1963.

Sparkman RS: Rupture of the spleen in pregnancy. Am J Obstet Gynecol 76:587, 1958.

Stapp JP: Human tolerances to severe abrupt deceleration. *In* Gauer OH, Zuidema GD: Gravitational Stress in Aerospace Medicine. Boston, Little, Brown, 1961.

Theurer DE, Kaiser IH: Traumatic fetal death without uterine injury. Obstet Gynecol 21:477, 1963.

Tourin B, Garrett JW: Safety belt effectiveness in rural California automobile accidents. *In* Annual Report to the Commission on Accidental Trauma of the Armed Forces Epidemiological Board. New York, Automotive Crash Injury Research of Cornell University, 1960.

Van Kampen LTB, Edelman A: Lap belts and three-point belt: a comparison of effectiveness. Voorburg. The Netherlands, Institute for Road Safety (SWOV), 1975.

Chapter 7

THERMAL BURNS

James W. Taylor

Definition of Terms and an Overview
of Therapy of the Major Burn Injury

Since the care of major thermal injuries is usually the province of general surgeons or plastic surgeons, the initial portion of this chapter will deal with the definition of terms and will briefly describe the clinical presentation and management of the patient with a major thermal injury.

A burn wound results when a person's skin is exposed to an excessive amount of thermal energy. How deeply the skin is burned is determined by two factors: the temperature of the heat source and the duration of the exposure. Therefore, a scald produced by boiling water at 100° C will be a less severe injury than a burn produced by exposing the skin for exactly the same period of time to hot oil at 200° C. Similarly, a flash burn, which is produced by the instantaneous exposure of the skin to a great amount of heat, is usually a less severe burn than one caused by the ignition of clothing, in which case the flames are held in contact with the skin for prolonged periods of time.

One generally classifies a burn as first degree, second degree, or third degree. A first degree burn is essentially an epidermal injury, which is characterized by erythema and pain. The common sunburn is an example of such an injury. A second degree burn is more significant. Pathologically, the second degree burn is characterized by death and destruction of portions of the epidermis and dermis with the retention of enough viable epidermal elements in the skin so that healing is possible from those elements without the need for skin grafting. A third degree burn is a still deeper injury, in which all the epithelial elements are destroyed or killed. In such a burn, the involved areas must ultimately be grafted with skin taken from another portion of the patient's body. An alternative terminology, which is more descriptive, calls the second degree burn a partial thickness burn and a third degree burn a full-thickness burn.

Certain clinical characteristics allow one to distinguish the second degree burn from the third degree burn. A typical second degree or partial-thickness burn presents clinically as a blistered, moist injury, which is red or mottled in color and is quite painful. The typical third degree or full-thickness injury is characteristically dry, pearly white, or charred, and because all the nerve endings have been destroyed, such a burn is anesthetic. There is also an intermediate type of injury, which is called either a deep second degree burn or a deep dermal burn and which is clinically difficult to distinguish from a third degree burn. With such burns even the best observers find great difficulty in deciding and correctly estimating the depth of the injury. The only absolute method of determining the depth is to wait and observe the healing characteristics of the burn wound.

MORTALITY STATISTICS

In determining the prognosis at the initial time of injury, the depth of the burn injury is much less important a factor than the extent of the injury. The prognosis is statistically related to the total area of second and third degree burns. The vast majority of patients with burns covering less than 30 per cent of their total body surface will survive. Roughly speaking, approximately half of the patients with 50 per cent of their total body surface burned will die, and only an occasional patient with burns of 80 per cent of the total body surface will survive. Statistics from The National Burn Information Exchange indicate that women fare worse than men, and that the extremes of youth or age decrease the chances of survival (Feller et al., 1976). The extent of the burn injury can be estimated using one of several charts available in most emergency rooms, which assign a percentage of the surface area to various portions of the body. Using such a chart, one could easily tell that a burn which involved all of one hand would be equivalent to 2.5 per cent of the total body surface. Without such a chart the less accurate "rule of nines" can furnish a reasonably accurate estimate. The "rule of nines" divides the body into sections covering 9 per cent of the surface area; the head and the arms each make up 9 per cent of the total body surface area; each leg equals 18 per cent; and the anterior and posterior surfaces of the body each equals 18 per cent. The sum of these is 99 per cent, with the remaining 1 per cent being routinely assigned to the perineum.

BURN SHOCK AND RESUSCITATION

Before the days of intravenous fluid therapy, patients with extensive burns usually died in shock during the first 24 to 48 hours. We now understand that a burn injury is accompanied by a generalized change in capillary permeability that leads to a loss of both electrolytes and colloid-containing fluids from the intravascular space into the subcutaneous tissues. If the lost intravascular fluid is not vigorously replaced, the patient will die in shock. Various empirical methods of burn resuscitation have been developed. Most regimens differ primarily in the amount of colloid administered and the timing of administration. All resuscitation formulas prescribe large volumes of sodium-containing fluids, the most popular being Ringer's lactate. At present the most commonly used formula is 4 ml of Ringer's lactate per kilogram of the patient's body weight times the percentage of the body surface which is burned, administered over the first 24 hours. This obviously is a massive amount of fluid. For example, a 70 kg man with a 50 per cent total body surface burn would require 14 liters of Ringer's lactate to be administered during the first 24 hours ($4 \times 70 \times 50 = 14{,}000$ ml). In the actual clinical setting, most resuscitations are carried out by beginning with such a formula and initially administering fluid at the prescribed rate, then altering that rate so as to maintain a urine output between 30 and 50 ml per hour. During the burn resuscitation the urine output will be the most valuable guide to the adequacy of therapy. The central venous pressure measurement is of limited value in detecting the overly vigorous resuscitation. The pulmonary wedge pressure determination has, however, proved to be more reliable as a guide to the status of left ventricular function. It is, there, strongly recommended that a Swan-Ganz catheter be used to follow the pulmonary wedge pressure in cases of complex resuscitation where it is feared that the patient has an impaired cardiovascular status and might not tolerate overly vigorous fluid administration.

COMPLICATIONS OF BURN INJURIES

Respiratory Problems: The respiratory problems in burns can be grouped into three overlapping categories: inhalation injuries, carbon monoxide poisoning, and pneumonia. At the time of the initial injury the patient may inhale fire, smoke, and various products of combustion. Flame and heat can produce oral and upper airway injuries, but dry air cannot conduct adequate amounts of heat to produce significant thermal injuries to the trachea and lungs. Steam can, however, produce such injuries. Smoke and other products of combustion can produce chemical irritation and chemical burns within the lungs. Upper airway burns can easily lead to obstruction, and such burns can readily be diagnosed by inspection and should be treated with an endotracheal tube if there is a threat of upper airway obstruction. A tracheostomy should be avoided initially as the endotracheal tube can frequently be adequate with a temporary obstruction, and a tracheostomy in a burned patient may become a source of sepsis.

A chemical pneumonitis is more difficult to diagnose than an upper airway burn. The patient will usually give a history of sustaining the burn in a closed space. Not infrequently there will be perioral burns with singed nasal hairs, and the patient will usually be coughing up carbonaceous sputum. Diagnosis of such an injury can be confirmed by bronchoscopy or by radioactive xenon lung scans. X-rays are of little value in the early course of such an injury, but should be obtained for their value as a baseline determination. The chest x-ray in a patient with a chemical pneumonitis will usually be free of infiltrates. X-ray changes usually become apparent in such patients within 3 to 5 days after the injury. After the diagnosis of an inhalation injury is made, vigorous supportive therapy is indicated.

The patient may also inhale large amounts of carbon monoxide in certain types of fires. When carbon monoxide becomes bound to hemoglobin, the ability to transport oxygen is severely diminished. There is recent evidence that the effects of carbon monoxide are more marked on fetal hemoglobin than on normal adult hemoglobin, and thus carbon monoxide exposure is potentially a significant hazard to an unborn child (Longo, 1976).

Finally, we shall mention pneumonia as a "catchall." Pneumonia may be a late sequela of inhalation injury, the result of aspiration in a severely injured patient, or a manifestation of sepsis and a generalized impairment of the normal host defenses.

METABOLIC COMPLICATIONS AND CHANGES

It has long been known that a large amount of water is lost through evaporation in the presence of a burn wound. Studies indicate that evaporative water loss occurs in a range of approximately 4000 ml per square meter of burn per day. It is also well known that 576 kilocalories are required to change 1000 ml of water to water vapor. The bulk of this energy must be supplied by the patient and this, of course, accounts for a great portion of the increased metabolic requirement of the burn victim.

In addition to this, Wilmore and associates have shown that a normal response to burn injury is a readjustment of the metabolic rate which appears to be regulated in the hypothalamus and is mediated by an increased output of catecholamines. Thus, the hypermetabolism of burns cannot be eliminated by merely placing the patient in a warm environment, although this can reduce the metabolic rate. Wilmore and co-workers (1974) showed that the increase in metabolic rate is proportional to the extent of the burn injury up to a level of approximately 40 per cent of the total body surface burned. After that point the metabolic rate no longer increases linearly with the burn size, but rather levels off at a metabolic rate of approximately twice the normal rate.

Most investigators believe that this augmented metabolic rate is somehow beneficial to the patient, and that therapeutically attention should be turned to providing the patient with enough calories in the form of both carbohydrates and amino acids so that he or she can maintain his own weight in the face of increased catabolism. If the patient is not supported adequately, the body proteins will be selectively catabolized, and the individual will lose weight steadily. There is a level of weight loss (generally set somewhere around 40 per cent of the body's weight) that is almost invariably associated with a fatal outcome.

COMPLICATIONS RELATED TO ALTERED HOST DEFENSES

The vast majority of patients with burns of less than 30 per cent of the total body surface will survive, and most with burns of greater than 70 per cent of the total body surface will die. Provided that the patient has a good resuscitation and is managed according to modern techniques, most of the deaths in burn cases will occur between the second and fourth week after the injury, and most of these deaths will be related either directly or indirectly to overwhelming sepsis. Sepsis can originate in a multitude of sites. The source can be the wound itself, infected veins that have been cannulated for intravenous infusions, pneumonia, or a variety of less common causes.

One of the basic and necessary steps in the cellular defense of the body is the attraction of leukocytes to targets where they can be beneficial. This property is called chemotaxis. Warden and co-workers (1974) presented evidence that leukocytes from patients with large burns show a significant depression in their ability to respond in vitro to a standard chemotactic agent. This depression, seen during the first 48 hours, was directly correlated with the extent of the patients' burns. Furthermore, significantly depressed leukocyte chemotaxis present more than 48 hours after the burn correlated highly with ultimate mortality. That is, those patients with very poor leukocyte chemotaxis usually died. Some other abnormalities in the patient's leukocyte function have been demonstrated. These include decreased bacterial killing, as was shown by Alexander and Wixson (1970). Thus, at least one of the major problems seen in burns resides in altered and impaired function of the patient's host defenses. Greater research into these abnormalities may ultimately provide us with means of enabling patients with huge burns to survive their injuries.

BASIC BURN WOUND MANAGEMENT

Although we do not know the cause of many of the complications seen in burned victims, we have observed that the metabolic rate returns to normal and other complications become less serious or disappear when the burn wound heals or is covered with skin grafts. Before this healing or coverage can occur, the eschar or burned skin must be separated from the burn wound. In small burns (that is, those covering less that 15 per cent of the total body surface), this can be done quite successfully by excising the burned skin and applying skin grafts. Periodically enthusiasm is revived for attempts at grafting larger burns, but these have failed routinely except in children who have been covered with skin grafts from another person and who have been enabled to accept this transplanted skin for long periods by the suppression of their immune systems. Such therapy has not yet been successfully carried out in adults and even for children is not routinely available. The best standard care of burn wounds involves controlling the level of bacterial proliferation in the eschar by means of topical antibiotics. These antibiotics include silver sulfadiazine, mefenide acetate, povidone-iodine, gentamicin, and silver nitrate. Regardless of what topical antibiotic one uses, the burned eschar will ultimately separate. When it becomes loose, it is debrided so as to prevent any pockets of infection from developing beneath it. This is done in periodic stages in the operating room or in smaller daily stages on the ward or in the whirlpool tank. The care of burn patients is greatly aided if the physician can depend on hydrotherapy and the support of an active physiotherapy department.

When it happens that some of the burn wound has separated and become ready for grafting but significant areas are not yet ready, homografts (that is, split-thickness skin taken from a cadaver) or xenografts (split-thickness skin taken from another species, such as a pig) can be applied to the burn wound. These biological dressings will adhere to the areas that are ready for grafting and will reduce the quantitative bacterial count from those areas of the burn wound to which they stick. Such dressings can preserve the burn wound in a satisfactory condition for grafting. The homografts must be changed every four to five days. Otherwise, they will "take" only temporarily and be rejected later, producing another eschar which would require debridement and cleaning.

When ultimately the burn wound is ready for grafting it should be grafted with split-thickness skin, which must be taken from the patient himself. Numerous methods for grafting exist; many produce comparable results and some have been devised to deal with specific problems in grafting. The scope of this chapter does not permit a detailed description of these methods.

REVIEW OF REPORTED SERIES OF BURNS DURING PREGNANCY

Despite the fact that the records of most major burn units contain cases of pregnant women with major thermal injuries, the literature on this subject is extremely limited. Mulla (1958) reported a case in which a patient with a 50 per cent total body surface burn at approximately seven and a half months' gestation spontaneously began labor three days after the injury. The infant survived, despite the fact that the mother later died. Schmitz (1971) reported six pregnant patients with burns. His series appeared to indicate that pregnant women with burns in excess of 35 per cent of their total body surface are in jeopardy of premature labor soon after their injury. Ten to 15 per cent burns did not predispose to premature labor. Tica and colleagues (1969) reported a single case of abortion following a 30 per cent burn, and they considered the direct cause to be an increased serotonin concentration in the blood. Merger and associates (1963) reported two cases of burns in pregnancy in which they used "spasmolytics" to prevent premature labor. Stage (1973) reported three cases. In one case, a 36 year old patient with 40 per cent second and third degree burns delivered a macerated fetus three months after her injury. She was not known to have been pregnant. The second case involved a 37 year old with a small burn who delivered at term without complications. The third case was a 21 year old with a 50 per cent burn, described as first and second degree. In that case, since she was at 41 weeks' gestation at the time of injury, labor was initiated with intravenous Pitocin. Both mother and infant did well. Stage further suggested that the single abortion he recorded and the other reported premature initiations of labor seen during the first week after injury might be related to the synthesis of prostaglandin E (PGE) resulting from the burn injury itself. Anggard and Jonsson (1972) reported that a substance, which subsequently was identified as PGE II, was present in the peripheral lymphatics of a scalded dog's paw. Human skin obtained from fresh surgical specimens has also reportedly shown the capability of producing PGE II after scalding.

In contradiction to the above noted reports, Ryan and co-workers (1962) described two pregnant patients with 65 and 75 per cent third degree burns in early pregnancy, who not only delivered live infants at term, but who also had such good healing as to suggest that pregnancy might in some way improve the healing of a mother's burns. Ryan was, however, unable to substantiate this impression in laboratory animal studies. Lastly, Dalla-Villa (1967) reported from Argentina 19 cases of pregnant women with burns. He reported an 80 per cent mortality rate when the burns occurred during the first trimester, but unfortunately the report contained too few details to analyze the cause of these findings. Thus, it can be seen that the previously reported series cannot be interpreted as representative. Most of the reports are extremely brief and give no information about the presence of fluid and electrolyte imbalance, hypoxia, acidosis, or sepsis. None detailed the fluid resuscitation used, and shock in the postburn period was noted in only one case. The paucity of published data on the specific problems of the burned pregnant woman has made it difficult to determine the most effective care for these patients. Therefore, we have reviewed the data collected at the U.S. Army Institute of Surgical Research between 1951 and 1974, which will provide the basis for our discussion in this chapter.

THE U. S. ARMY INSTITUTE OF SURGICAL RESEARCH SERIES OF BURNS DURING PREGNANCY

Between 1951 and 1974, 258 women of reproductive age were admitted to the burn unit of the U.S. Army Institute of Surgical Research. Nineteen were pregnant (Table 7–1). No doubt many of these patients were referred specifically to the Army Burn Center because they were pregnant, and therefore it is probably misleading to assume that the sampling is representative and that the percentage of burned women of reproductive age who are expected to be pregnant is 7 or 8 per cent. All of the burns were caused by flames or explosion; there were no scalds or electrical injuries. Eleven of the 19 patients were burned when flammable liquids or gases ignited, five when household appliances ignited their clothing, two when they were trapped in burning buildings, and one when she was involved in an aircraft accident. Two of the patients burned with flammable liquids were American Indians who had used gasoline as a means of committing suicide; their pregnancies were apparently the reason for the suicide attempts.

The extent of their patients' burns ranged from 6 to 92 per cent of the total body surface (mean 42.5 per cent), with the third degree component ranging from 0 to 83.5 per cent of the total body surface (mean, 22.4 per cent). The patient's ages ranged from 16 to 37 years; three were older than 30 and two were younger than 18. Their parity ranged from 0 to 5; eight were primigravidas. The duration of pregnancy at the time of the burn injury varied from 5 to 36 weeks. Seven patients were in the first trimester, nine in the second, and three in the third. Such a distribution of burns among the trimesters is not surprising, since in the third trimester a woman is often less active and tends to engage in fewer activities that might be considered dangerous. On the other hand, one might expect burns to be somewhat more common during the third trimester, since a woman at this stage might find it harder to escape from a fire or remove burning clothing.

The early treatment included fluid resuscitation, tetanus prophylaxis, pain relief, and escharotomy when indicated. The initial fluid resuscitation usually followed the Brooke formula, but there was variability because fluid administration was initiated in referring hospitals. After its introduction in 1964, mafenide acetate (Sulfamylon) was used as the topical antibiotic of choice. Wound care included frequent, periodic debridement, and in one case a major excision of the burn wound.

Frequent determinations were made of the patient's hematocrit, arterial blood gases and serum electrolytes, and, when indicated clinically, x-ray examinations and blood cultures were also obtained. Serum lipid and prostaglandin studies were not performed on any of these patients. The patient data are summarized in Table 7–1.

The most striking feature of the Institute of Surgical Research study of the 19 burn victims in pregnancy was that the outcome of the pregnancy was primarily determined by the extent of the mother's burn injury and by the ultimate fate of the mother. Seven of the 19 women died; all had burns covering more than 60 per cent of the total body surface. The remaining 11 patients, all of whom had burns over *less than* 60 per cent of the total body surface, survived. In six of the seven lethally burned patients the pregnancies terminated prior to the patients' deaths. One patient aborted at 2 days following the burn injury and another aborted at 36 days after the burn; four of the women delivered living infants weighing 680, 850, 1150, and 2500 gm, respectively, from the sixth to the fourteenth day after they were burned. Only the 2500 gm infant survived. The seventh patient died before the stillborn infant was delivered, and in her case there was clinical evidence of intrauterine death on the fifth postburn day, although the patient herself lived until the tenth postburn day. Of the 12 women who survived, 10 were discharged with their wounds healed and the pregnancies intact. One patient delivered, on the day after injury, a 2295 gm infant who did well. One other patient, a 37 year old primigravida, delivered a stillborn infant weighing 1105 gm, which had an apparent intrapartum uterine demise. This occurred coincidentally with a severe burn wound cellulitis. We would thus gain the impression that maternal survival is usually accompanied by fetal survival and that, if the mother's injury is lethal, the pregnancy will usually terminate spontaneously prior to her death.

BURN COMPLICATIONS THAT MAY CONTRIBUTE TO THE LOSS OF PREGNANCY

In the series of patients from the Army Burn Unit, five categories of burn complications were identified, which were related in time to the termination of pregnancy. It must, of course, be remembered that frequently more than one of these complications coexisted in the same patient, and that in a few patients the burn complications, the pregnancy loss, and the maternal demise followed one another in rapid succession.

Hypotension

The complication that may be most easily remedied is that of hypotension and inadequate cardiac output resulting from a delayed or inadequate early fluid resuscitation. Since the urine output has proven to be the single most useful method of assessing fluid resuscitation in a burned patient, the presence of anuria or oliguria in this series was taken as evidence for an inadequate or delayed early fluid resuscitation. Anuria or oliguria was seen in three patients. One patient, who was oliguric for 24 hours, developed numerous complications and had an intrauterine fetal demise on her fifth postburn day. Another patient was anuric for 14 hours and aborted on her second postburn day. The third

TABLE 7–1 **Patient Data and Outcome for 19 Pregnant Women with Thermal Injuries***

				Extent of Burn			
Patient Number	Age	Gravity/ Parity	Week of Gestation	Total (%)	3° (%)	Cause of Burn	Pregnancy Outcome
1	22	5/3	20	6	0	Apartment fire	Discharged pregnant
2	22	2/1	26	8.5	0	Gas heater explosion	Discharged pregnant
3	30	4/2	19	15	0	Oil stove explosion	Discharged pregnant
4	24	4/3	26	15	10	Clothes ignited by heater	Discharged pregnant
5	37	1/0	29	24.5	8.5	Clothes ignited by heater	Stillborn, 1105 g (intrapartum demise) PBD 4
6	22	1/0	15	26	12	Clothes ignited by heater	Discharged pregnant
7	18	1/0	5	28.5	4.5	Clothes ignited by stove	Discharged pregnant
8	21	3/2	36	29.5	3	Cleaning fluid fire	2295 g infant, delivered PBD 1, survived
9	15	1/0	8	30	28	Kerosene fire (suicide attempt)	Discharged pregnant
10	16	2/1	28	31	10.5	Fire bomb	Discharged pregnant
11	36	6/5	15	39.5	6	Kerosene stove explosion	Discharged pregnant
12	19	1/0	10	43	20	Clothes ignited by heater	Discharged pregnant
13	29	5/4	15	60.5	26.5	Kerosene fire (suicide)	Spontaneous abortion PBD 36
14	18	1/0	35	68	42	Gasoline explosion	2500 g infant, delivered PBD 8, survived
15	20	1/0	25	73	58.5	Aircraft accident	680 g infant, delivered PBD 14, neonatal death
16	37	6/5	26	74.5	24	Church fire	Intrauterine demise PBD 5, undelivered
17	16	1/0	22	86	40	Gas heater explosion	850 g infant, delivered PBD 8, neonatal death
18	26	3/2	16	90	35	Propane tank explosion	Aborted PBD 2
19	27	4/3	25	92	83.5	Gasoline fire	1150 g infant, delivered PBD 6, neonatal death

TABLE 7–1 Patient Data and Outcome for 19 Pregnant Women with Thermal Injuries *Continued*

MATERNAL OUTCOME	COMPLICATIONS PRIOR TO DELIVERY
Discharged PBD 2†	None
Discharged PBD 17	None
Discharged PBD 25	None
Discharged PBD 67	None
Discharged PBD 56	Burn wound cellulitis PBD 3, psychiatric illness.
Discharged PBD 67	None
Discharged PBD 65	*Staphylococcus aureus* septicemia on PBD 6 secondary to suppurative thrombophlebitis of the cephalic vein treated with appropriate antibiotics and vein excision.
Discharged PBD 53	None
Discharged PBD 83	Pleural effusion treated with thoracentesis.
Discharged PBD 48	None
Discharged PBD 76	None
Discharged PBD 104	None
Died PBD 37	*Pseudomonas and Providencia* septicemia PBD 19. Invasive *Pseudomonas* burn wound sepsis in both legs treated by excision of the burn wound on the legs. Bilateral bronchopneumonia. Serum sodium was 123 mEq/L and pO$_2$ was 47 mm Hg on PBD 36. Diabetes detected PBD 14.
Died PBD 57	Dilutional hyponatremia PBD 8, Na was 123 mEq/L.
Died PBD 15	Dilutional hyponatremia PBD 14 (Na, 121 mEq/L). *Staphylococcus* and *Aerobacter* septicemia PBD 7. *Providencia* septicemia PBD 14. Bilateral bronchopneumonia with pO$_2$ of 65 mm Hg on PBD 13. Acute fatty liver of pregnancy; pancreatitis diagnosed at the postmortem. *Providencia* (10^7 organism/gram) in placenta.
Died PBD 10	Pneumothorax secondary to tracheostomy. Bilateral bronchopneumonia; pO$_2$ of 60 mm Hg on PBD 5.
Died PBD 10	Bilateral bronchopneumonia PBD 8. Patient had respiratory arrest 6 hr after birth of infant. Blood cultures grew *Klebsiella, E. coli, Providencia* PBD 8.
Died PBD 8	Anuria for 14 hr after burn injury occurred. Dilutional hyponatremia on PBD 2 (Na 118 mEq/L).
Died PBD 26	Anuria for 12 hr after burn injury occurred. Vaginal bleeding and uterine contractions began on PBD 2 and recurred intermittently until PBD 6.

*From Taylor JW, et al: Obstet Gynecol *47*:434, 1976.
†PBD = postburn day.

patient was anuric for 12 hours and on the second postburn day developed vaginal bleeding and uterine contractions which recurred intermittently until she delivered a 1150 gm infant 6 days following burn injury. Furthermore, we speculate that some of the premature deliveries and abortions noted during the first burn week in studies of Merger and associates (1963), Schmitz (1971), and Stage (1973) may simply reflect the effect of insufficient fluid resuscitation and prolonged hypotension. Animal research has demonstrated the effect of maternal hypotension on the fetus. Romney and co-workers (1963) found that acute blood loss may decrease the uterine blood flow as much as 46.2 per cent, with a resultant drop in fetal tissue pO_2. Boba and associates (1966) routinely induced fetal bradycardia and hypotension by producing graded maternal hemorrhage. Furthermore, Greiss (1966) noted that following acute hemorrhage, which produced no maternal blood pressure alteration, the uterine blood flow can be compromised as much as 10 to 20 per cent. We believe that the hypovolemia and hypotension seen as a result of inadequate burn shock resuscitation might have an effect on uterine blood flow analogous to that seen in hemorrhagic shock. Thus, although a healthy adult may tolerate a delayed or inadequate resuscitation, the resultant hypotension may lead to fetal death or the initiation of labor. For this reason, an even greater than normal vigilance in fluid replacement and resuscitation of the burned pregnant woman is required, in order to insure prompt correction of intravascular deficits and to maintain satisfactory tissue perfusion. This is best monitored by careful attention to the rate of urine output; intravenous fluid should be administered to maintain a urine rate between 30 and 50 ml per hour.

Hypoxia

As we noted earlier, respiratory complications frequently accompany major burn injuries. Respiratory distress and hypoxia were temporally associated with the termination of pregnancy in four patients in the U.S. Army series. When she aborted, one patient had bilateral bronchopneumonia with an arterial pO_2 of 47 mm Hg. Another had bronchopneumonia with an arterial pO_2 of 65 on her thirteenth postburn day. She delivered a 680 gm infant on the fourteenth postburn day and died the next day. A third patient had a large pneumothorax and bronchopneumonia with arterial pO_2 of 60 mm Hg prior to the death of the fetus in utero. The fourth patient had bilateral bronchopneumonia when she delivered an 850 gm infant. Although blood gases were not measured at that time, the patient suffered a respiratory arrest six hours after her infant was born.

Animal studies by Dilts and associates (1969) have demonstrated how hypoxia can increase uterine vascular resistance to a greater extent than it increases systemic resistance. Such a change in the relative vascular resistance results in a proportional drop in the uterine blood flow and decreased fetal tissue oxygenation. In the U.S. Army series several patients simultaneously suffered hypoxia and hypotension; since both hypoxia and hypotension lower the uterine blood flow, the deleterious effect on the fetus is compounded. From a therapeutic point of view, an adequate degree of maternal oxygenation must be maintained. This is particularly true when the patient is being transported by air and when she develops respiratory complications. At those times oxygen must be supplied promptly. In milder instances nasal oxygen may be sufficient. At other times, mechanical respiratory support, including positive end-expiratory pressure (PEEP), will be required. The pregnant patient's oxygenation can often be improved by placing her in a semi-sitting position.

Sepsis

Overwhelming systemic infection and septic shock are frequent terminal events in patients with major burns. In the Army series, septicemia was diagnosed in five patients in a close temporal relationship to the termination of pregnancy. In one patient, *Providencia* and *Pseudomonas* were demonstrated in blood cultures on the nineteenth postburn day. She subsequently developed invasive *Pseudomonas* burn wound sepsis and persisted in a septic course until she aborted on the thirty-sixth day. Another patient had blood cultures showing *Staphylococcus aureus* and *Aerobacter* on her eleventh postburn day and *Providencia* on the fourteenth postburn day. The next day she delivered an immature infant. The placenta was cultured and grew *Providencia stuartii* at 10^7 colonies per gram of tissue. Another patient was hypotensive and clinically septic when the fetus died in utero. Her blood culture subsequently grew *Pseudomonas*. Blood cultures from the fifth patient showed growth of *Klebsiella*, *Escherichia coli*, and *Providencia* on the day she delivered an immature infant.

Sepsis can interfere with pregnancy through two mechanisms. The first is indirect: maternal hypotension produced by septic shock can lead to a reduction in the uterine blood flow. The second mechanism is direct: infection of the placenta itself, which was documented in one of the patients.

Sepsis in the burn patient must be treated vigorously. Constant vigilance must be maintained for the early signs of sepsis, which include changes in the level of consciousness, deterioration of normal gastrointestinal function, hypothermia, and impaired processing of glucose. When sepsis is suspected, blood cultures must be obtained, both to document its presence and to ascertain which antibiotics may be most effective. In addition to treating the infection with antibiotics to which the bacteria are sensitive, the physician must seek out the source of the sepsis and eliminate it. Common sources of sepsis are the burn wound itself, pneumonias, and infected sites in previously cannulated veins. It should be stressed that one of the patients in the Army series developed septicemia with *Staphylococcus aureus*, with the source of sepsis being an infected vein. The vein was excised and the patient treated with appropriate antibiotics. She and her fetus survived.

Electrolyte Imbalance

Patients as sick as those with major burn injuries frequently develop abnormalities in their electrolyte balance. Dilutional hyponatremia was associated with termination of pregnancy in three women in the U.S. Army series. It is impossible to say whether dilutional hyponatremia contributed directly to the onset of labor in these patients, because two had other complications concurrently. In the third patient the dilutional hyponatremia may also have been unrelated to the spontaneous delivery of her 2500 gm infant, since the mother was in her thirty-seventh week and may have needed no extraordinary stimulus to initiate labor. Even so, extreme vigilance over the electrolyte and fluid balance is at least as important in the burned pregnant patient as in the nonpregnant burn patient.

Fatty Liver

An unfortunate complication that contributed to the loss of the fetus in one of the patients in the U.S. Army series was fatty liver of pregnancy. One patient was treated for sepsis with tetracycline, a drug that has been implicated as the cause of fatty degeneration of the liver during pregnancy. Fatty liver of pregnancy has often been associated with abortion and maternal death. This complication should be totally avoidable, since tetracycline is rarely, if ever, the preferred antibiotic for use in an infected burn patient. The side effect of tetracycline introduces a larger problem of drug-related complications in pregnancy. A burn patient receives many drugs. It is sufficient to say that the physician should routinely check every drug given to a pregnant woman for potential harmful side effects.

GUIDELINES FOR THE MANAGEMENT OF THE BURNED PREGNANT WOMAN

The U.S. Army series indicates that the best therapy for the seriously burned pregnant woman is good routine burn care. Any changes made in the routine burn care should be in the direction of greater vigilance in the fluid resuscitation, greater attention to maternal oxygenation, more prompt correction of any electrolyte imbalance, and careful checking of any drug given to the woman to make sure that it is safe for use during pregnancy.

INDICATIONS FOR OBSTETRIC INTERVENTION

The U.S. Army data indicated that maternal survival is usually accompanied by fetal survival. Intervention in such cases would unnecessarily endanger the mother. Furthermore, when the mother has a lethal injury, the fetus is most frequently delivered live before the mother dies. Whether the infant then survives is related primarily to its maturity. We therefore recommend reserving obstetric intervention for the severely burned third-trimester patient who develops sepsis, hypotension, or hypoxia, and who has not yet delivered spontaneously.

REFERENCES

Alexander JW, Wixson D: Neutrophil dysfunctional sepsis in burn injury. Surg Gynecol Obstet *130*:431, 1970.
Anggard D, Jonsson CE: Formation of prostaglandins in the skin following a burn injury. *In* Ramwell P, Phariss B: Prostaglandins in Cellular Biology. Vol I. Palo Alto, Plenum Press, 1972.

Artz CP, Moncrief JA: The Treatment of Burns. 2nd Ed. Philadelphia, WB Saunders, 1969.

Boba A, Linkie DM, Plotz EJ: Effects of vasopressor administration and fluid replacement on fetal bradycardia and hypoxia induced by maternal hemorrhage. Obstet Gynecol 27:408, 1966.

Dalla-Villa JL: Serious burns in pregnancy. Panminerva Med 9:378, 1967.

Dilts PV Jr, Brinkman CR III, Kirschbaum TH, Assali NS: Uterine and systemic hemodynamic interrelationships and their response to hypoxia. Am J Obstet Gynecol 103:138, 1969.

Duma RJ, Dowling EA, Alexander HC, Sibrans D, Dempsey H: Acute fatty liver of pregnancy. Ann Intern Med 63:851, 1965.

Feller I, Flora JD, Bawol R: Baseline results of therapy for burned patients. JAMA 236:1943, 1976.

Greiss F: Uterine vascular response to hemorrhage during pregnancy. Obstet Gynecol 27:549, 1966.

Kunelis CT, Peters JL, Edmondson HA: Fatty liver of pregnancy and its relationship to tetracycline therapy. Am J Med 38:359, 1965.

Longo LD: Carbon monoxide effects on oxygenation of the fetus in utero. Science 194:523, 1976.

Lynch JB: Current status of treatment of burns. South Med J 69:1085, 1976.

Merger R, Barrar J, Nicholas A: Contribution to the study of grave burns in pregnancy. Gynecol Obstet (Paris) 62:101, 1963.

Mulla N: Labor following severe thermal burns. Am J Obstet Gynecol 76:1338, 1958.

Romney SL, Gavel PV, Takeda Y: Experimental hemorrhage in later pregnancy. Am J Obstet Gynecol 87:636, 1963.

Ryan RF, Longenecker CG, Vincent BW: Effects of pregnancy on healing of burns. Surg Forum 13:483, 1962.

Schmitz JT: Pregnant patients with burns. Am J Obstet Gynecol 110:57, 1971.

Stage AM: Severe burns in the pregnant patient. Obstet Gynecol 42:259, 1973.

Taylor JW, Plunkett GD, McManus WF, Pruitt BA: Thermal injury during pregnancy. Obstet Gynecol 47:434, 1976.

Tica A, Tica D, Baciu G, Georgescu D: Cu privire la interferenta biologica sarcina-arsura. Obstetrica si Ginecologica 17:443, 1969.

Warden AD, Mason AD, Pruitt BD: Evaluation of leukocyte chemotaxis in vitro in thermal injured patients. J Clin Invest 54:1001, 1974.

Wilmore DW, Long JM, Mason AD, Skreen RW, Pruitt BA: Catecholamines: mediator of the hypermetabolic response to thermal injury. Ann Surg 180:653, 1974.

Chapter 8

FRACTURES IN PREGNANCY

J. Albright, B. Sprague, G. El-Khoury, and R. Brand

A changing center of gravity as well as a tendency for nausea, fatigue, and orthostatic episodes might be considered factors that increase the risk of fracture in the pregnant woman. However, a survey of busy midwestern orthopaedic surgeons and radiologists indicates that expectant mothers are at less risk of sustaining skeletal trauma than are nonpregnant women. The search for case reports to illustrate the nature and significance of fractures occurring during pregnancy revealed few cases considering the large population of expectant mothers and their theoretically significant risk factors.

Thus, the apparent risk factors must be counterbalanced by the toughness of the youthful skeleton and to voluntary reduction in physical activity and even self-imposed confinement to a more protective home environment. The last trimester awkwardness created by the enlarged fetus does not seem to predispose to any particular patterns of fractures. In a search through the discharge diagnoses of pregnant patients cared for within the Department of Orthopaedics at the University of Iowa, we found that many more patients complained of lower back pain than presented with a fracture of any type.

The low back pain complaints were rarely related to specific trauma. Instead, most patients described an insidious onset during the last few months of gestation. Pain was usually associated with direct compression of the lumbosacral plexus or with mechanical strain secondary to an exaggerated lordosis.

Most of the fractures recorded in the survey were located in the extremities. Hospitalization was required for 20 women who had pelvic, spinal, or femoral fractures. These 20 fractures were usually one of multiple injuries. In neither of the two surveys was any fracture site or mechanism of injury found to be peculiar to the pregnant state. Thus, it appears that a pregnant woman suffers fewer fractures than the rest of the population. While the older medical literature contains references to delayed fracture healing in pregnancy (Buchsbaum, 1968) and one animal study suggested impaired healing of fractures in late pregnancy (Buchsbaum, 1970), our clinical experience does not support this.

From the standpoint of general treatment, the management of fractures in expectant mothers remains virtually unchanged from those that are routine to the orthopaedist. Treatment should yield a good bony union and complete restoration of function. Instances may arise in which the existing pregnancy mandates the choice of one course of therapy over another. In this instance, the choice is usually based on estimates concerning which management program would be likely to manifest the fewest complications for which the pregnant woman is at risk.

The following is a basic discussion of our approach to the management of common fractures occurring in pregnant women. Optimal care depends upon the availability of an orthopaedic surgeon for consultation.

THE SPINE

Despite their rarity, fractures of the axial skeleton are discussed first because they are potentially the most hazardous to the health of both mother and fetus.

The primary function of the spine is to provide stable but mobile protection for the spinal cord. To allow the spine to twist and bend and provide mobility, the spinal column is broken up into a series of bony links. Providing a coil-like shock absorber for the protection of the mobile and vulnerable spinal cord are the resilient discs, the pliable ligaments, and the muscles.

According to White (1976), "instability occurs when there is sufficient disruption of the architecture of the spinal column to produce a likelihood of neurological injury either immediate or eventual." The management of such injuries is influenced greatly by our understanding of the existence of such spinal instability. That a spine is unstable may be obvious; an example is the case of the fracture-dislocation productive of complete paralysis. On the other hand, occult instability can also be manifest solely on a positional basis. In instances such as a severe neck sprain from performing on a trampoline, disruption of the soft tissue is sufficient to lead to subsequent neurologic deficit if the position of instability is resumed. It is important to realize that a severe sprain with dislocation, followed by spontaneous reduction, can go unrecognized if there is no deformity at the time of the routine x-rays. Here the key to successful management is early detection, particularly prior to delivery. Detection depends on the establishment of a routine in which motion x-rays are obtained even with an otherwise normal radiographic series.

Cervical Spine

The neck is the most mobile, as well as the weakest, portion of the spine. It is relatively easy to disrupt and hard to repair. Particularly in this region, the radiographically apparent degree of skeletal damage may not relate directly to the extent of the neurologic damage. Thus, treatment of these patients must be aggressive, as if instability did exist, until it is proved otherwise. In the emergency room, this includes detailed neurologic examination, splinting by gentle head traction (in line with the long axis of the spine) and rapid radiographic assessment of the injury.

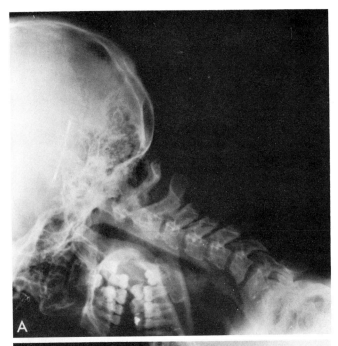

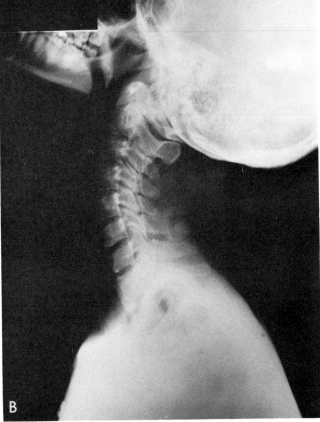

Figure 8–1 Occult instability of the cervical spine is commonly seen in forced flexion-distraction injuries causing posterior ligament sprains without fracture. Both flexion and extension lateral x-rays are needed to demonstrate this pathology. Exaggerated angulation and translation of one vertebra on another, as seen here at C-6, 7, should be looked for.

All the emergency room x-rays, including anteroposterior, lateral, oblique, and open mouth views, can be taken without moving the patient from the supine position. The lower cervical spine (C-5, 6, 7 and T-1) is the area most frequently injured and must be well visualized. Prior to discharge abnormal patterns of motion should be looked for with flexion-extension lateral views of the erect patient (Fig. 8–1).

Most fractures of the cervical spine (Fig. 8–2) are stable and require only symptomatic treatment. The well fitting hard collar, as well as the cervical brace, is very effective in preventing flexion and extension of the neck. The soft collar serves mainly as a reminder to restrict motion in its wearer. As such, its main use is for muscular strains.

A clinically unstable cervical fracture requires maximum attention to detail. The most important factor in deciding on management is the expectancy that the injury will repair to a point of stability without need for surgical fixation. Here, the existence of pregnancy will rarely enter into the list of factors that determine the choice of treatment. Facet dislocations, bursting fractures, and

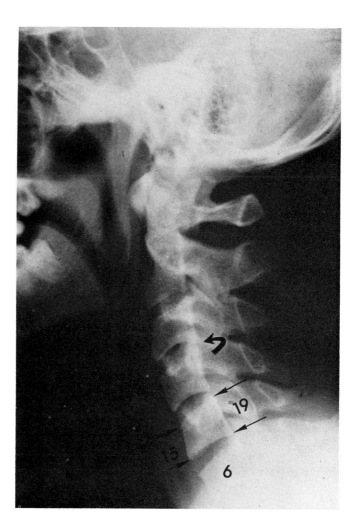

Figure 8–2 Compression fractures of the cervical spine exist when there is greater than a 3 mm difference in the adjacent vertebral body heights. Also note the posterior osteophytic ridge that resulted from this 2 year old injury.

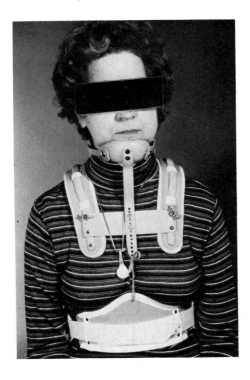

Figure 8–3 Cervical braces are effective for most neck injuries, if control of the sagittal plane position affords stability. The abdominal extension of this brace can be modified to fit the patient in the second and third trimesters of pregnancy.

other injuries with neurologic deficit are likely to do best with internal fixation prior to delivery. In most instances well fitted body casts or braces can be used to allow the patient to be up and about without surgery. Braces are most effective at restricting flexion and extension (Fig. 8–3). Thus, they are usually adequate for most cervical spine injuries, if control of position of the neck affords stability. Braces are not helpful where gross bony damage exists or where control or rotation is of utmost importance. In injuries of the C-1, 2 complex (Fig. 8–4), a plaster Minerva body cast is indicated as an alternative to surgical fixation. Either a headband or a halo skeletal fixation apparatus must be included because of the rotational instability involved (Fig. 8–5). It is essential that this body cast extend down onto the iliac crest for the ultimate stabilization. Even then, healing is difficult to achieve in this area without surgery, and any compromise in the fixation apparatus will guarantee a nonunion.

When the body cast is used in a woman in her second or third trimester, the abdominal wall of the cast may be impractical if the injury has occurred prior to the gross changes in abdominal shape, because too many cast changes would be needed before termination of pregnancy. It is also very likely that, for some somatotypes, the protuberance of the abdomen may preclude the use of a body cast at any time because the iliac crest cannot be reached and used for support. In this situation, skeletal traction may be used during delivery; however, if time permits, operative fixation is preferred. C-1, 2 wire fixation and grafting may be the best approach (Griswold et al., 1978) in the pregnant patient. However, surgery does not preclude casts or braces postoperatively.

When cervical spine instability exists at the time of delivery, it is especially

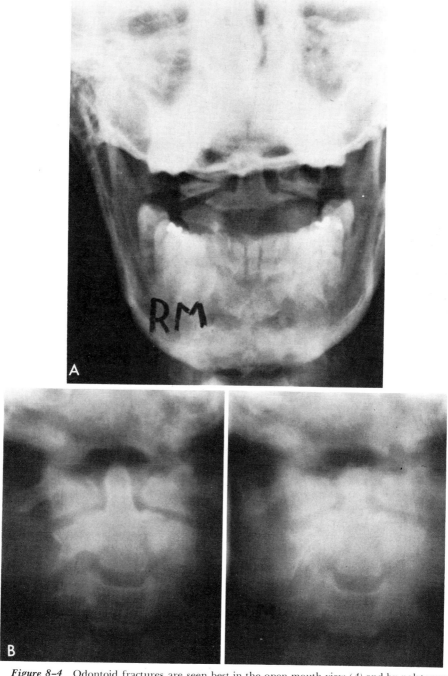

Figure 8–4 Odontoid fractures are seen best in the open mouth view *(A)* and by polytomography *(B)*. The resulting displacement and instability can be detected on lateral flexion-extension views.

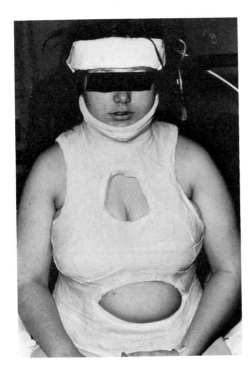

Figure 8–5 The Minerva jacket offers one nonoperative method of achieving maximum control in the grossly unstable C-12 complex occurring in odontoid fractures. The head band helps control rotation. The attachment of a halo pin fixation device to the body of this cast would afford even better control.

important to remember that it is better to "overtreat" in order to prevent later spinal disruption. During the violent contractions of delivery, it is possible that complete disruption of the unstable spine may occur without warning if the neck is not immobilized. White and associates (1976) demonstrated that when the various ligaments are sectioned one at a time in a laboratory, only small increments of abnormal motion are seen up to the critical point when complete disruption suddenly is manifested. The value of cesarean section must be weighed against the anticipated difficulty in delivery and the degree of instability of the fracture.

Thoracolumbar Spine

Fortunately, most fractures in this area of the spine are also stable and require only symptomatic treatment. Most common is the anterior wedge compression fracture that is located between T-10 and L-2 (Fig. 8–6). Usually, these fractures are stable from both a neurologic and an architectural standpoint. A concomitant reflex ileus is commonly found as a complication. Intravenous fluids and nasogastric suction may be required until peristaltic function returns. In 4 to 5 days, the patient is usually comfortable enough to stand up and to move about in bed. Walking can then be initiated with the aid of crutches. External support is usually unnecessary for the healing of this fracture, but complete comfort is not expected to occur for some 3 to 6 weeks. Occasionally, a Jewett hyperextension brace may be of benefit if it can be effectively modified to accommodate the protuberant abdomen. Prolonged bed rest is the alternative of

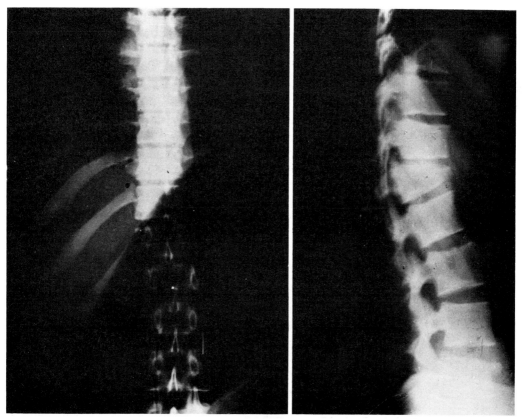

Figure 8-6 Wedge compression fracture of the thoracolumbar spine resulted from a fall onto the victim's buttocks, which created a flexion-compression injury.

last resort for relief of pain in such patients. Antiembolism stockings and early ambulation help maintain a good venous return and can obviate the need for anticoagulant therapy to prevent thrombophlebitis.

The more severe thoracolumbar spine fractures will often result in a spinal cord deficit. Injuries of this magnitude should initially be treated on a Foster or Stryker turning frame, followed by operative reduction and internal fixation if the day of confinement is near. The strong muscular contractions of delivery could be expected to enhance the neurologic deficit.

Lumbosacral Spine

Lumbosacral spine and pelvic fractures in the childbearing years frequently result from the violent trauma of automotive accidents in which the victim may be either a pedestrian or a passenger. Such injuries are of special importance in the expectant mother because they may directly affect maternal and fetal morbidity and mortality. Common complications occurring in the mother include hypovolemic shock, paraplegia, sacral plexus and sciatic nerve palsies, urinary retention, and pelvic infections. These complications occur in only 1 of 10 patients with such injuries, but they can be life-threatening if each problem is not

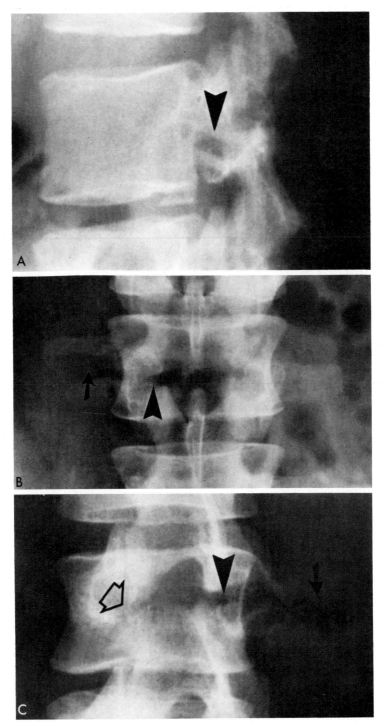

Figure 8–7 Unstable "Chance" fracture resulted from a lap-type seat belt injury. Neurologic deficit and severe soft tissue injury to the abdomen should be suspected. Ideally, the seat belt should be worn at the level of the iliac crest to protect the abdomen.

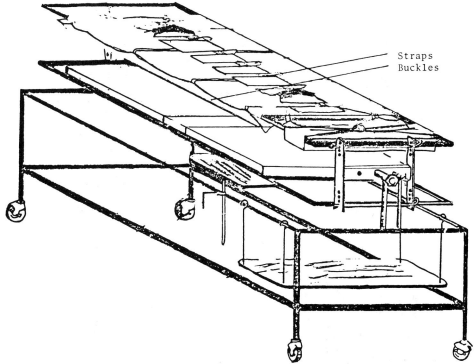

Straps
Buckles

Figure 8–8 The multiple strap support for the Foster frame allows for easy adaptation to the contours of the protuberant abdomen even in the prone position.

anticipated and treated effectively (Norrell, 1975). In terms of survival, the fetus appears to be amazingly resilient in utero. We could find no record of fetal mortality in our multiple-injury patients. However, the fetus too will be vulnerable if the forces of the injury are of sufficient magnitude. The likelihood of fetal injury can be estimated by assessing the severity of the fractures and the forces necessary to produce them (Fig. 8–7).

Patients with unstable fractures must be managed on a turning frame to protect the unstable spinal column while the patient is being turned to prevent pressure sores. Both the Foster and Stryker frames are well suited for adapting to the contours of the protuberant abdomen (Fig. 8–8).

Antiembolism stockings should be used to help prevent the venous pooling and subsequent thrombophlebitis that can occur in the recumbent pregnant patient. If the spine does not require surgical reduction and stabilization, external immobilization with a modified Jewett brace or molded body shells would allow the patient to be put in a regular bed and possibly even be started on a walking program.

Operative intervention in the paraplegic is desirable when spinal column stability needs to be reestablished. If delivery is expected soon after the accident, consideration should be given to operative fixation if the patient's general condition is such that she would tolerate such a procedure. Spinal stability is essential for vaginal delivery. If the stability cannot be achieved prior to delivery, cesarean section should be considered as an alternative to avoid further injury from the violent contractions of the last stages of labor.

THE PELVIS

As in the spine, the most common pelvic fractures do not affect the stability of the pelvis and are not contraindications to early weight-bearing.

The healing times of pelvic fractures vary from 3 to 6 weeks up to a period of months, and the prognosis is usually good unless the sacroiliac joint or acetabulum is fractured or unless there is significant soft tissue injury. Fractures with soft tissue or visceral injury carry the prognosis associated with those particular injuries, and if there is involvement of the sacroiliac or acetabular joints the patients will be predisposed to develop late traumatic degenerative arthritis.

Stable pelvic fractures require only symptomatic treatment and readily unite within 6 weeks. Even fractures of the pubis or the ischium acquired late in pregnancy do not contraindicate vaginal delivery.

However, at least a regional anesthetic will be required during labor for the extreme musculoskeletal pain level that might otherwise be experienced. Fractures of the rami should raise the index of suspicion for associated injuries to the lower urinary tract. Hematuria or difficulty in passing the urethral catheter should prompt investigation of the integrity of the bladder and the urethra by intravenous pyelography and cystourethrography.

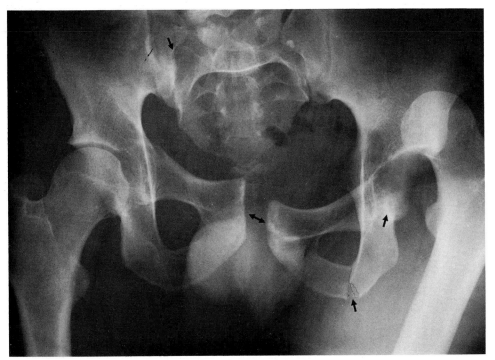

Figure 8-9   An unstable pelvis exists when the fracture interrupts the weight transmission from the spine to the lower extremity. In this case, bilateral instability exists because of the pubic and sacroiliac joint diastasis on the right. Despite the ramus fractures on the left, the side will be stable once the left hip is relocated. Retrograde cystography and intravenous pyelography were performed because of the severity of the injury and difficulty passing a catheter.

Major trauma to the abdomen and pelvis, of sufficient magnitude to produce unstable pelvic ring fractures (Fig. 8–9), may result in maternal and/or fetal death. The associated soft tissue damage within the retropelvic space is tremendous. Hypovolemic shock secondary to retroperitoneal hemorrhage is to be anticipated as a rule (Kane, 1975). A loss of five units of blood is not uncommon, especially when one of the pelvic ring fractures involves the iliac wing. During the routine exploration of the abdomen no attempt should be made to enter the pelvic area simply to investigate where the bleeding is coming from. This converts a closed space into an open one which will bleed profusely from multiple sites. This is especially true in the advanced stages of pregnancy when the pelvic veins are distended. After the hypovolemic shock has been reversed, and the disruption of the lower urinary tract has been treated, attention can be given to the musculoskeletal system. Also, neurologic deficit due to traction injuries of the lumbar plexus are not uncommon and should be looked for.

In the presence of pelvic instability, maintenance of the reduction of a pelvic ring fragment must often be accomplished by the constant forces applied by skeletal traction. A Steinmann pin can be placed in the distal femur ipsilateral to the unstable pelvic fragment and left in place for 4 to 12 weeks (Fig. 8–10). Decubital ulcers are of concern with this method when the fragments are highly unstable because of the pain produced when the patient turns any great amount. To avoid this, the patient should be turned slightly (i.e., 20 to 40 degrees) every 2 or 3 hours. Pelvic slings, binders, plaster shells, and skeletal fixation devices can also be considered for maintenance of the reduction. These skeletal fixation devices can also prove to be of great benefit when the fetal movement or spontaneous abdominal contractions cause the mother excessive pain. They have the disadvantage of providing the potential for infection.

Once the 2 to 3 week initial soft tissue healing time has passed, vaginal delivery can be accomplished even when the fractures are major ones and the patient is in balanced suspension system, without danger of recurrent major tissue damage. In this instance, cesarean section offers little overall advantage, as it carries with it an increased chance of infection.

When the fetus survives the pelvic injury and delivery is not expected for a few months, a plaster "mini-spica cast" can be used with or without a femoral pin left intact. This method does allow the patient more mobility than skeletal traction, but may not permit ambulation. In this instance, the cast is cut low enough to keep the abdomen free.

When severe diastasis of the pubic symphysis exists, significant residual pain and disability are uncommon and the presence or absence of an anatomic reduction does not necessarily relate to the final functional result. Even when immobilization is thought to be the most appropriate treatment, it may have to be abandoned if there is a need to mobilize the patient for important pulmonary care. Interestingly, many of these ambulating patients also experience spontaneous closure of the diastasis.

Alterations of the configurations of the pelvic ring can affect natural delivery if there is narrowing of the inlet. Although x-ray pelvimetry may often be of little value in predicting the adequacy of the pelvis, it may still be worth doing to look for gross alterations postfracture. The best assessment of the inlet can be obtained with the use of the computerized axial tomography (CAT) scan of

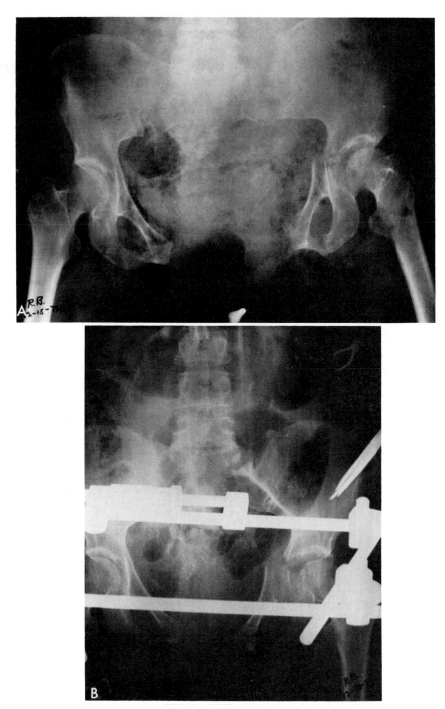

Figure 8–10 Marked diastasis of the pubic symphysis was seen in a severe pelvic injury *(A)*. Reapproximation was achieved *(B, C)* via threaded pinned fixation of the ileum and an external compression apparatus. (Courtesy of Dr. James Turner, Cedar Rapids, Ia.)

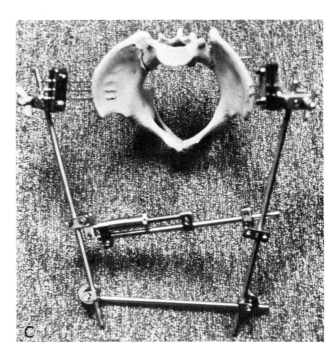

Figure 8-10 Continued

entire pelvis. When there is a serious question about inlet adequacy, it is likely that the radiation exposure risk to the fetus would be small compared to the trauma of a "trial by labor."

THE EXTREMITIES

Lower Extremities

Recumbency may be the biggest clinical problem in the treatment of fractures of the lower extremity. As in the pelvis, most of the immediate complications of lower extremity fractures are not strictly musculoskeletal. Fat emboli, blood loss, shock, and nerve injuries are also extremely important to the welfare of the patient. We prefer a management plan that promises the earliest possible ambulation for the patient. It is hoped that this can be accomplished nonoperatively, since infection is an all too common problem in the lower extremities. As in other areas, the specific nature and location of the fracture will dictate which treatment can be used effectively.

THE FEMUR

Hip Dislocations. Dislocations and fracture-dislocations of the hip are usually the result of a fall from a height or a motor vehicle accident. About 90 per cent of hip dislocations are posterior, with the patient characteristically assuming a posture of flexion, adduction, and internal rotation. The presence of associated acetabular fractures may be an important factor in dictating the type of treatment used (Fig. 8–9).

Normally dislocations or fracture-dislocations of the hip are managed by a closed reduction under suitable anesthesia as soon as possible after injury. If the relocated hip does not tend to dislocate again within a limited range of motion and if fracture fragments have resumed an adequate position, the patient is treated with bed rest for a period of 3 to 6 weeks with the hip held in extension to allow for soft tissue healing. The patient is then told to use crutches for a variable period of time.

If the hip is unstable, or fracture fragments are not in acceptable position, open reduction and internal fixation are usually required, after which patients are usually treated with bed rest for 3 to 6 weeks. This is followed by crutch walking, unless there are extenuating circumstances. Neither the pregnancy nor the proximity of the estimated date of confinement would have any bearing on the treatment of these injuries.

The major complication of a dislocated hip is aseptic necrosis, which may not become apparent until many months or even years after the injury. Aseptic necrosis follows 10 to 40 per cent of fracture-dislocations. Either internal stabilization of the fracture or cesarean section should be performed if early delivery is expected. The prognosis for simple dislocation without fracture is very good if the aseptic necrosis does not develop. However, with fracture-dislocations, degenerative joint disease secondary to the acetabular fracture is a common sequela and the prognosis is somewhat guarded.

Femoral Head and Neck Fractures.   Complications of fractures to the femoral head and neck include a high rate of avascular necrosis as well as the potential for nonunion (Albright and Weinstein, 1975). These fractures are usually treated with closed reduction and internal fixation. In most instances, at least partial weight-bearing should be achievable in the early postoperative period.

Femoral Shaft Fractures.   Fractures of the femoral shaft are relatively common injuries but are seen more often in men than in women. They are most commonly due to falls from a height, industrial accidents, or motor vehicle accidents. These injuries are occasionally associated with damage to the nerves or blood vessels, and perhaps 10 to 20 per cent of them are open injuries. Blood loss may be quite significant if the injury is closed, and as much as several liters of blood may be sequestered in the soft tissues around the femoral shaft.

At the University of Iowa Hospitals, these fractures are treated most often by skin or skeletal traction for a period of days to weeks followed by some form of casting until the fracture is healed. Quadrilateral socket cast-braces that allow weight-bearing and motion of the joint as well (Fig. 8–11) are commonly used.

Loss of the fracture fragments should not be a major problem if the cast has been applied adequately. The quadrilateral socket mechanism, which is needed to control rotation, can cause some discomfort in the perineal region. This factor is especially important if delivery is imminent, since adequate preparation of the perineum would be impossible. If the fracture is not amenable to cast-bracing, the pins-in-plaster technique is an acceptable alternative; in this method, pins placed above and below the fracture site are incorporated into a cast. These pins are then removed after 4 to 6 weeks and replaced by the more usual type of cast.

In the patient with multiple injuries who has a femoral shaft fracture, balanced suspension with skeletal traction is the preferred method in the initial

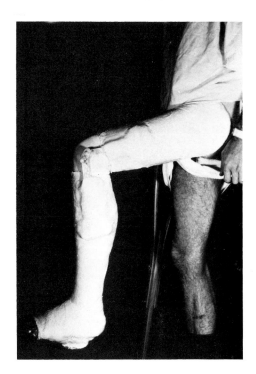

Figure 8–11 Cast-braces offer alternatives to traction or operative fixation for femoral and tibial shaft fractures.

period. This allows the patient to be managed without much fear of further complication from mishandling of the fracture sites. As with the pelvis, fractures of the femur are often a result of severe trauma. Thus, prompt diagnosis and treatment of fat emboli, shock from blood loss, and possible nerve injury is extremely important. In those cases in which more than a few rib fractures accompany the femoral fracture, the death rate secondary to pneumonia is very high unless the patient is made to get up as soon as possible. Depending upon the method of treatment, it may be 6 weeks before the patient can be made ambulatory.

In many centers throughout the world, operative reduction followed by internal fixation is used exclusively. This approach is acceptable in the early stages of pregnancy, provided that the patient understands the chances of nonunion and the risks posed by the anesthetic agent itself. Whether the technique involves compression plates, intermedullary rods, or cast-braces, the ultimate goal is a stable reduction that permits early ambulation and good joint motion while the fracture is healing. The healing times vary between 10 and 20 weeks.

The major complications of femoral shaft fractures are malunion and nonunion. The incidence of nonunion is nearly 5 per cent. Malunion also occurs in 5 to 10 per cent of patients with excessive shortening, malrotation, or excessive angulation. Limitation of knee motion may also be a problem, especially if the fracture is fairly close to the knee joint. Scarring between the quadriceps and the fracture callus is one of the major causes of limited flexion or an extensor

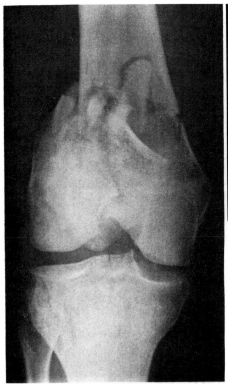

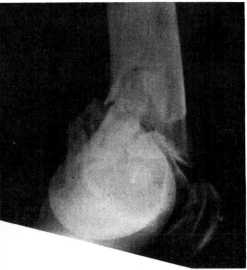

Figure 8–12 Supracondylar fracture of the femur. Note the flexion of the distal fragment due to the pull of the gastrocnemius.

lag. The cast-brace appears to minimize some of these problems, particularly limited motion and nonunion.

Supracondylar and Intercondylar Fractures. These fractures are occasionally associated with injury to neurovascular structures (Fig. 8–12). If displaced, they are frequently angulated posteriorly, owing to the pull of the gastrocnemius on the distal fragment.

The treatment is usually dictated by the degree of displacement and whether or not the fracture extends into the joint. Fractures not encroaching on the joint can ordinarily be managed by a combination of traction, long leg cast, and cast-brace. Fractures that do extend into the joint and exhibit significant displacement frequently require internal fixation. The healing time of these fractures varies between 10 and 16 weeks.

The incidence of nonunion of supracondylar and intercondylar fractures is relatively low, and the prognosis is good unless the injury extends into the joint. In the latter case, the primary early problem is joint stiffness. Later problems include the development of degenerative arthritis secondary to trauma and to the final alignment of the articular surfaces.

Tibial Fractures. In persons in the childbearing age group, tibial shaft fractures not uncommonly result from skiing injuries (Fig. 8–13). When these fractures are complicated by severe displacement, open wounds with tissue loss, or infection, malrotation and nonunion are likely. Open fractures are sometimes treated by skeletal traction to the distal tibia or calcaneus with suspension of the

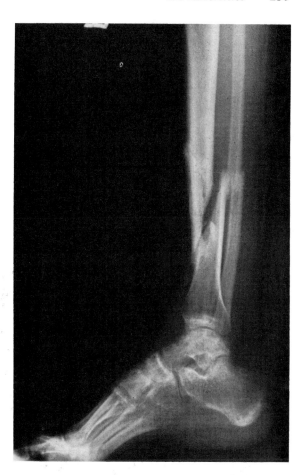

Figure 8–13 Fractures of the tibial shaft are most often treatable with a cast-brace or short leg patellar tendon weight-bearing walking cast.

extremity on a metal frame to facilitate care of the soft tissues. For specific tibial shaft fractures, in which there is difficulty in maintaining satisfactory position, pins may be placed above and below the fracture site and incorporated into a cylinder cast following closed reduction. With simple cylinder circular plaster treatment, shortening of 1 or 2 cm is common and considered acceptable. The major complication of a closed tibial shaft fracture is delay or nonunion; it may require 6 to 12 months or longer to heal in adults.

The fractures are most often treated by a closed reduction in either a cast-brace or a combination of long followed by short leg casts. The patients are usually put on a nonweight-bearing regimen and progress through a period of partial to full weight-bearing. It is now common practice to apply a long leg cast for several days to weeks followed by a special type of short leg cast called a patellar tendon weight-bearing cast. This type of cast is well molded around the proximal tibia and provides a hydrostatic column–like effect on the fracture fragments. These casts allow knee motion and even ankle motion depending on particular design. Regardless of the severity of the initial injury, it is no longer necessary to immobilize the knee and the ankle for prolonged periods.

Patients should be encouraged to exercise daily with the cast on in order to avoid the much prolonged rehabilitation that occurs as a result of muscle weakness and joint stiffness. In the early post-injury period the combination of exercises with weight-bearing activity and elevation of the extremity will significantly reduce the incidence of thrombophlebitis and pulmonary embolus.

Other Lower Extremity Fractures.   The remaining types of fractures about the foot and ankle all require specific treatment but essentially are not affected by the existence of pregnancy. Exercise and ambulation are important in fracture healing and maintenance of the patient's health.

Ankle.   Fractures about the ankle are among the most common fractures seen by general orthopaedists. They involve either the medial, lateral, or posterior malleolus, or combinations of the three (Fig. 8–14). Perhaps the two most

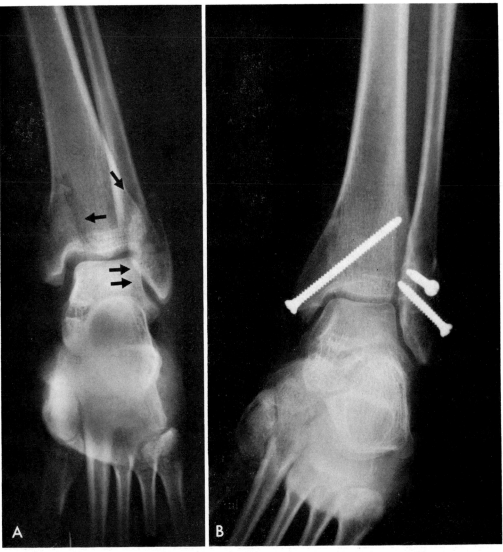

Figure 8–14   Trimalleolar fracture of left ankle resulted from a fall off a stepladder onto this extremity with the foot externally rotated and everted. Anatomic reduction was achieved by open reduction and long leg nonweight-bearing cast for 3 months.

common ankle fractures are the simple inversion injury with avulsion of the lateral malleolus or an eversion external rotation injury in which there are a spinal fracture of the distal fibula and a fracture of the medial malleolus or tear of the deltoid ligament medially. Ordinarily there is no neurovascular injury. Occasionally, however, the posterior tibial tendon may be displaced into a medial malleolar fracture and prevent reduction. The fractures of the posterior malleolus are frequently associated with a posterior subluxation of the talus on the tibia, particularly if the fracture involves more than 20 to 30 per cent of the joint surface when viewed on the lateral x-ray.

Fractures of the ankle require accurate reduction of the fragments and restoration of the normal position of the talus and the tibial mortise. In many of these ankle fractures an acceptable position cannot be obtained by closed reduction, and an open reduction is needed. Fractures in this area ordinarily require casts for periods of 6 to 12 weeks.

Perhaps the most significant complication is a secondary degenerative arthritis due to a failure to accurately reduce the fragments and restore the normal anatomy. Fractures of the medial malleolus have a 15 per cent incidence of nonunion. However, a large long-term follow-up study of cases of nonunion of the medial malleolus indicates that they ordinarily are not symptomatic. The more severe injuries may result in some stiffness of the ankle joint with permanent loss of motion.

Talus. Fractures of the talus are somewhat uncommon injuries and usually occur across the neck (Fig. 8–15). Most of these fractures are nondisplaced or minimally displaced but occasionally may be dislocated from the ankle, the subtalar joint, or both. They are not usually associated with other soft tissue injuries except with the severe dislocations, in which there may be major damage to the ankle ligaments or other surrounding soft tissues.

The more common nondisplaced injuries are usually treated with a short leg nonwalking cast for 3 to 6 weeks, followed by a walking plaster cast for a total of 8 to 12 weeks. The severely displaced or dislocated injuries may require open reduction and internal fixation, followed by a period of casting for 8 to 12 weeks.

Calcaneus. Fractures of the os calcis (Fig. 8–16) are relatively common injuries and are usually due to a fall from a height with the subject landing on his or her heels. They are occasionally bilateral and are frequently associated with a compression fracture of the lumbar spine owing to acute forward flexion when the patient lands on the heels.

Severe swelling is quite common in these injuries owing to crushing of the soft tissues and it is therefore important to prevent swelling by elevating the extremity for the first 3 to 5 days or longer. Ordinarily, such fractures may be treated without immobilization and perhaps better overall function is gained if the patient begins plantar flexion, dorsiflexion, inversion, and eversion of the foot within a few days after injury. Following the initial period of elevation, patients may be treated with crutches and nonweight-bearing (or weight-bearing as tolerated) or a short leg plaster for several weeks. Prolonged plaster immobilization is not advised in the comminuted fractures involving the joint surfaces owing to the fact that it seems to prolong swelling and incur greater stiffness in the foot. The time for bony union ordinarily is 8 to 10 weeks, although the soft tissues may require considerably longer to heal.

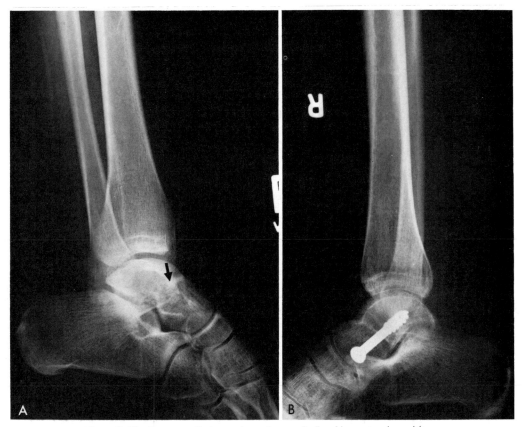

Figure 8-15   Fracture of talar neck was internally fixed in anatomic position.

While simple os calcis fractures (not involving the joint surface) have a very good prognosis, the more severe injuries may be quite disabling. They are often associated with long-term pain, swelling, and poor function. This is particularly true if the injury is bilateral. Late degenerative arthritis of the subtalar joint is a common accompaniment of those fractures that extend into the subtalar joint.

Metatarsals.   Fractures of the metatarsals are fairly common injuries in young adults. The fractures of the base of the fifth metatarsal where the peroneus brevis tendon inserts are perhaps most common. This injury is often called a "dancer's fracture." The mechanism of injury is severe inversion with simultaneous contraction of the peroneus brevis attempting to put the foot into eversion. Normally, isolated metatarsal fractures are not associated with significant injury to other structures. Fatigue fractures of the second metatarsal, or "march fractures," have been seen in pregnancy. In two instances they occurred during prolonged physical exertion in otherwise inactive women. Because x-rays are often not obtained until callus is present, this fracture is sometimes mistaken for an osteogenic sarcoma (Fig. 8–16).

Most metatarsal fractures, including those at the base of the fifth metatarsal, may be treated symptomatically by prevention of swelling followed by crutches and weight-bearing as tolerated or with a short leg walking cast. They normally heal within 6 to 10 weeks, but the period of immobilization need not be that long.

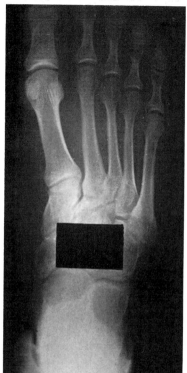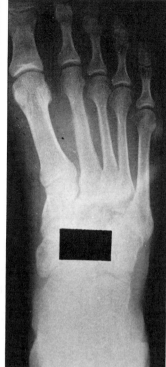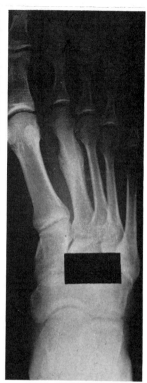

Figure 8-16 Radiographic sequence of healing "march fracture." Note appearance of callus at 6 weeks (*center*), which could be mistaken for periosteal osteogenic sarcoma.

The fractures of the base of the fifth metatarsal frequently are uncomfortable for many weeks.

Phalanges. Fractures of the toe phalanges are common injuries and are usually due to an individual's stubbing his or her toe against a hard surface.

These injuries may be treated symptomatically in most cases by elevating the foot and immobilizing the fractured toe by taping it to the adjacent digit. Such fractures heal quite predictably within 3 to 6 weeks and complications are unusual unless they are open fractures.

Upper Extremities

With few exceptions, upper extremity fractures have no effect on, and are not affected by, pregnancy. Therefore, only a few specific fractures will be covered.

Because fracture complications are more noticeable in the upper extremities, it is important for both the physician and patient to be aware of the possible problems. Often slight angulation and bayonet apposition of long bone fractures are unavoidable and must be accepted. Fractures that communicate with the joint may give rise to stiffness and arthritis. Stiffness may occur in joints adjacent to the fracture as a result of the immobilization. Usually this is temporary; however, with fractures of the upper extremity permanent partial stiffness may be present to some degree. In any fracture that requires pinning or open reduction and internal fixation, the incidence of this stiffness is higher. Also, infections and nonunions do occur after pinning and plating. The goal of successful treatment for any fracture is to obtain an osseous union of the fracture fragments in a successful anatomic and functional position. Another goal is to restore the functional capacity of that extremity with regard to joint motion. Frequently it is difficult to achieve both goals because of the need for both immobilization and motion. The treatment varies with the fracture location. When the return of function of the extremity is more important than the anatomic fracture alignment (e.g., impacted humeral neck fracture), motion takes priority over fracture immobilization.

Humeral Shaft Fracture.   This is the only upper extremity fracture we have seen to carry any implications for the pregnant female (Fig. 8–17). It is produced by falls on the outstretched hand or by direct trauma to the upper arm. Direct trauma produces a comminuted or transverse type of fracture. The indirect type of trauma produces a spiral or oblique fracture. Fracture of the midshaft of the humerus may also have associated radial nerve palsy. Enclosed fractures of the humerus and associated radial nerve palsy are usually due to a contusion of the nerve, producing a physiologic block. Ninety per cent of radial nerve palsies of this nature will regain function with time. Hence, initially the humeral shaft fracture is to be treated as though there were no neurologic deficit. The usual

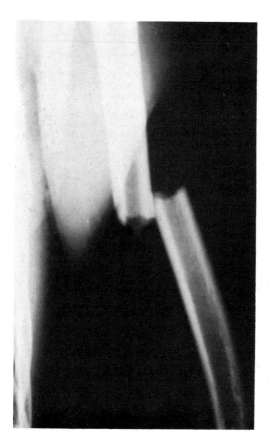

Figure 8–17   Treatment of fracture of humeral shaft can present problems since the hanging arm cast may be difficult to manage during pregnancy when the abdomen is protuberant.

treatment of the humeral shaft fracture in the pregnant or nonpregnant patient is a hanging arm cast. This cast is a long arm cast with the elbow flexed to 90 degrees and the forearm held in a neutral position relative to pronation-supination. A plaster loop is formed at the wrist for suspension of the cast from the neck by a sling. There is no support for the cast at the elbow; thus, the weight of the cast produces traction on the fracture fragments and aligns them as well. For this cast to work correctly, the patient must be in an upright position — sitting, standing, or in the semi-Fowler position. Consequently, the patient must sleep in a reclining chair or propped up in bed and cannot sit in chairs with arms which may prevent the cast from hanging free at her side. These requirements may prove quite impossible in the second and third trimesters because of the protuberant abdomen. As an alternative, a double sugar-tong splint can be used with difficulty. If the patient is not ambulatory, the fracture should be immobilized by overhead traction using a Steinmann pin inserted through the proximal ulna. Nonunion is rare unless open reduction and internal fixation are attempted. The fracture usually heals enough to discontinue the cast within 8 weeks. The first signs of new regeneration of the forearm will be contractions of the brachioradialis muscle. If no recovery is apparent by the time of cast removal, careful electromyographic documentation of progress and location of the block will be helpful in deciding whether or not the nerve should be explored.

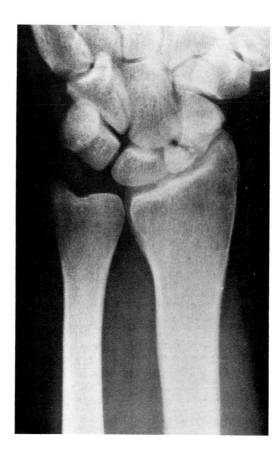

Figure 8–18 Navicular fracture of wrist.

Wrist and Hand Fractures. Although they carry no implications for pregnancy, two fractures appear to us to be possibly more common in the third trimester in physically active but somewhat awkward females. The Colles fracture is the most common fracture of the wrist in adults. It is produced by falls onto the outstretched hand, with dorsiflexion and supination being forced as the momentum of the body carries it over the planted hand. In treating a young patient, it is very important to first maintain a good anatomic reduction. Pins in plaster are frequently used toward achieving this goal. Finger motion is encouraged but immobilization is not discontinued until the fracture site has healed. By using the skeletal fixation the extreme plantar flexion–ulnar deviation position necessitated by the cast is avoided.

Navicular fractures are seen mostly in young healthy and athletically vigorous men and women who have had their wrists forced into dorsiflexion and radial deviation by a fall or blow. There are pain and tenderness in the anatomic snuffbox and limited dorsiflexion and radial deviation on examination. Anteroposterior, lateral, and oblique x-rays of the wrist should be obtained whenever this fracture is suspected. Even if the initial x-rays are negative, the patient could be immobilized in a volar splint or short arm cast and returned for repeat x-rays in 2 weeks' time. At that time a navicular fracture that was not obvious on initial x-rays may sometimes be seen subsequent to resorption at the fracture site. If this fracture is diagnosed early and treated properly, it can heal within 8 to 10 weeks. Nonunion and aseptic necrosis of the proximal fragment are of major concern here.

REFERENCES

Albright JP, Weinstein SL: Treatment for fixation complications: femoral neck fractures. Arch Surg *110*:30–36, 1975.

Buchsbaum HJ: Accidental injury complicating pregnancy. Amer J Obstet Gynecol *102*:752, 1968.

Buchsbaum HJ: Healing of experimental fractures during pregnancy. Obstet Gynecol *35*:613, 1970.

Griswold DM, Albright JA, Schiffman E, Johnson R, Southwick WO: Atlanto-axial fusion for instability. J Bone Joint Surg *60-A*:285–292, 1978.

Kane WJ: Fractures of the pelvis. *In* Rockwood CA, Green DP (eds): Fractures. Philadelphia, JB Lippincott Company, 1975.

Norrell HA: Fractures and dislocations of the spine. *In* Rothman RH, Simeone FA (eds): The Spine. Philadelphia, WB Saunders Company, 1975.

White AA, Southwick WO, Panjabi MM: Clinical instability in the lower cervical spine. Spine *1*:15–27, 1976.

Chapter 9

OCCUPATIONAL HAZARDS

Robert B. Wallace and Valerie A. Wilk

This chapter considers some of the proved and potential medical problems of pregnancy related to the work environment. It describes the current status of pregnant women in the work force, the general types of occupational hazards, a review of the known or potential occupational hazards to the pregnant worker and her fetus, delineation of specific agents and jobsites of current interest, the occupational evaluation of the pregnant worker, and the relationship between the clinician managing a pregnant worker and the respective industry. There is much yet to be learned about the dangers of the workplace. It is assumed that the pregnant woman deserves to have the opportunity — and has the desire — to continue to work as long as she is able without undue risk to herself, her fetus, or others around her. Not included in this discussion, but perhaps equally important to medical considerations, are the legal, administrative, financial, regulatory, civil rights, and disability issues related to the pregnant and potentially pregnant worker.

WOMEN IN THE WORK FORCE

Between 1950 and 1977 the number of women employed outside the home in the United States more than doubled, to a total of nearly 38 million, constituting about 40 per cent of the nation's workers. In November 1977 nearly 50 per cent of all women 16 years of age and over were gainfully employed (U.S. Department of Labor, 1977). Since the early 1960's the sharpest increases in participation rates in the labor force have occurred among women in the age groups 20 to 24 years and 25 to 34 years of age, when most pregnancies occur. In 1977, 68 per cent of women 20 to 24 years old and 61 per cent of those 25 to 34 years old were in the labor force. These two age groups composed 41 per cent of all employed women.

According to the National Survey of Family Growth (U.S. Department of Health, Education, and Welfare, 1977), an estimated 41.5 per cent of about 3,034,000 women who had a live birth during a 12 month period in 1972–73

**TABLE 9–1 Major Occupation Groups of Employed Women
16 Years and Older, November 1977***

Major Occupation Group	Number (in Thousands)	Per Cent Distribution
Professional, technical	6057	16.0
Managers, administrators	2276	6.0
Sales	2564	6.8
Clerical	13,201	34.8
Craft and kindred	610	1.6
Operatives	4450	11.7
Nonfarm laborers	430	1.1
Service workers	7844	20.7
Private household	1188	3.1
Other	6655	17.6
Farm workers	452	1.2
TOTAL	37,884	100.0

*U.S. Department of Labor, Bureau of Labor Statistics: Employment and Earnings, December 1977.

worked during their pregnancy, highlighting the potential problem in work-related hazards. Such pregnant workers composed about 8.8 per cent of the estimated 14,357,000 ever-married women of reproductive age in the labor force at the time. Over 53 per cent of the pregnant working women were between 15 and 24 years of age. Of all women who worked during pregnancy, 16.1 per cent were nonwhite. The survey further showed that the rate of unwanted children was slightly higher among mothers who were full-time workers as opposed to those not in the labor force (15.1 versus 12.3 per cent). Among married women, those in the labor force expected to bear fewer children in the future compared to nonworking women. One fourth of those women working during their pregnancies returned to work within 4 months of delivery, and approximately 50 per cent returned within one year.

Table 9–1 shows the number and per cent distribution of women workers by major occupational groups in November 1977. More than three fifths (64 per cent) of the women were employed in white-collar jobs. About one fifth (21 per cent) were service workers, while 15 per cent were blue-collar workers, and fewer than 2 per cent were farm workers. This contrasts with the distribution for men, of whom 41 per cent were white-collar workers and nearly half (46 per cent) blue-collar workers. Nine per cent of male workers were in service jobs and 4 per cent were farm workers (U.S. Department of Labor, 1977).

THE HAZARDOUS OCCUPATIONS

A general perspective on those industries associated with the highest rates of injury, illness, and lost workdays will alert the physician with a pregnant patient to intensify inquiry into job conditions. These rates, shown in Table 9–2, are directed more to maternal than fetal risk. In 1974, construction, manufacturing, and transportation and public utilities were the industries with the highest incidence of work-related injury and illness. Forty-five per cent of all male workers and 24 per cent of all female workers were employed in these industries.

**TABLE 9–2 Incidence of Occupational Injury and Illness
in the Private Sector by Industry, 1974***

	INCIDENCE PER 100 FULL-TIME WORKERS†		
	Total Cases	Lost Workday Cases	Nonfatal Cases Without Lost Workdays
Private Sector	10.4	3.5	6.9
Agriculture, forestry, and fisheries	9.9	4.5	5.3
Mining	10.2	5.1	5.0
Contract construction	18.3	5.9	12.4
Manufacturing	14.6	4.7	9.9
Transportation and public utilities	10.5	4.8	5.7
Wholesale and retail trade	8.4	2.8	5.6
Finance, insurance, and real estate	2.4	0.8	1.6
Services	5.8	1.9	3.9

*U.S. Department of Labor, Bureau of Labor Statistics: Employment and Earnings, December 1977.
†Incidence represents the number of injuries and illnesses per 100 full-time workers and was calculated as: (N/EH) × 200,000, where N = number of injuries and illnesses; EH = total hours worked by all employees during calendar year; and 200,000 = base for 100 full-time equivalent workers (working 40 hours per week, 50 weeks per year).

It is, of course, possible that within these industries some women may have less hazardous tasks, but specific information is lacking. The two industries that employ the most women, services and wholesale and retail trades, have relatively lower illness and injury rates.

Of all the categories of job-related illness, skin diseases or disorders were the

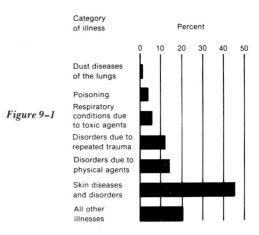

Percent Distribution of Illnesses, by Category of Illnesses, United States, 1973

Figure 9–1

U.S. Dept. of Labor
Bureau of Labor Statistics
1975

most frequent. Agriculture, forestry, and fisheries had the highest rates for this category; manufacturing industries also had a high rate. As shown in Figure 9–1, nearly 50 per cent of all occupational illnesses are skin diseases and disorders, a proportion possibly exaggerated because they are easily recognized and frequently appear soon after contact with the irritant. Unfortunately, chronic exposures that lead to chronic illness after several years are not so easily attributable to the workplace.

GENERAL CONSIDERATIONS OF OCCUPATIONALLY RELATED PROBLEMS IN PREGNANCY

Preconception Issues and Fertility

As stated above, working women may differ in regard to their desires for children and in their concern over fertility from those not in the labor force. These attitudes may also be reflected in differences in contraceptive practices and in readiness for therapeutic abortion. Various environmental and occupational exposures may alter menstrual function and the ability to conceive. An increased frequency of polymenorrhea was observed in women in the chemical industry in Eastern Europe (Alekperov et al., 1969). Ovarian and adrenocortical alterations have been observed in women occupationally exposed to organochlorine pesticides (Blekherman and Illyina, 1972). Women chronically exposed to carbon disulfide at work may have a greater incidence of general gynecologic problems (Finkova et al., 1973), a situation also reported for chlorinated hydrocarbons (Mukhametova and Vozovaya, 1972). An association has recently been proposed between 1,3-dichloropropene and decreased sperm count (Center for Disease Control, 1978). All of this suggests that the work environment can affect fertility adversely, both psychologically and physiologically, and that the occupational history of both sexual partners should be part of any infertility evaluation.

Fetal Development and Outcome

ABORTION, PREMATURITY, PRENATAL MORTALITY. Epidemiologic studies linking employment to pregnancy outcome are quite diverse regarding populations, work sites, and analytic techniques, such as controlling for the general effect of variations in social class or race. Studies by the U.S. Department of Labor in the early part of the twentieth century, which focused mostly on infant mortality, showed significantly higher rates among employed women. This may have been related to concomitant poverty, exceedingly poor hospital conditions, and conditions in the home after the mother returned to work. More recently, Diddle (1970) reviewed six studies performed in the 1950's and 1960's. One found increased prematurity, stillbirths, and neonatal mortality among employed women, though none of the work was unusually exacting or dangerous. The other five observed diverse groups and found prematurity and perinatal mortality rates unaffected by the employment status of the mother. One of these latter studies, apparently encompassing the entire United States national experience for one year, actually found prematurity rates higher among the un-employed. At this point, it is probably best to conclude that although there appears to be no overall marked adverse effect of employment during gestation on the outcome of pregnancy, there are undoubtedly many specific agents to which pregnant women may be exposed that may be conducive to these prob-lems; some will be discussed later in this chapter. Although most of the pregnant women in the work force may not be exposed to them, the increasing number of women continuing to work later in gestation, the trend for women to hold more hazardous jobs, and the evolution of new work environments demand continued epidemiologic surveillance and clinical alertness.

TERATOGENESIS, MUTAGENESIS, AND CARCINOGENESIS. There is paramount concern that work exposures, whether physical, chemical, or psychosocial, may lead to adverse effects on the fetus through a wide variety of biological mechan-isms. The spectrum of these effects may range from fetal wastage and congenital defects to childhood cancer, behavioral alterations, and a wide variety of long-term physiologic disorders. Damage to germinal cells may not become evident until subsequent generations. Some postulated pathophysiologic mechanisms include induced mutation, chromosomal breaks and nondisjunction, mitotic interference, altered nucleic acid function, lack of appropriate biosynthetic precursors and substrates, altered energy sources, enzyme inhibition, osmolar imbalance, and altered membrane characteristics (Wilson, 1973).

At the clinical level, proving associations between environmental exposures and subsequent disease is often difficult. At the work site exposures are multiple and inadequately characterized. Quantifying doses and duration is complex. Extrapolation of data from experimental animals may be hazardous and con-troversial, though often it is useful. Individuals may differ in susceptibility to the putative agents for both genetic and environmental reasons. Collection and characterization of fetal, infantile, and childhood illnesses are incomplete. There are statistical and epidemiologic limitations on establishing associations, particu-larly if the number of exposures or cases is small. Some environmental agents are so disseminated that it is difficult to find a nonexposed "control" group. The easiest environmental pathogens to incriminate are often the most persistent and cause the most overt damage.

It should be noted that while exposure to certain occupational teratogens, mutagens, or carcinogens may be limited to the work site (such as physical agents), the pregnant woman and her fetus may encounter other agents in diverse ways. The worker tends to live near her place of employment and may receive added exposure to some agents through the water or air. Offending substances can be brought home by the worker or other household members via soiled clothing or implements. Many industrial agents are also contained in products intended for household use. An infant may receive continued expo-sure by these same mechanisms and also from maternal breast-feeding.

Some drugs have been implicated as being embryotoxic, but relatively few have been shown to be teratogenic in humans (Wilson, 1977). However, it is difficult to prove such an effect if there is only a slight increase in the incidence of defects. The general subject of adverse drug exposure is not always directly relevant to the work site and is beyond the scope of this discussion. Nevertheless, a few comments are necessary. A drug with a chemical structure similar to an industrial agent may have important implications if shown to be toxic or teratogenic. In addition, a drug with therapeutic benefit to the pregnant woman may be toxic to the fetus or newborn (Apgar, 1966). It is conceivable that a drug may alter the persistence or metabolism of an internalized occupational agent, with adverse consequences. A pregnant woman may be exposed to a drug inadvertently if she participates in its manufacture. Finally, inadequate attention has

TABLE 9–3   General Categories of Proved or Possible Teratogenic and Embryotoxic Agents

CATEGORY	EXAMPLES OF SPECIFIC AGENTS	REMARKS
PHYSICAL AGENTS		
Radiation	Ionizing	From diagnostic x-rays, radioisotopes. Probable long-term carcinogenic, growth-retarding, behavioral effects.
	Microwaves	Mechanism may partly be hyperthermia; human data inadequate.
	Ultrasound	Embryotoxic in animal models. No evidence it is harmful in human diagnostic uses.
Temperature Extremes	Hypothermia	Fetal wastage and malformations in animals.
	Hyperthermia	Human evidence inadequate; some work sites (e.g., laundries, foundries) may elevate body temperature.
CHEMICAL AGENTS		
Heavy Metals	Lead	Wide variety of human reproductive defects suggested. Protection of pregnant worker important.
	Cadmium	Mainly animal evidence.
	Mercury	Definite human evidence of embryotoxicity.
Altered Atmospheric Gases	Hypoxia	Animal evidence.
	Carbon Monoxide	Pregnant women more sensitive to effects.
	Hypercapnia	Teratogenic in animals.
	Sulfur Dioxide, Nitrogen Oxides	Common air pollutants with demonstrated general clinical reactions. No teratogenicity noted.
Environmental Chemicals	Anesthetic Gases	See text.
	Vinyl Chloride	See text.
	Insecticides	Organochlorines, organophosphates, carbaryl, DDT, etc. Essentially animal evidence and rare human case reports.
	Herbicides, Fungicides	Essentially animal data.
	Polychlorinated Biphenyls (PCB's)	Intrauterine growth retardation in animals. Present in wide variety of industrial products. Linked to human fetal disease.
	Industrial Solvents	Benzene (possibly leukemogenic); perchloroethylene, xylene, tetrachloroethylene implicated in animal studies.
	Naturally occurring substances	Various plants (e.g., jimsonweed, locoweed), mycotoxins (e.g., aflatoxins, ergotamine), minerals (selenium), alkaloids and extracts (e.g., quinine, colchicine). Acute poisoning more likely than chronic exposure.
BIOLOGICAL AGENTS		
Infectious Agents	Rubella, Cytomegalovirus, Herpes virus, *Toxoplasma gondii*	Wide variety of agents, some related to laboratory work or other industrial exposures. See text.

been paid to the fact that many drugs commonly used during pregnancy have sedative properties, which may impair work performance or be a potential cause of injury to those working with machinery. As the number of pregnant workers increases, the routine use of these agents must be reevaluated.

Table 9–3 reviews the general classes of actual or putative teratogens and embryotoxins related to occupational exposures. Some specific agents will be discussed in more detail later in this chapter. The list of actual and suspect agents is burgeoning as clinical and experimental reports multiply. Exhaustive reference catalogs of implicated agents are available and are relatively up-to-date (Shepard, 1976; Weinstein, 1976). The table is not exhaustive, and most evidence is from animal studies, which are presented to alert the clinician to potentially hazardous occupational settings. Drugs and hormones that may have adverse effects on the fetus are omitted. Also omitted are the nutritional deficiencies and excesses that may be implicated in experimental studies. It is unclear whether these occur in sufficient severity and frequency in humans to be important, but nutritional alteration may interact with other environmental agents.

Despite abundant experimentation using animal models, the number of proved human fetal transplacental carcinogens is small. Two agents receiving recent attention are x-irradiation, which has been linked to subsequent leukemia (Stewart et al., 1958), and maternal consumption of synthetic estrogens, leading to vaginal adenocarcinoma (Herbst et al., 1971). Other suspect agents exist, particularly drugs (Fraumeni and Miller, 1972). Exposure to chemical carcinogens may not be limited to the prenatal period. A woman returning to the same job may continue to transmit the agents via contaminated clothing or breast milk. It is possible that many environmental teratogens are also carcinogenic, and relationships between cancer and congenital malformations have been described in humans. In occupational situations, when either carcinogens or teratogens are suspect, heightened monitoring for the other seems important.

BEHAVIORAL AND NEUROLOGIC EFFECTS. Although extremely difficult to evaluate, it is possible that prenatal occupational exposures may have adverse effects on subsequent behavioral and neurologic function (Weiss and Spyker, 1974). Recent work has particularly focused on heavy metals. A striking example is the neurologic syndrome (Minamata disease), which causes incomplete brain development and cerebral palsy–like symptoms in infants born to mothers exposed to methyl mercury. Structural or chemical lesions may remain dormant over a major part of the life span only to become manifest, perhaps with other superimposed insults, later in life. It is conceivable, though unproved, that occupationally induced changes in maternal behavior may affect the infant owing to altered mother-child interactions. The entire problem needs further exploration.

Maternal Considerations

It is not within the scope of this discussion to describe all the adverse effects of occupational situations on women of reproductive age, but rather to review some job-related problems relevant to the normal pregnant worker. Concomitant medical or surgical conditions may drastically alter tolerance to work exposures, and, therefore, clinical management and employment recommendations.

The basic presumption is that a normal woman with a normal fetus and an uncomplicated pregnancy in a job that presents no greater potential hazards than those encountered in normal daily life may continue to work until the onset of labor. It is then the duty of the clinician to continually assess the status of the pregnancy at each prenatal visit and to recommend (1) continued adherence to this presumption, (2) modification in work environment, or (3) cessation of work. These latter recommendations cannot be made casually as there is growing evidence of adverse physical and psychosocial health consequences associated with forced job termination (National Institute for Occupational Safety and Health, 1977a). Much of the following is based on an excellent review of pregnancy and work produced by the American College of Obstetricians and Gynecologists (1977).

GENERAL SYMPTOMS.   There are a wide variety of complaints that may occur more frequently during pregnancy, including nausea and vomiting, fatigue, breast swelling and tenderness, headache, frequency of urination, constipation, backache, peripheral edema, dizziness and syncope, and insomnia. These may have several consequences. Increased absenteeism or impaired work efficiency may jeopardize a woman's job. There may be increased danger of injury from machinery or other situations. A stressful work site with a hot environment, prolonged standing, or inadequate restroom facilities can increase the likelihood of such problems developing. Pregnancy-related emotional changes may lead to friction with co-workers and make the work site more stressful.

HABITS.   The work environment may perpetuate behavioral patterns that have special significance during pregnancy. A long commuting trip may increase physical discomfort or fatigue. Social pressures or situations may facilitate smoking or alcohol consumption. Some work sites may not have adequate nutritious food available. Work schedules may prevent the patient from taking medication at the prescribed times and even from attending prenatal clinics. It has been suggested that some working women may not seek prenatal care until the second trimester for fear of losing employment (Hunt, 1975).

EFFECT OF PHYSIOLOGIC ALTERATIONS OF PREGNANCY ON WORK.   The progressive physiologic alterations during gestation may impair the capacity for strenuous work or, in some instances, enhance susceptibility to environmental agents. However, confirmatory studies at various work sites are generally lacking.

Pregnancy is characterized by progressively increasing blood volume, heart rate, stroke volume, and cardiac output, at least into the third trimester (Ueland, 1977). As pregnancy advances there is a progressive decline in exercise tolerance and cardiac reserve (Ueland et al., 1969), which should be considered in certain occupational settings. Further, cardiac dynamics are related to body position, in part because of pressure on the vena cava from the enlarging uterus. This may have implications for postural requirements during work. Fetal heart rate changes after application of a standardized exercise have been measured (Pokorny and Rous, 1967). The fetal rate varied from practically no change in some subjects to a gradual rise over 3 min, suggesting that fetal oxygenation may be compromised in some women during exercise and that women vary in their degrees of physical conditioning. Relative heart volume, plasma volume, and total hemoglobin level increase with exercise and are positively correlated with physical fitness in pregnancy (Erkkola and Makela, 1976). There may be an increase in the energy cost of work and a prolonged recovery from a fixed work load, with adjustment by slowing the work pace (Blackburn and Calloway, 1976). Since mothers with a small heart or with diminished cardiac reserve due to mild heart diseases tend to have smaller babies, grading of the work load to physical conditioning may be useful, particularly for those with strenuous jobs.

The hemoglobin concentration declines during pregnancy, and there is evidence that physical fitness is in part dependent on the total hemoglobin (Erkkola and Makela, 1976). Aside from the nutritional anemias, any industrial exposure that limits the oxygen-carrying capacity of the blood, such as carbon monoxide, methylene chloride, or hydrogen cyanide, or that causes hemolysis or decreased hematopoiesis may markedly interfere with exercise capacity.

Physiologic changes in the pulmonary system during pregnancy may have relevance to work. Minute ventilation, respiratory rate, and tidal volume are elevated during gestation in response to increased oxygen demand and basal metabolic rate. A 17 to 20 per cent decline in functional residual capacity and a 4 per cent reduction in total lung capacity at term have been reported (Leontic, 1977). This may contribute in part to the declining work capacity late in pregnancy. It is possible that the decreased functional residual volume during pregnancy accelerates the rise in alveolar concentration of adventitious gases inspired (Moya and Smith, 1965), making the worker more susceptible in certain occupational settings. During pregnancy, capillary enlargement throughout the respiratory tract results in mucosal edema and hyperemia in the nasopharynx and tracheobronchial tree, causing voice changes and impaired nose-breathing. These symptoms may be aggravated by dusts, pollen, and airborne irritants.

Musculoskeletal changes during pregnancy are relevant to certain occupational settings. There is accentuated lumbar lordosis and dorsal kyphosis as the enlarging uterus moves the center of gravity backward in the lower portion of the spine and forward in the neck region. This may increase the risk of falls and result in some loss of balance (American College of Obstetricians and Gynecologists, 1977) and in lower back discomfort late in pregnancy (Pritchard and MacDonald, 1976). There is increased mobility of the sacroiliac, sacrococcygeal, and pubic joints, which may lead to pain and tenderness. Coccygodynia may occur in thin women who must sit on hard surfaces because of the backward tipping of the pelvis.

During the third trimester it is recommended that women wear low-heeled shoes to lessen the shift of the weight-bearing angle (American College of Obstetricians and Gynecologists, 1977), and high heels should be avoided because of the risk of falling. Shoes should offer good support. Although the amount of heavy lifting during pregnancy should probably be reduced, the size, shape, and position of the load are also important. Lifting loads in front becomes more difficult as term approaches. Body balance is also important in lifting and carrying, and after the twenty-fourth week capacity may diminish if the load requires good balance or strained posture. The potential for even minor blows to the protruding abdomen should be avoided. Belts and automobile safety harnesses usually present no difficulty if they are not constrictive. Because of the softening and extensibility of the abdominal musculature and pelvic ligaments, these structures may be more vulnerable to physical damage. Thus, pregnant women should not work in areas with inadequate protection against slips and falls.

SPECIFIC OCCUPATIONS AND EXPOSURES

This section considers selected work sites and occupation-related environmental agents which have been linked to adverse health effects on the pregnant worker, focusing on those in which recent experimental, clinical, or epidemiologic findings have emerged.

Anesthetic Gases and the Operating Room

The effects of exposure to anesthetic gases have been sought since an unusually high incidence of headache, fatigability, irritability, nausea, pruritus, and spontaneous abortion was reported among Russian anesthesiologists (Vaisman, 1967). The similarity in chemical structure of some of these agents to known or suspected human carcinogens strengthened the plausibility of the association (Corbett, 1975). A United States nationwide study of occupational diseases among operating room personnel (Cohen et al., 1974) found that women exposed to anesthetics had a significantly higher incidence of spontaneous abortion, congenital abnormalities among live-born offspring, cancer, and liver disease than did the control group. The children of male anesthesiologists whose wives were unexposed to these gases also had a higher risk of congenital abnormalities. Another study has reported a twofold increase in infertility among operating room personnel (Knill-Jones et al., 1972). These findings raise the question of the safety not only of operating room personnel but also of pregnant patients given inhalation anesthesia. Reduction in operating room contamination by use of waste-gas scavenging equipment and decreasing the duration of exposure are recommendations to minimize these hazards.

Pesticides

In general, there is a dearth of epidemiologic studies relating the wide variety of chemicals called pesticides to cancer, birth defects, or fetal loss, and these relationships have by no means been proved. Aside from their untoward effects on the environment, pesticides have been shown to affect human health largely through acute toxicity, with wide-ranging effects on the nervous system, liver, kidneys, and other organ systems. Fatalities from acute poisoning are all too common. The potential for pesticide exposure may be as great in the home as in agricultural or related occupational settings.

There have been reports on the possible association between exposure to chlordane-based compounds and related chlorinated hydrocarbon pesticides and blood dyscrasias, such as aplastic anemia and leukemia in humans (Infante and Epstein, 1977). Chlordane and heptachlor cause hepatic tumors in animals (Infante and Newton, 1975). Other chlorinated hydrocarbons (aldrin, dieldrin,

DDT, Kepone, and lindane), the organophosphate esters (Diazinon, dimethoate, and Dipterex), and carbamates (MBC [methyl-2-benzimidazolecarbamate], dithiocarbamates) have been carcinogenic in test animals. DDT and its metabolites and analogues, lindane, heptachlor epoxide, and dieldrin have been detected in adipose tissue, the liver, adrenals, lungs, heart, brain, kidneys, and spleen of stillborns and of infants dying in the early neonatal period as well as in the cord blood of normal neonates (Curley et al., 1969), indicating transplacental passage. Chlorinated hydrocarbon pesticides have also been found in human milk.

Radiation Exposure

Industrial radiation exposure may potentially occur in a wide variety of settings where x-ray machines, accelerators, radionuclides, nuclear reactors, or radiation-containing ores are in use. Occupational studies of workers exposed to ionizing radiation have shown an increased incidence of leukemia, lung cancer, and other cancers (United Nations, 1972).

Radiation also affects the fetus. The most frequent abnormalities among offspring are small size at birth and markedly stunted growth, microcephaly, mental retardation, microphthalmus, pigmentary degeneration of the retina, genital and skeletal malformations, and cataracts (Dekaban, 1968). The resulting injury depends to a certain extent on the stage of development at the time of irradiation. Many organs and systems are very sensitive to irradiation between 3 and 12 weeks' gestation. Surviving children may have marked abnormalities of the brain, eyes, and genital and skeletal systems, as well as stunting of growth. Some suffer recurrent seizures. There is evidence that even small intrauterine exposures may reduce the child's intelligence (Miller and Blot, 1972). Eye anomalies may be caused by irradiation before as well as during pregnancy (Jacobsen and Mellemgaard, 1968). It has also been reported that an increased number of children with Down's syndrome were born to mothers exposed to abdominal radiation (Uchida et al., 1968).

Radiation may be leukemogenic to the developing fetus (Cooper and Cooper, 1966). Leukemia and malignancies developed twice as often in children born to women subjected to x-ray pelvimetry during pregnancy than in those not receiving radiation *in utero* (Russell and Russell, 1952). Experimental evidence indicates the absence of a threshold for the development of childhood cancer and leukemia (Garland, 1964). Besides the risk of producing somatic injury to the fetus there is also the risk of causing genetic damage as a result of radiation of the maternal and fetal gonads (Cooper and Cooper, 1966).

Vinyl Chloride

Vinyl chloride monomer (VCM) is used in the production of vinyl chloride and polyvinyl chloride, and in the manufacture of plastic wrappings and other plastic products. A significant increase in fetal loss was observed among wives of workers exposed to VCM. The cause was thought to be germ cell damage in the fathers through direct exposure to VCM (Infante et al., 1976). Exposure to vinyl chloride has been linked to a marked increased risk of angiosarcoma of the liver (Monson et al., 1974). Further human and animal data suggest a possible increased risk for cancers of the brain and central nervous system, the respiratory system, and the blood-forming organs (Ducatman et al., 1975).

Chloroprene (2-chlorobutadiene) is chemically related to vinyl chloride and is used as the starting material for synthetic rubber. In animal studies it was found to have chronic effects on the lungs, nervous system, liver, kidneys, and heart muscle (von Aettingen et al., 1936). Functional disruption of spermatogenesis was found in males occupationally exposed to chloroprene for less than or up to 10 years. Morphologic disruption of spermatogenesis in men having greater than 10 years of exposure has been reported, as well as a threefold increase in miscarriage among the wives of these workers (Sanotsky, 1976). A high incidence of chromosomal aberrations in the lymphocytes of male workers exposed to chloroprene has also been reported (Katosova, 1973). With more women entering the rubber and plastics industries, further studies of the effects of chloroprene on pregnancy will most certainly be needed.

Estrogens

Prolonged contact with estrogenic preparations during their production and processing sometimes causes systemic disorders in workers, especially in women and children. Estrogen may be absorbed through the skin, inhaled, or swallowed while being handled during production. Women working in a drug company producing stilbestrol complained of irregular and copious menstrual bleeding, pain and swelling of the breasts, edema of the ankles, nausea, and sensations of abdominal distention (Pacynski et al., 1971). Children of both male and female workers have been contaminated by estrogen dusts carried home by parents on their clothing or on other articles. Exposure results in sore and enlarged breasts and possibly early puberty (Prouty, 1952; Green, 1958) and accelerated skeletal growth. Leukorrhea has also been reported (Pacynski et al., 1971).

Evidence suggests that diethylstilbestrol is a transplacental carcinogen that causes vaginal and cervical cancer in female offspring (Herbst et al., 1974) and abnormalities in the semen and genital tract anatomy in males (Gill et al., 1977). Estrogens taken during pregnancy may be related to congenital defects (Janerich et al., 1974).

Infectious Agents

There is evidence that women are more susceptible to infection during pregnancy than at other times and that this susceptibility increases as gestation progresses (Blattner, 1974). A high percentage of cases of overt or subclinical maternal viral infection result in fetal wastage, congenital defects, or neonatal illness resulting in early death or permanent disability (Haldane et al., 1969). Transplacental transmission is probably the most common means of access of pathogens to the fetus, although there is also evidence of ascending infections from cervical lesions (Blattner, 1974).

A wide variety of infectious agents have been implicated. Maternal rubella can cause deafness, cataracts, and cardiac lesions in the fetus. Neonatal cytomegalic inclusion disease results in defects such as intracerebral calcification and microencephaly. Primary endocardial fibroblastosis has been associated with mumps, one form of Down's syndrome with infectious hepatitis, and congenital cataracts with herpes zoster and varicella (Haldane et al., 1969). Herpes simplex virus, Coxsackievirus B, influenzavirus, adenovirus, and echovirus 7 are also suspected of causing congenital defects. Some viruses such as measles, variola, vaccinia, and poliomyelitis tend to produce abortion or acute disease in the neonate rather than congenital defects. It has been presumed that abortion results from death due to widespread necrosis in the fetus. However, this may also occur from side effects of the maternal illness, such as fever, toxins, or placental changes (Blattner, 1974).

The laboratory technician and the hospital worker exposed to infected patients or their secretions belong to two occupations that probably carry greater risk of acquiring damaging infections. A 1969 Canadian study found a higher incidence of congenital defects among the offspring of nurses who had cared for premature or congenitally defective infants during their pregnancies or who had themselves had some infection during pregnancy than among nurses without such exposure or illness (Editorial, 1970). The increased risk of hepatitis among hospital personnel, especially in some specific locations such as hemodialysis units, is well recognized. Pregnant women with hepatitis B infection may transmit this to their infants, and it has been recommended that seronegative pregnant women be transferred to low-risk work areas (Center for Disease Control, 1976). Similarly, there may be nosocomial transmission of group B streptococci, which is associated with low birth weight and prematurity (Aber et al., 1976).

Laboratory workers, including those handling animals and blood products, probably have a substantial incidence of laboratory-acquired infections (Yager, 1973), including hepatitis. A guide to the management of such biohazards has been published by the National Institutes of Health (1974).

Heavy Metals

Heavy metals can alter enzyme specificity and efficiency. Pathogenicity can be related to interactions with other exposures. A trace metal excess may be influenced profoundly by a concomitant excess of another or by a deficiency in an essential trace substance or other nutrient (Louria et al., 1972).

MERCURY.   Both inorganic and organic mercury are transmitted across the placental barrier. Inorganic mercury used in the treatment of syphilis has been reported to be an abortifacient, and mercury has been found in the stillborn babies of treated mothers (Hunt, 1975). Methyl mercury is highly dangerous because of its ability to penetrate the blood-brain barrier, thus causing injury to the central nervous system of adult and fetus (Gerstner and Huff, 1977). There is preferential concentration of methyl mercury in the fetus, whose tissues are more sensitive to its toxic effects, resulting in affected infants even when the mothers are asymptomatic (Matsumoto et al., 1965; Snyder, 1971). Congenital mercury poisoning may result in central nervous system defects, mental retardation, convulsions, seizures, defective vision, or cerebral palsy.

Dental assistants are exposed to mercury vapor in dental offices during preparation of amalgam fillings. Mercury is also used in the manufacture of electrical and scientific instruments, light switches, fluorescent lamps, metal alloys (amalgams), pigments, dyes, pesticides, germicides, batteries, and a wide variety of chemicals. The effect of long-term low-dose exposure on reproductive outcome is unclear.

CADMIUM. Cadmium has toxic effects on the hepatic, renal, hematologic, cardiovascular, and pulmonary systems. Emphysema and proteinuria due to renal damage are the abnormalities most often found in workers exposed to cadmium for a prolonged period. The photographic, plating, rubber, motor, aircraft, and battery industries all use cadmium, and it is a byproduct in zinc smelting (Louria et al., 1972).

Cadmium is detectable in the human fetus, suggesting that the metal crosses the placenta and is retained in the fetus (Flick et al., 1971). Animal studies have shown that cadmium has a site-specific teratogenic effect, which may be due to both a direct effect on embryonic tissue and to changes in maternal metabolism that secondarily affect embryogenesis (Buell, 1975). This teratogenic effect is apparently dependent on alterations in the cadmium-zinc ratio (Louria, 1972). Cadmium has also been implicated in bronchogenic and prostatic cancer.

LEAD. There is evidence that women are more susceptible to the toxic effects of lead during adolescence and pregnancy (Rom, 1976; Boulos, 1976). Studies on human populations have associated lead exposure with sterility, menstrual disorders, birth defects, increased prematurity, and increased chromosomal aberrations. Women of childbearing age exposed to lead on the job (e.g., in the pottery, rubber, and storage battery industries) and in the general environment (through food and in the ambient air) are thus at special risk (Muir, 1977). Lead may cause abnormal spermatogenesis, a possible reason for the high fetal wastage among wives of lead workers. Iron and calcium deficiencies may increase the susceptibility to lead toxicity, and during pregnancy lead may be mobilized from the skeletal storage sites (Rom, 1976).

Lead has been found in the umbilical cord blood of newborns as well as in other fetal tissues and in breast milk. Some studies show higher lead concentrations in the fetus than in the mother (Angle and McIntire, 1964). The effects of lead on the fetus may be due to its necrosing effect and to disturbance in the fetal blood supply, which can result in abortion (Boulos, 1976). Experimental and clinical findings indicate that the fetus is most susceptible to lead toxicity during the stage of most active growth, i.e., early pregnancy (Angle and McIntire, 1964). It is possible that there is no threshold level for adverse effects of lead on the development of the human fetus.

NICKEL. Although an increased risk of lung and nasal cancer has been reported among nickel workers (Doll, 1958; Sunderman, 1968), little is known about the toxic effects of nickel on the pregnant woman. Embryotoxic hazards may be comparable to those of other heavy metals (Sunderman, 1977).

Vibration

The effects of whole body or localized vibration (frequencies of less than 20 cps, or 20 Hz on the pregnant woman or fetus are not known (American College of Obstetricians and Gynecologists, 1977). However, among pregnant concrete layers, who run the risk of developing high frequency vibration disease, there was a higher percentage of late toxemia and abnormal labors with quick delivery

(Gratsianskaya et al., 1974). There were also increased frequencies of large-sized infants, neonatal asphyxial complications, and perinatal mortality.

Carbon Monoxide

Aside from its obvious presence in tobacco smoke, excess carbon monoxide (CO) may be present in polluted community or industrial environments to which mother and fetus may be exposed. Under steady state conditions, fetal carboxyhemoglobin concentration is 10 to 15 per cent greater than the mother's, and fetal elimination occurs more slowly than in the mother. Pregnant women are probably more sensitive to CO than those not pregnant. Acute CO poisoning has caused fetal and combined maternal-fetal deaths. Chronic moderate CO exposure has caused decreased birth weight and increased neonatal mortality in rats. The overall effect of chronic low level exposure on fetal and newborn growth and development is not clear, and much more work is needed (Longo, 1977).

Airline Industry Employment

The most pervasive problem faced by flight attendants is tiredness. Factors contributing to fatigue include cumulative sleep deficiencies, time changes, physical work load, levels of temperature, humidity, oxygen content, noise, personal discomforts, problems with food and liquid intake, upset circadian rhythms, tension, and emotional disturbances (Wofford, 1977). Although altered circadian rhythms have physiologic consequences, the effects on the developing embryo are unknown. In addition, the known factors in gas exchange in early embryonic life do not provide any concrete evidence that maternal hypoxia of as low a degree as would occur in the aircraft cabin would have any adverse effect on the embryo (Cameron, 1973). Although it is recommended that flight attendants be allowed to fly during the first trimester of pregnancy (Cameron, 1973), further research is needed concerning the possible hazards of working during the second and third trimesters.

Miscellaneous Organic Compounds

ORGANIC SOLVENTS. The aromatic hydrocarbons benzene, toluene, and xylene may affect the central nervous system and under certain circumstances be myelotoxic (National Institute for Occupational Safety and Health, 1977b). In terms of reproductive function, these agents have been associated with prolonged and intense menstrual bleeding. Benzene crosses the placenta, but it is not clear whether it causes an increased rate of congenital defects or of miscarriages in humans. Benzene and toluene have been associated with chromosomal aberrations.

The halogenated hydrocarbons are most often associated with hepatorenal toxicity. Trichloroethylene (TCE), chloroform, and carbon tetrachloride cause cancer experimentally. In animals, carbon tetrachloride can pass through the placenta and damage the liver of the fetus. TCE diffuses across the placenta rapidly and is concentrated preferentially in the fetal blood (Laham, 1970).

NITROSAMINES. These agents are used in the electrical, rubber, and dyestuff industries as well as in the manufacture of explosives, insecticides, fungicides, and lubricating oils. *N*-Nitroso compounds are toxic, mutagenic, teratogenic, and carcinogenic. These compounds include dialkyl, alkyl aryl, diaryl, and various cyclic nitrosamines as well as a number of nitrosamides (Magee, 1972). Dialkylnitrosamines are highly toxic to the liver. The nitrosamides are highly carcinogenic locally, inducing tumors of the skin, subcutaneous tissues, and stomach. These compounds (e.g., *N*-nitrosoethylurea) can induce nervous system tumors in up to 100 per cent of the offspring when mother animals are injected on the fifteenth day of pregnancy (Ivankovic and Druckrey, 1968).

CARBON DISULFIDE.   A solvent used in the manufacture of rubber, viscose rayon, and other diverse chemicals, carbon disulfide can affect the reproductive functions of both men and women. Menstrual irregularities, decreased fertility, and frequent miscarriages have been reported among women (Ehrhardt, 1966); decreased libido and sperm abnormalities have been reported in men (Lancranjan, 1972).

POLYCHLORINATED BIPHENYLS (PCB's).   These are used as cooling fluids in capacitors, transformers, and other industrial products and are also used as heat transfer agents and plasticizers for waxes and adhesives. Known toxic effects include chloracne, skin pigmentation, and eye discharges. In animals PCB's cause liver cancer and reduced fertility. PCB's have been found in human tissues and milk. In Japan, nine pregnant women who had used cooking oil contaminated with tetrachlorobiphenyl gave birth to babies with dark brown staining of the skin ("cola-colored babies") (Miller, 1971). Two of the infants were stillborn; one of these was premature and died from intrauterine knotting of the umbilical cord. Five of the seven liveborn infants were small-for-date. While laboratory tests showed no abnormalities and the skin discoloration faded within a few months, the possibility of late-occurring effects remains (Miller, 1974).

EVALUATION AND PREVENTION FOR THE PREGNANT WORKER

It should be obvious from the foregoing discussion that much is yet to be learned about the adverse physical, psychologic, and social health effects of work on all persons, including pregnant women. The problem must be pursued using basic research, clinical observation, and epidemiologic surveillance to better understand the nature of work hazards and to construct appropriate preventive measures and standards of allowable exposure. It has been argued that there should not be separate standards for pregnant women, as the work environment should be safe for all. This latter goal should prevail, but occupational exposures to hazardous agents or situations are continually occurring; protective measures may be unavailable or misused, and many hazards are inadequately understood. It seems likely that some environments will never be made safe for the pregnant worker and her fetus, and difficult decisions will have to be made. There must be a balance between protecting the mother and fetus and preserving the woman's right and desire to work while avoiding pregnancy discrimination.

Clearly, the decision to work during pregnancy is tempered by many other considerations besides health, including permissive or restrictive legislation, company work policies, obstetric care availability and funding sources, unemployment benefits, and liability and workmen's compensation issues. These are extremely important, but are beyond the scope of this chapter. The following paragraphs will outline an evaluation and a preventive plan that will assist the clinician in managing the pregnant worker and that interface with existing industrial medicine programs.

Placement of Women in High Risk Areas

A program of prevention might begin with initial avoidance of high risk areas for fertile women of childbearing age. This leaves open the possibility of real or perceived job discrimination and implies that the work site is not truly safe. Larger companies with occupational medicine programs or consultation may have preemployment examinations and placement programs with varying regulations. Some may proscribe working in areas with known or suspected teratogens or carcinogens. At the very least, the worker should be educated to the potential problems of, and means of self-protection from, environmental agents. Smaller companies may have no such organized placement and educational activities.

A related question is whether evaluation for pregnancy ought to be done as part of the initial preemployment evaluation of the worker. An industry may request this not only to avoid potential untoward exposures but also for medicolegal purposes (Pyle, 1970). For example, a fetus is not a worker and cannot receive workmen's compensation, and a worker cannot bind her unborn child from liability (Lerner, 1976). In any case, it is clear that in many instances effective prevention must begin prior to conception. If a pregnancy occurs while employed, a woman may have reason to suppress this information for fear of transfer to a lower-paying job or dismissal. Industry should encourage early recognition and reporting of pregnancy and, if necessary, provide satisfactory employment alternatives without penalty so that preventive measures can be taken early.

Evaluation of the Pregnant Worker

When the pregnant worker presents herself for prenatal care, the acquisition of information about past and current occupational exposures is paramount. Without neglecting the usual medical, social, and environmental history, the physician should focus on data likely to be important in management. Job titles may be misleading or unrevealing. The type of industry, length of employment, specific types of processes, and materials handled or exposed to should be elicited. Physical conditions at work, including temperature, posture, exercise requirements, noise, and radiation, should be determined. The physical state of chemicals (gas, liquid, solid) and potential routes of exposure (skin, lungs, oral cavity, etc.) are also important. The industrial hygiene and safety practices of the company, as well as the availability and regular use of protective devices, will assist in the development of employment recommendations. An inquiry into health problems of other employees may give clues to potential occupational hazards (Imbus, 1975).

If the physician has a patient with a condition suspected of being work-related or wishes to identify noxious influences for preventive purposes, identifying the putative agent(s) can be difficult and time-consuming. Often the patient cannot specifically identify workplace hazards. The next most practical recourse is to contact the place of employment. In large industries the occupational physician or industrial hygienist should be consulted. In smaller industries that have many persons employed, the best resource is the plant manager. Inquiry here can be quite helpful, but adequate information may not be forthcoming for many reasons, including inadequate knowledge, fear of legal or regulatory proscription, incomplete characterization of industrial contaminants or chemical byproducts, or protection of the identity of product constituents by proprietary laws. Many hazardous substances are labeled as such, but many others are not because they have been processed or transformed. If a union exists, assistance may be obtained from its personnel.

There is no unitary statutory or public health authority to mandate identification of industrial agents or to provide for chemical analyses. If one suspects a class of agents, such as a pesticide, aromatic hydrocarbon, infectious agent, or heavy metal, the regional public health or environmental laboratory may assist in identification. The local poison control center may have product constituent information. If a maternal, infant, or fetal death has occurred due to suspected accidental occupational exposure, the local medical examiner may assist in evaluation. When a clear and imminent occupational hazard exists, intervention by the regional health department under general public health statutory authority is possible. Assistance can also be provided by notification of the nearest office of the federal Occupational Safety and Health Administration (OSHA), particularly if it appears a worker is being inadequately protected from industrial exposures. Nearby institutions with training programs in occupational medicine, environmental health, or industrial hygiene may provide necessary expertise on a formal or informal basis.

It is crucial to keep good records of occupational exposures, not only for immediate clinical purposes, but also for future scrutiny if workplace hazards are ever to be fully identified and controlled (Amdur, 1977). A standardized occupational history form may be useful and time-saving. One example is available from the American College of Obstetricians and Gynecologists.

Laboratory Evaluation

The management of the pregnant worker includes a thorough physical examination with special attention to those systems potentially affected by identified work hazards. Laboratory tests may also provide useful information (Imbus, 1975). For general health assessment, the routine complete blood count, urinalysis, and electrocardiogram are important. A chest x-ray, with appropriate shielding, may be indicated for exposures to certain respiratory agents. Nonspecific tests of exposure include the readily available liver, renal, and pulmonary function tests. In certain circumstances, objective tests of muscle strength or exercise tolerance may be useful for baseline evaluation and subsequent placement. Some tests measure increased susceptibility to conditions potentially caused by work exposures: serum antitrypsin assay for pulmonary obstructive disease, glucose-6-phosphate dehydrogenase for chemically induced hemolysis, and immunologic tests which screen for agent hypersensitivity (Stokinger and Scheel, 1973). Finally, specific tests exist for the agents or their metabolites, such as blood levels of heavy metals.

Occupational Medicine Programs and the Community Physician

It is crucial that the community physician managing a pregnant worker become conversant with the facilities, policies, and personnel of the industry's occupational medicine program. This is not easy because of the wide variety and changing nature of such programs. Small businesses may have no organized programs at all or contract for services with nearby physicians, hospitals, and clinics (National Institute for Occupational Safety and Health, 1977c). Larger firms may have medical, nursing, and clinical facilities to provide much interim care and evaluation.

Communication with an industry's occupational medicine personnel will benefit clinician and worker. It may be the easiest way to identify and quantify potential work hazards and to understand the company's preventive measures and recommendations. Arrangements may be made for prenatal visits, flexible work schedules, and serial clinical observations; special safeguards or other considerations may be requested. Definitive information can be obtained about industrial hygiene, occupational health nursing, first aid, educational programs, pre- and intra-employment screening practices, available counseling and referral practices, and pertinent government regulations.

CONCLUSIONS

The pregnant woman and her fetus are clearly at special risk from a variety of occupational hazards, because of both the nature of the hazards and the physiology of gestation. The full impact of many work exposures is unclear and requires more basic research, skillful clinical observation, and complete epidemiologic surveillance, particularly since the number of women entering potentially hazardous occupations is increasing. Without neglecting the nonwork environment or usual obstetric management principles, attention must be paid to the physical, chemical, and social work exposures which are of potential danger. In many instances, a preventive program will be effective only when initiated prior to conception. At the same time, the desires and rights of the pregnant worker must be considered.

REFERENCES

Aber RC, Allen N, et al: Nosocomial transmission of group B streptococci. Pediatrics *58*:346, 1976.

Alekperov II, et al: The course of pregnancy, birth, and the postpartum period in women working in the chemical industry: a clinical-experimental study. Tr Azerb Nauchino-Issled Inst Gig Tr Prof. Z *4*:52, 1969. Abstract reprinted in Hunt, 1975.

Amdur ML: Information gathering. *In* National Institute for Occupational Safety and Health: Occupational Safety and Health Symposia, 1976. Washington DC, US Department of Health, Education, and Welfare, Publication No. 77–179. 1977.

American College of Obstetricians and Gynecologists: Guidelines on Pregnancy and Work. Chicago, 1977.

Angle CR, McIntire MS: Lead poisoning during pregnancy. Am J Dis Child *108*:436, 1964.

Apgar V: The drug problem in pregnancy. Clin Obstet Gynecol *9*:523, 1966.

Blackburn MW, Calloway DH: Basal metabolic rate and energy expenditure of mature, pregnant women. J Am Diet Assoc *69*:24, 1976.

Blattner RJ: The role of viruses in congenital defects. Am J Dis Child *128*:781, 1974.

Blekherman NA, Illyina VI: Some ovarian and adrenal cortex hormonal function indexes in women working with organochlorine pesticides. Fiziol ZH (Kiev) *18*:268, 1972. Abstract reprinted in Hunt, 1975.

Boulos BM: Special proglems of lead in women workers. *In* National Institute for Occupational Safety and Health (BW Carnow, ed): Health Effects of Occupational Lead and Arsenic Exposure: A Symposium. Washington DC, US Department of Health, Education, and Welfare, Publication No. 76–134. 1976.

Buell G: Some biochemical aspects of cadmium toxicology. J Occup Med *17*:189, 1975.

Cameron RG: Should air hostesses continue flight duty during the first trimester of pregnancy? Aero Med *44*:552, 1973.

Center for Disease Control: Perspectives on the control of viral hepatitis, type B. Morbid Mortal Weekly Rep (Suppl) *25*:1, 1976.

Center for Disease Control: Possible long-term effects of 1,3-dichloropropene — California. Morbid Mortal Weekly Rep *27*:50, 1978.

Cohen EN, Bruce DL, et al: Occupational diseases among operating room personnel: a national study. Anesthesiology *41*:321, 1974.

Cooper G, Jr, Cooper JB: Radiation hazards to mother and fetus. Clin Obstet Gynecol *9*:11, 1966.

Corbett TH: Inhalation anesthetics — more vinyl chloride? Environ Res *9*:211, 1975.

Curley A, Copeland MF, Kimbrough RD: Chlorinated hydrocarbon insecticides in organs of still-born and blood of newborn babies. Arch Environ Health *19*:628, 1969.

Dekaban AS: Abnormalities in children exposed to x-radiation during various stages of gestation: tentative timetable of radiation injury to the human fetus. Part 1. J Nucl Med *9*:471, 1968.

Diddle AW: Gravid women at work. Fetal and maternal morbidity, employment policy, and medicolegal aspects. J Occup Med *12*:10, 1970.

Doll R: Cancer of the lung and nose in nickel workers. Br J Ind Med *15*:217, 1958.

Ducatman A, Hirschhorn K, Selikoff IJ: Vinyl chloride exposure and human chromosome aberrations. Mut Res *31*:163, 1975.

Editorial: Hazards for pregnant nurses. Lancet *1*:458, 1970.

Ehrhardt W: Experiences with the employment of women exposed to carbon disulphide. International Symposium on Toxicology of CS_2. Prague, 1966. Reprinted in Hunt, 1975.

Erkkola R, Makela M: Heart volume and physical fitness of parturients. Am Clin Res *8*:15, 1976.

Finkova A, et al: Gynaecologic problems of women working in an environment contaminated with carbon disulphide (author's transl.). Cesk Gynekol *38*:535, 1973. Abstract reprinted in Hunt, 1975.

Flick DF, Kraybill HF, Dimitroff JM: Toxic effects of cadmium: a review. Environ Res *4*:71, 1971.

Fraumeni JF, Jr., Miller RW: Drug-induced cancer. J Natl Cancer Inst *48*:1267, 1972.

Garland LH: A radiologist looks at radiation protection procedures. Radiology *82*:963, 1964.

Gerstner HB, Huff JE: Selected case histories and epidemiologic examples of human mercury poisoning. Clin Tox *11*:131, 1977.

Gill WB, Schumacher GFB, Bibbo M: Transplacental effects of diethylstilbestrol on the human male fetus: Abnormal semen and anatomical lesions of the male genital tract. *In* Society for Occupational and Environmental Health (E Bingham, ed): Proceedings of the Conference on Women and the Workplace. Washington, DC, Society for Occupational and Environmental Health, 1977.

Gratsianskaya L, Eroshenko E, Libertovich A: Influence of high frequency vibration on the genital region in females. Gig Tr Prof Zabol *18*:7, 1974; Excerpta Medica Sect. 35, *5*:301, 1975.

Green M: Gynecomastia and pseudoprecocious puberty following diethylstilbestrol exposure. Am J Dis Child *95*:637, 1958.

Haldane EV, van Rooyen EE, et al: A search for transmissible birth defects of virologic origin in members of the nursing profession. Amer J Obstet Gynecol *105*:1032, 1969.

Herbst AL, Ulfelder H, Poskanzer DC: Adenocarcinoma of the vagina. Association of maternal stilbestrol therapy with tumor appearance in young women. N Engl J Med *284*:878, 1971.

Herbst AL, Robboy SJ, et al: Clear-cell adenocarcinoma of the vagina and cervix in girls: analysis of 170 Registry cases. Am J Obstet Gynecol *119*:713, 1974.

Hunt VR: Occupational Health Problems of Pregnant Women. A Report and Recommendations for the Office of the Secretary, Department of Health, Education and Welfare, April 30, 1975. Order No. SA–5304–75.

Imbus HR: Clinical aspects of occupational medicine. *In* C Zenz: Occupational Medicine. Principles and Practical Applications. Chicago, Year Book Medical Publishers, 1975.

Infante PF, Newton WA: Prenatal chlordane exposure and neuroblastoma N Engl J Med *293*:308, 1975.

Infante PF, et al: Genetic risks of vinyl chloride. Lancet *1*:734, 1976.

Infante PF, Epstein SS: Blood dyscrasias and childhood tumors and exposure to chlorinated hydrocarbon pesticides. *In* Society for Occupational and Environmental Health (E Bingham, ed): Proceedings of the Conference on Women and the Workplace. Washington DC, Society for Occupational and Environmental Health, 1977.

Ivankovic S, Druckrey H: Z Krebsforsch *71*:30, 1968. Cited in PN Magee: Possibilities of hazard from nitrosamines in industry. Ann Occup Hyg *15*:19, 1972.

Jacobsen L, Mellemgaard L: Anomalies of the eyes in descendants of women irradiated with small x-ray doses during age of fertility. Acta Ophthalmolog *46*:352, 1968.

Janerich DT, et al: Oral contraceptives and congenital limb reductions. N Engl J Med *291*:697, 1974.

Katosova LD: Gig Tr Prof Zabol *10*:30, 1973. Cited in H Bartsch, C Malaveille, et al: Tissue-mediated mutagenicity of vinylidene chloride and 2-chlorobutadiene in *Salmonella typhimurium*. Nature *255*:641, 1975.

Knill-Jones RP, Rodrigues LV, et al: Anesthetic practice and pregnancy: controlled survey of women anesthetists in the United Kingdom. Lancet *1*:1326, 1972.

Laham S: Studies on placental transfer. Trichloroethylene. Ind Med Surg *39*:46, 1970.

Lancranjan I: Alteration of spermatic liquid — patients chronically poisoned by CS_2. Med Lav *63*:29, 1972. Cited in A Hricko: Working for Your Life: A Woman's Guide to Job Health Hazards. Berkeley, Calif: Labor Occupational Health Program and Public Citizen's Health Research Group, 1976.

Leontic EA: Respiratory diseases in pregnancy. Med Clin North Am, *61*:111, 1977.

Lerner S: Pre-employment examination and job placement of the pregnant woman. Occup Health Nurs *24*:15, 1976.

Longo LD: The biological effects of carbon monoxide on the pregnant woman, fetus, and newborn infant. Am J Obstet Gynecol *129*:69, 1977.

Louria DB, Joselow MM, Browder AA: The human toxicity of certain trace elements. Ann Int Med *76*:307, 1972.

Magee PN: Possibilities of hazard from nitrosamines in industry. Ann Occup Hyg *15*:19, 1972.

Matsumoto H, Koya G, Takeuchi T: Fetal Minamata disease. A neuropathological study of two cases of intrauterine intoxication by a methyl mercury compound. J Neuropathol Exp Neurol *24*:563, 1965.

Miller RW: Cola-colored babies: chlorobiphenyl poisoning in Japan. Teratology *4*:211, 1971.

Miller RW, Blot WJ: Small head size after in utero exposure to atomic radiation. Lancet *2*:784, 1972.

Miller RW: How environmental effects on child health are recognized. Pediatrics *53*:792, 1974.

Monson RR, Peters JM, Johnson MN: Proportional mortality among vinyl-chloride workers. Lancet *2*:397, 1974.

Moya F, Smith BE: Uptake, distribution and placental transport of drugs and anesthetics. Anesthesiology *26*:465, 1965.

Muir, W: Lead and women, a unique problem? *In* Society for Occupational and Environmental Health (E Bingham, ed): Proceedings of the Conference on Women and the Workplace. Washington DC, Society for Occupational and Environmental Health, 1977.

Mukhametova GM, Vozovaya MA: Reproductive power and incidence of gynecological disorders among female workers exposed to the combined effects of gasoline and chlorinated hydrocarbons. Gig Tr Prof Zabol *16*:6, 1972. Abstract reprinted in Hunt, 1975.

National Institute for Occupational Safety and Health: Termination: The Consequences of Job Loss. Washington DC, US Department of Health, Education, and Welfare (NIOSH) Publication No. 77–224, 1977*a*.

National Institute for Occupational Safety and Health: Working with Solvents. Washington DC, US Department of Health, Education, and Welfare (NIOSH) Publication No. 77–139, 1977*b*.

National Institute for Occupational Safety and Health: Seminar/Workshop Proceedings. Development of Clinic-Based Occupational Safety and Programs for Small Businesses. Washington DC, US Department of Health, Education, and Welfare (NIOSH) Publication No. 77–172, 1977c.

National Institutes of Health: Biohazard Safety Guide, 1974. Washington DC, US Government Printing Office Stock No. 1740–00383, 1974.

Pacynski A, Budzynska A, et al: Hyperestrogenism in workers in a pharmaceutical establishment and their children as an occupational disease. Polish Endocrinology 22:125, 1971.

Pokorny J, Rous J: The effect of mother's work on foetal heart sounds. *In* J Horky, ZK Stembera: Proceedings of the International Symposium on Intrauterine Dangers of the Foetus. New York, Excerpta Medica Foundation, 1967. Cited in Hunt, 1975, p. 40.

Pritchard JA, MacDonald PC: Williams Obstetrics. New York, Appleton-Century-Crofts, 1976.

Prouty M: Gynecomastia with pigmentation in a four year old male following stilbestrol exposure. Pediatrics 9:55, 1952.

Pyle LA, Jr: The use of a pregnancy test in preplacement medical evaluation. J Occup Med 12:26, 1970.

Rom WN: Effects of lead on the female and reproduction: a review. Mt Sinai J Med 43:542, 1976.

Russell LB, Russell WL: Radiation hazards to the embryo and fetus. Radiology 58:369, 1952.

Sanotsky IV: Problems of chloroprene toxicology (immediate and long-range effects). Symposium on potential environmental hazards from technological developments in rubber and plastics industry. National Institute for Environmental Health Sciences. Research Triangle Park, North Carolina, March 1–3, 1976. Cited by JK Wagoner, PF Infante, DP Brown: Genetic effects associated with industrial chemicals. *In* Society for Occupational and Environmental Health (E Bingham, ed), Proceedings of the Conference on Women and the Workplace. Washington: Society for Occupational and Environmental Health, 1977.

Shepard TH: Catalog of Teratogenic Agents. 2nd Ed. Baltimore, Johns Hopkins University Press, 1976.

Snyder RD: Congenital mercury poisoning. N Engl J Med 284:1014, 1971.

Stewart A, Webb J, Hewitt D: A survey of childhood malignancies. Br Med J 1:1495, 1958.

Stokinger HE, Scheel LD: Hypersusceptibility and genetic problems in occupational medicine — a consensus report. J Occup Med 15:564, 1973.

Sunderman FW, Jr: Nickel carcinogenesis. Dis Chest 54:527, 1968.

Sunderman FW, Jr: A review of the metabolism and toxicology of nickel. Ann Clin Lab Sci 7:377, 1977.

Uchida I, Holunga R, Lawler C: Maternal radiation and chromosomal aberrations. Lancet 2:1045, 1968.

Ueland K, et al: Maternal cardiovascular dynamics. IV. The influence of gestational age on the maternal cardiovascular response to posture and exercise. Am J Obstet Gynecol 104:856, 1969.

Ueland K: Pregnancy and cardiovascular disease. Med Clin North Am 61:17, 1977.

United Nations: Report of the Scientific Committee on the Effects of Atomic Radiation (UNSCEAR), Ionizing Radiation: Levels and Effects, Vols. I and II, August 1972.

United States Department of Health, Education, and Welfare: Pregnant workers in the United States. Advance Data No. 11, September 15, 1977.

United States Department of Labor, Bureau of Labor Statistics: Employment and Earnings, December 1977.

Vaisman AI: Work in operating theaters and its effects on the health of anesthesiologists. Eksp Khir Anesteziol 3:44, 1967. In Excerpta Medica Sect. 24, 3:1, 1968.

Vallee BL, Ulmer DD: Biochemical effects of mercury, cadmium, and lead. *In* EE Snell: Annual Review of Biochemistry, Vol. 41. Palo Alto, Annual Reviews Inc., 1972.

von Aettingen WF, Hueper WC, et al: 2-Chloro-butadiene (chloroprene): its toxicity and pathology and the mechanism of its action. J Ind Hyg Tox 18:240, 1936.

Weinstein L (ed): Teratology and Congenital Malformations. Vols. I, II, III. New York, IFI/Plenum, 1976.

Weiss B, Spyker JM: Behavioral implications of prenatal and early postnatal exposure to chemical pollutants. Pediatrics 53:851, 1974.

Wilson JG: Environment and Birth Defects. New York, Academic Press, 1973.

Wilson JG: Embryotoxicity of drugs in man. *In* JG Wilson, FC Fraser: Handbook of Teratology. Vol. 1 — General Principles and Etiology. New York, Plenum Press, 1977.

Wofford SK: Health problems in the airline industry. *In* Society for Occupational and Environmental Health (E Bingham, ed): Proceedings of the Conference on Women and the Workplace. Washington DC, Society for Occupational and Environmental Health, 1977.

Yager JW: Congenital malformations and environmental influence: the occupational environment of laboratories. J Occup Med 15:724, 1973.

Chapter 10

SPORTS INJURIES

James A. Nicholas

EPIDEMIOLOGY

According to the Women's Sports Foundation, over 50 million American females were actively engaged in some form of athletic recreation during 1975. With many of these women in their childbearing years, it is obvious that a significant percentage may be pregnant, some unknowingly. The physiologic changes brought about by pregnancy may expose this group to a greater risk of athletic injury. However, since no statistics are available at present on how many pregnant females perform which sports, data on injury must be extrapolated from data on sports-playing women in general.

Traditionally, the sports in which women have indulged were those unlimited by conditions of age and endurance. This pattern was due in part to the restricted opportunities that women possessed in team sports at least until the last decade. In recent years, however, women have participated with much greater frequency in sports requiring both strength and contact. Although in general they still do not compete directly with men, they now enjoy auto and motorcycle racing, hang gliding, roller derby, speed skating, skiing, horseback riding, surfing, soccer, and even ice hockey and football. It has been reported that more women are hurt in skiing than are men. Indeed, 60 per cent of all patients with skiing injuries are female — an important fact when one considers that the number of American skiers has grown from 10,000 in 1935 to 11 million today. Although it is not known how many pregnant women are included in these statistics, we have seen enough in our practice to suggest that there are considerable numbers. Noncontact sports, such as track and field, jogging, scuba diving, racquet sports of all types, throwing sports (such as bowling), fencing, mountain climbing and hiking, softball, all forms of rhythm dance (including jazz, ballet, and modern "disco"), basketball, and volleyball are equally popular among contemporary women.

Regardless of the sports that a pregnant woman plays, her risk of injury is influenced by the amount of time that she is able and willing to devote to athletics. For many women, essential activities (sleeping, eating, personal hygiene), educational pursuits, work, and child-rearing leave little time for sports except during vacations and on weekends. If a woman gives up working when she becomes pregnant, she will have much more opportunity for recreation. Many such women try to exercise and play sports. Although there are still no firm data on how many women fall into this category, it is reasonable to assume that the percentage of pregnant women at risk of athletic trauma is at least as high as, or possibly higher than, the percentage in the general female population. In our experience, many women have participated in jogging up to the time of delivery, and several have run marathon races up to the eighth month. In addition, the greater availability of transportation to distant sites means that accidents are occurring more often far from medical care.

Other factors governing the pregnant woman's risk of athletic injury are her age and the state of her health (Nicholas, 1975). By far the largest number of American females indulging in sports are adolescents between the ages of 10 and 17. However, the increasing tendency for women to marry and to have families at later ages means that more and more women over 30 will be subject to the stresses described in this chapter.

Normally it is not necessary to proscribe for the pregnant woman, at least during the first two trimesters, recreational activities that have been performed with enjoyment prior to pregnancy. (The exceptions, of course, are specific obstetric contraindications.) However, the physiologic changes associated with pregnancy — particularly the tendency to fluid accumulation — can inhibit recovery when injuries are sustained from sports. The differing responses of the male and female to hard impacts, falls, and direct trauma can (at least indirectly) present problems for the pregnant woman. Women have a higher incidence of foot and ankle sprains, especially of the smaller joints, perhaps owing to greater flexibility and generally shorter stature. (Inexperience in active recreation and inferior equipment may be other factors.) When such injuries are serious, anesthesia, surgery, and casts may be required, followed by extensive rehabilitation. Major fractures occurring during the eighth or ninth month of pregnancy may provoke problems during delivery. On the other hand, the loosening of the joints of the pelvic girdle and pubis may facilitate delivery — an effect that was recognized by Hippocrates more than 2200 years ago.

SOME PHYSIOLOGIC EFFECTS OF
ATHLETIC ACTIVITY DURING PREGNANCY

Body Build

Somatotyping has been used for almost 40 years to study the effects of sports performance on the human body (Sheldon, 1940). Such measurements may have some bearing on how an injury occurs. Especially in the last decade, the somatic differences between males and females of all ages have been studied extensively. Females have more body fat, are more flexible, and have relatively smaller bones. Studies of the changes in body composition with pregnancy are necessary to relate these differences to injury and prevention. Sheldon's concept of gynandromorphy (the degree to which a person possesses characteristics of the opposite sex) is also important in determining the prognosis of injury. Certain athletic injuries received during pregnancy may take longer to heal because of gynandromorphic characteristics. The available information should be used more frequently to predict the course (and even to define the treatment) of injuries occurring to women who are pregnant (Carpenter, 1941).

The Institute of Sports Medicine and Athletic Trauma has classified the different flexibility traits among male and female teenage gymnasts and ballet dancers. The females were found to be four times more flexible than the males. This continues throughout life and may be a significant factor in the predilection for certain types of injuries. The very tightly structured person is more apt to have disc disease of the neck and lower back, as well as muscle strains of the calf and hamstrings. However, he or she is less likely to have subluxation of the joints of the patella, shoulder, or ankle.

Exercise Testing

Athletic activity is more taxing on the cardiorespiratory system in females than in males, and their hearts therefore work at a higher rate due to higher energy expenditures (Knuttgen et al., 1974; Katch and McArdle, 1976). In exercises of 20 to 40 minutes' duration (such as vigorous cycling, running, rope jumping, or swimming), blood flow to the extremities has been reported to increase 18 times from the resting state, to about 22 liters per minute (Williams and Sperryn, 1976). There is a corresponding drop in the splanchnic and renal blood flow. In the healthy, nonpregnant female, these changes may be an advantage in that they enhance the important training effect of exercise. In pregnancy, however, peripheral blood flow is normally already increased to the ankles, feet, forearms, and hands. It is uncertain whether the training effects of vigorous exercise are desirable in this state. However, the few studies available at present have failed to establish that an uncomplicated pregnancy in a fit woman is threatened by exercise at any level.

Exercise may assist the pregnant woman by breaking down catecholamine metabolites stored in the heart and brain. Exercise performed every 72 hours is thought to be effective in degrading these substances, reducing their adrenergic effects, especially for individuals with hypertension (Bruce, 1974). Exercise is also reported to enhance the fibrinolytic activity of the serum of healthy pregnant women (Kovalcikova, 1975). Exercise may augment the physical work capacity of the mother and benefit her during labor (Erkkola, 1976). Both maternal and fetal heart beats are responsive to exercise and can probably be slowed by training (Eisenberg de Smoler et al., 1974).

Other studies, such as the respiratory response to exercise on a bicycle, have not been substantially informative.

Drugs

An indirect physiologic effect of high-class athletic competition is the influence of drugs administered to improve performance. Drugs have reportedly been used to stimulate performance both directly (amphetamines) and indirectly (i.e., the "disinhibiting" effect of alcohol in marksmen). The number of pregnant females involved in doping practices, especially before the pregnancy is officially diagnosed, has not been reported, perhaps because of the differences in personal, political, legal and moral values in different countries. Also, it is difficult to define by universal agreement what constitutes doping.

The use of hormones to suppress menstruation (and thereby eliminate biological disadvantage as a factor in competition) requires further study. Since artificially delayed menstruation is in effect a pseudopregnancy, the fact that it does not appear to compromise performance may shed new light on the relationship between the physiologic changes of pregnancy and athletic capacity.

PERFORMANCE FACTORS

In 1952, June Stover Irwin (Fig. 10–1) captured a bronze medal for the United States in the platform diving event, hurling herself at 30 miles an hour from 33.5 feet above the water. After the Olympics she let the women in on a secret: she was 3½ months pregnant. Just how many women have been pregnant and have won Olympic events is not known. However, it is reported that three of the gold medal winners at the 1956 Melbourne Olympics were pregnant. Margaret Court competed in world class tennis until she was 8 months pregnant. After delivery, she won the women's championship at Wimbledon, an event that had previously eluded her.

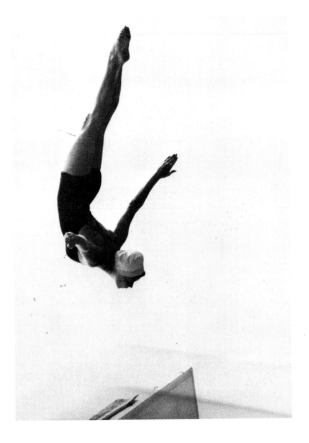

Figure 10–1 June Stover Irwin goes through her paces during the women's high diving event at the Olympic pool in Helsinki, Finland, August 1, 1952. After qualifying in this event she went on to take third place in the finals August 2. (Wide World Photos.)

Although comprehensive epidemiologic data are lacking, these anecdotes demonstrate that pregnant women can play sports well into the second and third trimesters without ill effects. What is needed is a specific correlation between various sports and their potential to injure the pregnant female.

A promising development is the formulation of such a classification for the population at large. Each of the more than 100 recreational activities challenges our bodies to a greater or lesser extent with 21 demands (Table 10–1). Thirteen of the 21 factors are *neuromuscular* (concerned with the body's neural, muscular, and skeletal components), and five are *psychometric* (concerned primarily with psychologic and behavioral components). In addition, three *environmental* demands affect individuals, whatever sport they play. Each performer's response to the demands also depends, as we have seen, on prior physical training, body composition, and state of health. Thus, we can quantify the demands, but not the individual's reaction to them.

Injuries result when the body fails to confront adequately the 21 demands of performance. Once it is known how the physiologic changes of pregnancy alter the pregnant woman's ability to meet the particular demands of each sport, the incidence of certain injuries (such as backache, tendon strains, and chronic sprains) can be reduced. The patient who wishes to continue her physical activity can be diverted to those sports that she can play with least risk. A 1 hour swim daily, for example, is safe throughout pregnancy and enhances flexibility, endurance, and aerobic training without the contact elements that create hazard.

Effect of Childbirth on Performance

Childbirth has been shown to have little effect on performance. Mothers and even grandmothers have demonstrated remarkable endurance and speed in Olympic competition. According to Williams and Sperryn (1976), athletic women have relatively quick deliveries, little pain, and a shorter period of convalescence. Moreover, upon resumption of athletic activity many improve their performance. Essentially, women can play all sports after delivery, if they are able to meet the imposed demands. What should be remembered, however, are the physiologic changes in the vascular system of the extremities. If a serious athletic injury does occur to a pregnant woman, she may have difficulty returning to her customary sport during the pregnancy, or even following the birth of her child.

MOTIONS IN SPORTS

As important to the pregnant woman as physiologic performance factors are the body movements required by each sport. Locomotion may be slowed during pregnancy because of increasing mass, altered upright posture, and increased fluid retention. Six main types of motion are used in sports (Table 10–2; see definitions). These are walking, running, jumping, kicking, throwing, and stance. It is of value to know which sports emphasize which motions. The body's physiologic response to pregnancy has a marked influence on a woman's capacity to perform certain skills. During the first and second trimesters, she is

TABLE 10–1

	NEUROMUSCULAR AND PHYSICAL FACTORS (A)															
	PERFORMANCE FACTORS															
SPORTS	Strength	Endurance	Body Type	Flexibility	Balance	Agility	Speed	Coordination	Sub-Total A1	Timing	Reaction Time	Rhythm	Steadiness	Accuracy	Sub-Total A2	Total A
1. Archery	1	1	0	1	2	0	0	2	7	1	0	1	3	3	8	15
2. Auto Racing	2	2	1	0	1	0	0	3	9	3	3	1	3	3	13	22
3. Badminton	1	2	1	2	2	2	2	3	15	2	3	2	2	2	11	26
4. Ballet	2	3	3	3	3	3	2	3	22	3	3	3	3	3	15	37
5. Ballroom Dance	1	1	1	1	2	2	1	2	11	2	1	3	1	1	8	19
6. Baseball	2	1	1	2	2	2	2	3	15	3	3	2	1	3	12	27
7. Basketball	2	3	3	2	3	3	3	3	22	3	3	2	2	3	13	35
8. Bicycling	2	2	2	1	2	1	1	1	12	1	2	3	2	2	10	22
9. Big Game Hunting	2	3	1	1	1	1	2	3	14	3	2	2	3	3	13	27
10. Billiards	0	0	0	0	2	1	0	2	5	2	0	3	2	3	10	15
11. Bobsledding	2	2	1	1	3	1	2	2	14	3	3	2	2	3	13	27
12. Bowling	1	1	0	1	1	0	0	1	5	2	1	3	2	3	11	16
13. Boxing	3	3	2	2	3	3	3	3	22	3	3	3	3	3	15	37
14. Bridge	0	1	0	0	0	0	0	0	1	3	1	2	2	3	11	12
15. Bull Fighting	3	3	2	3	3	3	3	3	23	3	3	2	2	2	12	35
16. Calisthenics	1	1	2	2	2	1	2	2	13	2	1	3	2	1	9	22
17. Canoeing	1	2	1	1	2	1	1	2	11	3	1	2	2	2	10	21
18. Camping	1	1	0	0	2	0	0	1	5	0	0	0	0	1	1	6
19. Circus Acts	2	2	1	3	3	3	2	3	19	3	2	2	2	3	12	31
20. Cricket	2	2	2	2	2	2	2	3	17	3	3	2	1	2	11	28
21. Curling	1	1	0	1	2	2	1	3	11	2	1	2	2	3	10	21
22. Diving	1	1	2	3	3	3	1	3	17	3	2	2	3	3	13	30
23. Equestrian	2	2	1	2	3	2	1	3	16	3	2	2	2	2	12	28
24. Fencing	2	3	1	2	3	3	3	3	20	3	3	3	3	3	15	35
25. Field Hockey	2	2	1	1	2	2	2	2	14	2	2	2	1	1	8	22
26. Figure Skating	2	2	1	3	3	3	3	3	20	3	3	3	2	3	14	34
27. Fishing (Deep Sea)	2	2	1	1	1	1	1	1	10	3	3	2	2	1	11	21
28. Football	3	2	3	2	3	3	3	2	21	3	3	3	3	3	15	36
29. Golf	1	1	1	2	2	0	0	3	10	3	1	3	3	3	13	23
30. Gymnastics	3	2	2	3	3	3	2	3	21	3	3	3	3	3	15	36
31. Handball	2	2	1	2	2	2	2	2	15	2	3	2	2	2	11	26
32. Hiking	1	2	1	1	1	0	0	1	7	1	1	1	1	0	4	11
33. Hockey	3	3	2	2	3	3	3	3	22	3	3	3	3	3	15	37
34. Ice Follies	2	2	2	3	3	3	3	3	10	3	2	3	2	3	13	33
35. Jai Alai	3	3	2	2	3	3	3	3	22	3	3	2	2	2	12	34
36. Jockey Riding	3	3	3	1	3	3	2	3	21	3	3	3	2	2	13	34
37. Judo	3	2	1	3	3	3	3	3	21	3	3	3	3	3	15	36
38. Karate	2	2	2	3	3	3	2	3	20	3	2	2	3	3	13	33
39. Lacrosse	2	2	1	1	2	2	2	3	15	2	2	2	2	2	10	25
40. Modern Dance	2	2	0	2	3	2	1	2	14	1	1	3	1	0	6	20
41. Motor Cycling	1	1	0	0	2	0	0	3	7	3	3	2	2	3	13	20
42. Mountain Climbing	3	3	1	2	2	2	1	2	16	3	3	2	3	2	13	29
43. Paddleball	2	2	2	2	2	2	2	3	17	3	3	2	1	2	11	28
44. Polo	2	2	1	1	3	3	1	3	16	3	3	2	2	3	13	29
45. Rodeo	3	3	1	2	3	2	1	3	18	3	3	2	3	3	14	32
46. Racing	3	3	2	2	2	1	1	2	16	3	2	3	3	3	14	30
47. Rugby	2	3	1	2	3	3	3	3	23	3	3	2	1	2	11	34
48. Sailing	1	2	0	0	1	2	0	2	8	2	3	2	2	3	12	20
49. Scuba Diving	1	2	0	1	2	1	0	2	9	2	3	2	2	2	12	21
50. Skiing	1	2	1	2	3	3	1	3	16	1	2	2	2	1	8	24
51. Snowmobiling	2	2	0	0	2	2	0	3	11	2	2	2	2	2	10	21
52. Soccer	2	3	1	2	3	3	3	3	20	3	3	2	2	2	12	32
53. Surfing	2	3	2	0	3	3	0	3	16	3	3	2	3	3	14	30
54. Swimming	2	2	2	2	2	1	2	2	15	2	2	3	2	3	12	27
55. Table Tennis	1	1	1	1	1	2	2	2	11	3	3	2	1	3	12	23
56. Tap Dance	2	2	1	1	2	2	1	3	14	3	2	3	2	3	13	27
57. Tennis	1	2	1	2	2	3	2	3	16	2	2	2	2	2	10	26
58. Tumbling	1	2	2	3	3	2	2	3	19	3	2	2	2	3	13	32
59. Volleyball	2	2	2	2	3	3	2	3	19	3	3	2	1	3	12	31
60. Water Polo	2	2	2	2	1	3	2	3	17	3	3	2	1	2	11	28
61. Yachting	2	3	1	0	2	2	0	3	13	3	2	1	3	3	12	25
Performance Totals	111	124	76	97	139	121	91	153		156	139	135	128	146		

TABLE 10-1 *Continued*

SPORTS	Total A	MENTAL AND PSYCHOMETRIC FACTORS (B) PERFORMANCE FACTORS							ENVIRONMENTAL FACTORS (C)				FINAL TOTAL A + B + C
		Intelligence	Creativity	Alertness	Motivation	Discipline	Sub-Total B	Total A + B	Playing Conditions	Equipment	Practice	Sub-Total C	
1. Archery	15	1	0	2	1	3	6	21	2	2	3	7	28
2. Auto Racing	22	2	3	3	3	3	14	36	3	3	3	9	45
3. Badminton	26	0	1	2	1	2	6	32	3	3	2	8	40
4. Ballet	37	1	3	3	3	3	13	50	1	1	3	5	55
5. Ballroom Dance	19	1	2	2	1	1	7	26	0	0	1	1	27
6. Baseball	27	1	1	3	2	2	9	36	3	2	3	8	44
7. Basketball	35	1	1	3	3	2	10	45	1	1	3	5	50
8. Bicycling	22	1	2	2	1	2	8	30	2	2	2	6	36
9. Big Game Hunting	27	2	2	3	2	3	12	39	1	3	2	6	45
10. Billiards	15	0	2	1	1	1	5	20	2	2	3	7	27
11. Bobsledding	27	1	1	3	2	2	9	36	0	0	3	3	39
12. Bowling	16	0	2	2	2	2	8	24	1	2	2	5	29
13. Boxing	37	1	0	3	3	3	10	47	0	1	3	4	51
14. Bridge	12	2	2	3	2	2	11	23	0	0	3	3	26
15. Bull Fighting	35	2	3	3	3	3	14	49	1	2	3	6	55
16. Calisthenics	22	1	2	2	2	2	9	31	0	0	2	2	33
17. Canoeing	21	1	2	2	2	2	9	30	3	2	2	7	37
18. Camping	6	1	2	2	2	2	9	15	3	3	2	8	23
19. Circus Acts	31	1	2	2	3	3	11	42	1	2	3	6	48
20. Cricket	28	1	1	2	2	2	8	36	2	3	3	8	44
21. Curling	21	1	2	1	2	2	8	29	2	2	3	7	36
22. Diving	30	1	2	2	3	2	10	40	1	1	3	5	45
23. Equestrian	28	1	2	3	2	2	10	38	2	3	3	8	46
24. Fencing	35	1	0	3	3	3	10	45	0	2	2	4	49
25. Field Hockey	22	1	1	2	2	2	8	30	2	2	2	6	36
26. Figure Skating	34	1	1	3	3	3	11	45	2	1	3	6	41
27. Fishing (Deep Sea)	21	1	0	3	2	3	9	30	0	1	2	3	33
28. Football	36	2	1	3	3	3	12	48	2	3	3	8	56
29. Golf	23	1	2	1	2	3	9	32	2	2	3	7	39
30. Gymnastics	36	0	0	3	3	3	9	45	1	1	3	5	50
31. Handball	26	0	1	2	2	2	7	33	1	1	2	4	37
32. Hiking	11	0	2	1	1	2	6	17	1	0	0	1	18
33. Hockey	37	0	0	3	3	3	9	46	2	3	3	8	54
34. Ice Follies	33	1	2	2	2	2	9	42	3	2	3	8	50
35. Jai Alai	34	1	2	3	2	2	10	44	2	3	3	8	52
36. Jockey Riding	34	1	3	3	3	3	13	47	1	2	2	5	52
37. Judo	36	1	1	3	3	3	11	47	1	0	3	4	51
38. Karate	33	2	3	3	2	3	13	46	0	1	3	4	50
39. Lacrosse	25	1	0	2	2	2	7	32	2	2	2	6	38
40. Modern Dance	20	1	3	2	1	0	7	27	0	0	1	1	28
41. Motor Cycling	20	1	2	3	2	2	10	30	2	3	2	7	37
42. Mountain Climbing	29	2	0	3	3	3	11	40	2	2	3	7	47
43. Paddleball	28	0	2	2	2	2	8	36	2	2	2	6	42
44. Polo	29	1	3	3	2	3	12	41	3	3	3	9	50
45. Rodeo	32	1	0	3	3	3	10	42	2	2	3	7	49
46. Racing	30	0	1	3	3	3	10	40	2	2	2	6	46
47. Rugby	34	1	2	3	2	3	11	45	2	2	3	7	52
48. Sailing	20	2	3	3	3	3	14	34	3	3	3	9	43
49. Scuba Diving	21	1	1	3	2	2	9	30	2	3	2	7	37
50. Skiing	24	1	1	2	2	2	8	32	3	3	3	9	41
51. Snowmobiling	21	1	2	2	2	2	9	30	3	3	2	8	38
52. Soccer	32	0	0	3	3	2	8	40	1	1	2	4	44
53. Surfing	30	1	3	3	3	3	13	43	3	1	3	7	50
54. Swimming	27	1	0	3	2	2	8	35	1	0	3	4	39
55. Table Tennis	23	0	2	2	2	2	8	31	0	1	2	3	34
56. Tap Dance	27	0	1	2	2	2	7	34	0	1	2	3	37
57. Tennis	26	1	2	2	2	2	9	35	2	2	3	7	42
58. Tumbling	32	0	1	2	2	2	7	39	2	1	3	6	45
59. Volleyball	31	0	1	3	1	2	7	38	2	2	2	6	44
60. Water Polo	28	1	2	2	2	2	9	40	1	0	3	4	44
61. Yachting	25	2	3	3	2	2	12	37	3	3	3	9	46
Performance Totals		55	94	151	134	142			96	105	154		

TABLE 10–2

DEFINITION OF TERMS:

WALKING — A form of bipedal locomotion in which the alternate support phases of the legs are usually linked by a transitional phase when both feet contact the ground. At no time are both feet off the ground simultaneously.

RUNNING — A form of bipedal locomotion in which the alternate support phases of the legs are linked by a float phase, when both feet are off of the ground.

JUMPING — A ballistic motion of the legs propelling the body away from, or over a weight-supporting surface.

KICKING — A ballistic motion of the lower extremity, whereby its center of mass (and/or that of an external object) is propelled about or away from the body's center of mass.

THROWING — A ballistic motion of the upper extremity whereby its center of mass (and/or that of an external object) is propelled about or away from the body's center of mass.

STANCE — Maintenance of a specific functional posture over a period of time.

COMPILATION OF MOTIONS USED IN VARIOUS SPORTS

INSTITUTE OF SPORTS MEDICINE AND ATHLETIC TRAUMA

ACTIVITY TOTAL	53	77	101	93	155	132	
SPORTS	WALK	RUN	JUMP	KICK	THROW	STANCE	TOTAL
·1. Archery	0	0	0	0	3	3	6
2. Auto Racing	0	0	0	2	3	3	8
3. Badminton	1	2	2	0	3	1	9
4. Ballet	1	2	3	3	2	3	14
5. Ballroom Dance	1	0	1	1	1	1	5
6. Baseball	1	3	2	1	3	3	13
7. Basketball	2	3	3	1	3	3	15
8. Bicycling	0	0	0	3	2	2	7
9. Big Game Hunting	2	1	1	0	3	3	10
10. Billiards	1	0	1	0	3	3	8
11. Bobsledding	0	0	0	2	3	3	8
12. Bowling	1	1	1	0	3	2	8
13. Boxing	2	2	1	0	3	2	10
14. Bridge	0	0	0	0	2	1	3
15. Bull Fighting	2	2	2	1	2	3	12
16. Calisthenics	1	1	1	1	1	2	7
17. Canoeing	0	0	0	1	3	1	5
18. Camping	2	0	0	0	1	0	3
19. Circus Acts	1	2	3	2	2	3	13
20. Cricket	1	3	1	0	3	2	10
21. Curling	1	2	1	0	2	2	8
22. Diving	0	1	2	3	3	3	12
23. Equestrian	0	0	2	2	3	3	10
24. Fencing	0	0	3	1	3	3	10
25. Field Hockey	1	3	2	1	3	2	12
26. Figure Skating	1	3	3	2	2	3	14
27. Fishing (Deep Sea)	0	0	0	0	3	2	5
28. Football	1	3	3	3	3	2	15
29. Golf	2	0	0	0	3	3	8
30. Gymnastics	1	1	3	2	2	3	12
31. Handball	1	2	3	0	3	1	10
32. Hiking	3	1	2	0	1	1	8
33. Hockey	1	3	2	3	3	2	14
34. Ice Follies	1	2	3	2	3	2	13
35. Jai Alai	1	3	3	2	3	2	14
36. Jockey Riding	0	0	2	2	3	3	10
37. Judo	1	0	2	3	3	3	12
38. Karate	1	0	2	3	3	3	12
39. Lacrosse	1	3	1	1	3	2	11
40. Modern Dance	1	2	1	2	1	2	9
41. Motor Cycling	0	0	0	3	2	2	7
42. Mountain Climbing	3	1	3	1	2	2	12
43. Paddleball	1	3	3	1	3	2	13
44. Polo	0	0	0	3	3	3	9
45. Rodeo	1	2	3	3	3	2	14
46. Racing (Running)	0	3	0	0	1	1	5
47. Rugby	1	3	2	3	3	2	14
48. Sailing	0	0	2	1	2	1	6
49. Scuba Diving	0	0	1	3	3	1	8
50. Skiing	1	2	3	3	3	3	15
51. Snowmobiling	0	0	0	1	3	2	6
52. Soccer	2	3	3	3	2	2	15
53. Surfing	0	0	2	3	2	3	10
54. Swimming	0	0	0	3	3	2	8
55. Table Tennis	1	1	2	0	3	1	8
56. Tap Dance	2	2	3	3	2	2	14
57. Tennis	1	3	2	1	3	2	12
58. Tumbling	0	0	3	2	2	3	10
59. Volleyball	1	2	3	2	3	2	13
60. Water Polo	0	0	3	3	3	1	10
61. Wrestling	2	1	1	1	2	2	9

0 = Little or No Involvement
1 = Mild Involvement
2 = Moderate Involvement
3 = Heavy Involvement

INSTITUTE OF SPORTS MEDICINE AND ATHLETIC TRAUMA, LENOX HILL HOSPITAL, 130 EAST 77th STREET, NEW YORK, N.Y. 10021 usually able to participate effectively and safely in sports with high requirements of stance and run. During the final months of pregnancy, however, these motions may result in severe fatigue or strain. With the advice of her physician, she can use the information in Table 10–2 to alter her recreational activities to meet her capabilities. Injuries are more likely in sports having high ratings in the run, kick, throw, and jump components of motion. Walk and stance demand less of the pregnant patient and therefore are safer and easier, though often less enjoyable. Our classification system allows the physician to give more objective advice to the pregnant woman who wishes to play sports. It also enables the physician to recognize those sports that increase the risk of injury owing to high motion and performance demands. In sum,

1. It is important to recognize that each case must be assessed individually.

2. Sports are healthful, useful, and of great value, but injury produced from sports during pregnancy is often characterized by a lengthy recovery period.

3. A more intensive rehabilitative effort may be required to make up the residual deficits of the patient who is injured during pregnancy.

TYPES OF INJURIES SUSTAINED DURING PREGNANCY

Injuries from sports are largely those involving the musculoskeletal system, with occasional trauma occurring to the nervous system, viscera, chest, head, and face.

Lacerations, Contusions, Abrasions, Blisters

These are the most common injuries seen in athletes. Although they are usually of the nuisance type, they demand early diagnosis to make sure that hemorrhage, infection, and injury to deeper structures do not supervene. A number of sports have a tendency to provoke these types of injuries, and the patient should be alerted to them. Jogging, mountain climbing, hiking, camping, long bicycle rides, water skiing, tennis, and other racquet sports often produce blisters on the feet and hands. Lacerations and abrasions from falls are common. Although these are relatively minor injuries, if edema persists in an extremity, or if infection occurs, they can become much more serious. For this reason protective equipment should be mandatory for pregnant females who insist on riding horses or motorcycles, or who ski or climb hilly terrains. Such protective equipment may include special shoes, helmets, goggles, elbow pads, and gloves.

Dislocations and Fractures

Dislocations and fractures in the pregnant woman should be treated as they are in a nonpregnant woman. However, a few sports injuries are of particular importance, especially those about the pelvis.

DISLOCATIONS.   In pregnant females, separation of the symphysis pubis is presumably a result of antepartum softening of most joints, including the sacroiliac joints. However, subluxation may be seen in both nonpregnant and pregnant females who participate in dance or in gymnastics. Falls occurring with the legs wide apart can separate the pelvis, injure the coccyx, or tear the adductor tendons. This mechanism of injury also occurs commonly in water skiing, snow skiing, and "splits" on a tennis court. Serious and painful disability of the involved joints often results. Rest is the treatment of choice. In some patients, surgery is necessary. It follows, then, that sports with higher risk for dislocation should be eliminated in the last trimester. In addition to those already mentioned, horseback riding, paddle ball, and any sports involving jumping from a height should be included on the list of avoided activities.

Pregnant women who complain of tenderness and pain over the pubic symphysis or in the sacroiliac or coccygeal joints without acute trauma should limit participation in jumping sports (see Table 10–2). In most cases, bed rest, a light support, some massage over the sacroiliac region, and heat will provide relief.

It has been reported that once pubic separation occurs, it is more likely to be recurrently symptomatic with certain injuries in the next pregnancy (Barber and Graber, 1974). Prevention of such symptoms (which can be aggravated in dance classes emphasizing hyperabduction) is extremely important. Specific hip flexor, abductor, and adductor exercises should be done postpartum in such instances.

FRACTURES.   Although fractures are discussed elsewhere (Chapter 8), there are specific fractures of the pelvis that occur in certain sports. It is best for the pregnant female not to participate in these sports. Unless the patient is accomplished in performance, pelvic fractures are especially likely when she is thrown while riding a horse, a motorcycle, or a bicycle. Even skateboarding — a rage in the United States at the present time — can produce pelvic fracture. It also occurs when jumping from a height, as in a poor high dive, a sky dive, or other new exotic sport.

The hazard in pelvic fractures is excessive callus formation, malaligning the pelvic canal. Hence, women who contemplate having a child should abandon competitive sports in which there is risk of falls from heights. Falls on the coccyx can, of course, occur to anyone, but in sports in which speed is required the danger of falls is greater. These include speed skating, figure skating, skiing, complicated modern dance and ballet jumps, and gymnastics using a beam. In spite of this, we know of a woman jockey who rode horses up to the seventh month of pregnancy without any difficulty. Hiking, mountain climbing, and horseback riding are associated with a higher incidence of pelvic fractures. Coccygodynia is a risk in marathon running and in bicycle and horseback riding. It is being seen with increasing frequency during pregnancy, owing to present popularity of these sports.

In any of these sports, a woman should be told not to ignore pelvic pain from a fall or from overuse, and should it be present, she should be examined early. X-rays are permissible but should not be taken unless the validity of the contemplated conservative treatment is questioned. Crepitus, severe swelling or ecchymosis, spasm, gait disturbance, and weakness of extremities all indicate that x-rays must be taken as part of an orthopedic examination. In some patients, pain is the only real symptom and may be due to a stress fracture. These are apt to occur in the neck of the femur, or in the tibia, fibula, or feet, and can cause prolonged pain if the patient is not instructed to rest. If pain occurs after athletic activity, a period of rest for several weeks is indicated, and the sport should be curtailed throughout the pregnancy. If the patient insists on activity, it is best restricted to aquatic sports.

Except for major displaced fractures (which must be managed surgically), conservative treatment is advocated. Extensive workup should be deferred, if possible, until the termination of the pregnancy. Surgery for a fractured hip, of course, may be necessary in a rare instance, but it should be done with the simplest method involving the shortest anesthesia, and in a manner in which the least amount of blood loss is sustained. At no time should x-rays be withheld if they are necessary for the accurate diagnosis and treatment of fractures or dislocations. *In sports injuries a careful history of the mechanism of the injury may obviate or reduce the necessity for x-rays.*

Sprains and Strains

The musculoskeletal system is the largest "organ" of the body. Since most sports injuries involve this system, it is important to recognize the soft tissue injuries that are common in sports. The physician should be aware that any trauma to the musculoskeletal system is likely to leave residual disability of a significant degree which the mother may not notice as long as she is relatively inactive. Rehabilitation is advocated as soon as possible after pregnancy, so that less residual weakness, loss of motion, instability, or incidence of re-injury occurs when the patient resumes her sporting activity. It is common to see in practice women who have tried to "firm up" and "go back to the sport of their choice" only to have injuries acquired prior to delivery resurface. Such recurring symptoms should be thoroughly investigated. Weakness of the thighs, contractures of the tendons, and increased instability must be identified and corrected.

It is not overstating the case to say that sprains and strains left untreated during pregnancy constitute a major problem for the sports orthopedist. The symptoms of these injuries may be ignored during the pregnancy by the primary physician. For this reason, it is pertinent to review what is meant by a sprain and a strain, and why they produce lasting effects.

SPRAINS (Nicholas, 1973a). Sprains are defined as injuries to joints in which the ligaments binding the joints together are torn or stretched to some degree. The residual potential of such injuries is to produce ligamentous and joint instability and weakness, as well as subsequent traumatic arthritis. Sprains in pregnant women are frequent. There is usually a history of a twist or fall, or even a relatively minor incident, followed by rather substantial swelling of a joint. Initial suspicion of a sprain (before a hematoma develops) requires a vigilant approach with examination. Treatment consists of immediate application of ice, elevation, compression, and immobilization until the sprain heals. Some sprains, such as those of the ankle joint, heal very slowly in females, often owing to poor initial management of the injury.

Characteristically, sprains may produce only a few minutes of pain. The pain then seems to resolve and the patient feels able to continue to run or jump, as when one plays tennis for a time. However, 12 hours later, the patient may be in great pain and have severe swelling. Such injuries may take months or even a year to resolve. The most important sprains seen in sports are: (1) to the neck, back and wrist from numerous causes, often associated with twists and bends; (2) to the ulnar collateral ligament of the thumb ("gamekeeper's thumb"), such as from bowling, excessive tennis, golf swinging with a loose grip, and many other sports in which the thumb is used in throwing and catching motions; (3) to the ligaments of the knee, necessitating early expert orthopedic opinion if possible; and (4) to the ankle and foot ligaments.

An appropriate period of immobilization, elevation, and exercise with a plaster cast or brace can and should be used to treat pregnant women for torn ligaments. Should this treatment prove unsuccessful, subsequent instability, if bothersome, can be corrected after delivery and after an attempt at rehabilitation. However, one must remember that edema is characteristic of pregnancy. Casts and braces may have to be split early, and the extremity may have to be elevated during rest periods throughout the pregnancy. A good way to do this is to raise the foot of the bed on 6 inch books or blocks.

In warm weather in the last trimester, what seem to be minor sprains of the foot can prove troublesome. Frequent elevation and continuous elastic compression are important. It may be necessary to elevate the extremity at night by raising the bed on blocks, since pillows may be insufficient. It is not uncommon to see sprains of ligaments incurred in the first trimester of pregnancy cause disabling inflammation throughout the rest of the pregnancy. Such residual edema can prove vexing and may lead to sympathetic dystrophy, as well as stiffness from contracture. Acute thrombophlebitis is also common. If such a condition occurs, a year of convalescence may be required. Nerve and lymphatic entrapment may result from fibrous proliferation or scarring. In athletically minded women, who look forward to resumption of their sports after delivery, this can be one of the most serious problems seen by the orthopedist. *Early motion after adequate immobilization — even walking with a cast—and elevation after proper diagnosis of sprain are the best ways to prevent this complication.* Corrective shoes, orthotics to prevent contracture, exercises, and occupational rehabilitation are important aids in such treatment.

In most patients, a brace or cast brace, crutches, and a long convalescence with rehabilitative effort will suffice. However, in pregnant women with acute knee instability, surgery may be necessary. Where there is a locked knee due to a displaced torn cartilage, it is not proper to allow the knee to lose its extension. Manipulation to restore extension of the knee is indicated, in our opinion, if it can be done simply and with minimal anesthesia. Surgery may be required if the knee cannot be unlocked.

With the availability of arthroscopy, a displaced torn meniscus can be maneuvered, sometimes under local anesthesia, so as to unlock the knee. In some patients, articular fractures occur and fragments may be removed with use of the arthroscope. These techniques permit postponement of surgery until after delivery, if extension can be recovered and held through the use of exercises and support. Arthrography with aspiration is useful when arthroscopy is not available, or when the knee is swollen and it is necessary to determine why it is locked.

Knee sprains and torn cartilages can be confused, especially in women, with the common condition of subluxing patella. The latter injury is characterized by a buckling episode, swelling, tenderness, and hemarthrosis. It should always be differentiated from the injured swollen knee as an emergency problem, requiring orthopedic consultation if possible. Examination of the opposite knee and of other joints for laxity, and a history of "growing pains" of the knee in the midteens, should lead to the suspicion of this most common of knee ailments in females.

Treatment, after diagnostic maneuvers, consists of splinting, traction, or bracing, combined with quadriceps exercises. A long convalescence should be expected to prevent recurrence, and exercises both for strength and for stretching are important.

STRAINS (Nicholas, 1973b).   Muscle-tendon tears are frequent after the age of 30 and are apt to occur in the shoulder, elbow, and fingers in throwing sports such as tennis and golf. Calf and hamstring tears (which occur in running) and shin splints are common in jumping sports, such as the various racquet games. Cramps of the calves and thighs, often experienced in pregnancy, can also signify to athletic pregnant women that these muscles are shortened and are possible sites of tears. The calf and thigh muscles should be stretched daily throughout gestation. Cramps can occur in the ankles and posterolateral compartment of the leg as well, owing to static contractures. The results may be pain on extended walking and night cramps of the calf, which are best relieved by persistent stretching and limbering massage. The subjects of motion, linkages of joints and their muscle relations, and exercise can be reviewed by the interested reader (Nicholas et al., 1977).

BACKACHE.   The most disabling and most difficult strain to treat is backache. The pregnant woman often acquires back pain while swimming or while playing golf or tennis. Fractures and nerve root irritation from disk protrusion must be ruled out. Back strain is extremely common in women who play contact and endurance sports.

Since acute back pain is frequent during pregnancy because of ligament laxity, muscle stretching, and changing mechanics of posture, it is easy to see why prolonged sporting activity can stretch or tear the muscles supporting the spine and pelvis.

Backache in the pregnant woman should not be treated trivially lest it become a chronic problem. It is important to pay prompt attention, make a correct diagnosis, and prescribe effective rest, support, and exercise.

Most back strains are related to stretching of contracted tissues of the low back and neck, because of excessive twisting motions or fatigue. Throwing, sudden stop and start movements, and walking and running with alternating pelvic rotation are the usual mechanisms of injury.

If pain radiates to the back of the thighs or below the knees, neurologic consultation is advisable, since the pain may be of neuropathic or of osseous origin.

The treatment of most ligamentous sprains and muscular strains is rest. An electric horizontal bed can be rented, if necessary. Moist warm packs, analgesics, and massage may help to alleviate muscle spasms. Some physicians utilize 1 per cent lidocaine (Xylocaine), injected into locally tender so-called "trigger zones."

This is permissible over the sacroiliac and spinous processes if they are believed to be the primary source of pain.

Stretching exercises, supports if tolerated, and heat are used until the pain has disappeared, but it is best to curtail twisting motions and the prolonged jarring of running in such patients until they have delivered their babies. They can be encouraged to stretch, walk, ride a bike, or swim for exercise instead of participating in the sports that produced the problem.

OVERUSE (IMPINGEMENT) SYNDROME.   One form of chronic strain is called the overuse syndrome, or impingement syndrome. This injury occurs in any of the hundreds of fibrous tunnels where tendons must glide, or under their sheaths. Thus, joggers can have pain in the extensor retinacula of the ankles and feet, whereas tennis players may develop impingement under the acromion. Tendinitis, as the condition is often called, can occur in tendinous segments throughout the body. The most commonly involved include the short flexors of the feet, the finger extensors, the Achilles tendon, the patellar tendon ("jumper's knee"), the gluteal tendons to the hip, the sacrospinalis attachments to the pelvis, and the rhomboid, latissimus, and serratus attachments to the scapula, rotator cuff, and dorsal spine ("swimmer's shoulder"). All of these tendons may be stretched and overused in athletic individuals, and the stretching is exacerbated by pregnancy.

Even mild sports, such as swimming, can produce neck and shoulder girdle pain. Pain during swimming calls for changing the stroke to a nonpainful movement, as is done in any other motion that produces pain.

OTHER INJURIES.   Trauma from high-impact sports can injure the large leg muscles as well as the rib cage, lungs, and viscera. Treatment must proceed as it would in any patient with internal bleeding. We should mention only that considering the large number of women who indulge in sports today, it is likely that more injuries to the lungs and other visceral organs will be seen. The best prevention is knowledge that sports can cause such injury. Even if the trauma was produced by a noncollision sport, it is best to obtain early medical and surgical opinions if the injury is suspected of producing internal hemorrhage.

CONCLUSION

Sports medicine is an increasingly comprehensive and multidisciplinary sector of medical science. Even so, study of athletic women is still in its infancy. Until sounder statistics are available on the ability of pregnant women to perform sports and on the specific injuries that sports may produce during pregnancy, it is difficult to provide substantial information on the physiologic effects of athletic activity on the pregnant female. Yet sports medicine — especially classifications, nomenclature, and characteristics of sports injuries commonly seen today — should be part of the medical training of the gynecologist.

The obstetrician must also recognize that an orthopedic surgeon (or other physician who has had experience in the care of athletic injuries) should be called in when an athletic pregnant woman is hurt. Patients today do not expect to stop being physically fit, and demand care that will allow them to return to the sports they love following the delivery of their babies. Fitness and freedom from recreational injury are important considerations to many women and their families.

In the next decade, the increased interest in sports among women of childbearing age should assert itself in the production of more information about obstetric and gynecologic sports medicine. It is hoped that this chapter has offered a perspective on the data that do exist, and on the work that remains to be accomplished.

REFERENCES

Barber HRK, Graber EA: Surgical Disease in Pregnancy. Philadelphia, WB Saunders, 1974, pp. 179–183.

Bruce RA: Progress in exercise cardiology. *In* Yu PN, Goodwin JF: Progress in Cardiology. Philadelphia, Lea & Febiger, 1974.

Carpenter W: Anthropometric study of masculinity and femininity of body build. Res Quart, Dec 1941, pp 712–719.

Eisenberg de Smoler P, et al: Maternal exercise and fetal heart rate. Arch Invest Med (Mex) 5:595, 1974 (English abstract).

Erkkola R: The physical work capacity of the expectant mother and its effect on pregnancy, labor and the newborn. Int J Gynecol Obstet 14:153, 1976.

Katch FI, McArdle WD: Nutrition, Weight Control and Exercise. Boston, Houghton Mifflin, 1976.

Knuttgen NG, et al: Physiological response to pregnancy at rest and during exercise. J Appl Physiol 36:549, 1974.

Kovalcikova J: Effect of physical exercise on the fibrinolytic activity of serum of healthy pregnant women. Cesk Gynekol 40:125, 1975 (English abstract).

Nicholas JA: Sprains and dislocations of joints and related structures. *In* Lewis D: Practice of Surgery. Orthopedics 2, Chapter 2. Hagerstown, Md, Harper & Row, 1973a.

Nicholas JA: Injuries to tendons, muscles and soft tissues. *In* Lewis D: Practice of Surgery. Orthopedics 2, Chapter 3. Hagerstown, Md, Harper & Row, 1973b.

Nicholas JA: Orthopedic surgery in pregnancy. *In* Barber HRK, Graber EA: Surgical disease in Pregnancy. Philadelphia, WB Saunders, 1974.

Nicholas JA: Risk factors, sports medicine and the orthopedic system: an overview. J Sports Med 3:243, 1975.

Nicholas JA, Grossman RB, Hershman E: The importance of a simplified classification of motion in sports in relation to performance. Orthop Clin North Am 8:499, 1977.

Sheldon WH: The Varities of Human Physique. New York, Harper Brothers, 1940.

Williams JGP, Sperryn PN (Eds): Sports Medicine. 2nd Ed. Baltimore, Williams & Wilkins, 1976.

Chapter 11

PSYCHOLOGIC TRAUMA AND STRESS

Anne M. Seiden

INTRODUCTION: THE PSYCHOSOMATIC APPROACH IN OBSTETRICS

Clear scientific evidence that psychologic trauma in pregnancy can have lasting effects on the fetus has been hard to establish. Nevertheless there is a long history of folk belief in such effects. Scientific observers may have been especially skeptical of such beliefs, because of the prevalence of folklore associating psychologic trauma with improbable anatomic damage to babies, as is illustrated by the following anecdote.

> A visiting cardiologist was being taken on rounds in a Scandinavian hospital, being shown cases of congenital heart disease which were his special field of expertise. Because of the frequent association of certain forms of congenital cardiac malformation with polydactyly, they showed him also a young man who had no known heart disease, but had six fingers and toes on each side. "Does anyone in your family have extra fingers and toes?" he was asked through an interpreter. "No, my condition isn't hereditary," he said, "it was caused because my mother had a terrible fright while she was carrying me." With unconscious intuition, the visiting professor happened to ask, not "What frightened her?" but *"Who* frightened her?" "Oh," said the young man, "it was really a fright. A neighbor of ours, who also has six fingers and toes, popped out on her suddenly behind the barn one day."

Thus, in prescientific eras teratogenesis, complications of pregnancy and labor, and even childhood temperament, were widely attributed to various kinds of psychologic trauma or symbolically significant nutritional practices during pregnancy. Indeed, a large part of prenatal practice in folk medicine consists of methods for protecting the psychologic well-being of the pregnant woman, along with rituals concerning foods to be eaten or avoided (Spencer, 1977). Certain psychologic experiences were to be cultivated or avoided, in hope of affecting the health or psychologic characteristics of the baby, and of bringing good labor, and plentiful milk (Mead and Newton 1967).

Perhaps in reaction to the oversimplified prescientific belief in psychologic transmission from mother to fetus, Western medicine for a time developed a belief in the relatively inviolate isolation of the fetus in an intact uteroplacental system. The belief in the so-called "placental barrier," which was thought to protect the fetus from most drugs given the mother, is perhaps the strongest example of an excess in the opposite direction.

Nevertheless, psychosomatic medicine almost from its beginning did allow for the possibility that psychologic experiences of the mother might affect the course of pregnancy. In its early form, this consisted of searches for possible conversion symptoms in the complications of pregnancy. Thus, hyperemesis gravidarum, and even the milder and more usual forms of nausea in pregnancy, were seen as unconscious wishes to reject the pregnancy (Deutsch, 1945).

Habitual abortion, prematurity, and even infertility were thus seen as rather literal translations into action of the mother's unconscious wishes. In general, these speculations did not yield useful clinical approaches, since the length of psychoanalytic therapy usually recommended for resolving such deep unconscious wishes is considerably longer than the length of gestation. More recently, the careless use of psychogenic explanations for problems of women has been effectively criticized (Lennane and Lennane 1973), but the issues cannot be ignored. The problem is a serious one. Discovery of a hitherto unrecognized psychogenic etiology for problems of pregnancy and birth would be of great benefit to women, insofar as it held out promise of effective treatment or prevention. When loosely and carelessly applied, however, the risks of iatrogenic complications carrying over into the child-raising period are great. The risk is twofold. If the disturbance is wrongly thought to be psychogenic, the proper medical treatment of a medical problem might not be provided. Beyond that, the physician is absolved from further search for effective treatment, and the woman is told that in effect the problem is her fault. It is implied that there is something wrong with her emotional responses to the pregnancy and to the anticipated baby. If she takes this seriously, her confidence in her spontaneous responses is undermined, her capacity for effective coping is diminished, and her likelihood of experiencing anxiety and depression is augmented.

Thus, the problem in psychophysiologic approaches to obstetrics has been similar to that in psychosomatic medicine in general. Loosely applied, psychosomatic concepts are potentially hazardous to patient care: they suggest a division of patients into some who are "normal" and some who are "crocks." The special difficulties of the latter can be defined as outside the purview of the physician who is not a specialist in the area. A kind of inappropriate moralizing can creep into the patient-physician relationship, deriving ultimately from an inappropriate emphasis on the mind-body dichotomy, introduced into Western medicine with the concepts of Cartesian dualism (Seiden 1978b). The answer will undoubtedly be found in a judicious combination of two approaches: first, far more specificity in studies of the actual mechanisms by which psychosocial stress affects somatic reactions, and second, a recognition of the ubiquity of these relationships. The recent draft of the American Psychiatric Association's Diagnostic and Statistical Manual III for psychiatric disorders has made a major step forward by dropping the category of psychosomatic illness, as such, in favor of a rating of the importance of psychosocial factors in the genesis of a particular patient's presenting situation (Looney et al., 1978). Nowhere should this be more obvious than in the case of pregnancy and its complications. Since pregnancy begins typically with an act of sexual intercourse (inherently a psychosocial event), and proceeds in a context of mounting psychosocial implications to the climactic events of labor, birth, and bonding — themselves highly sensitive to psychosocial stresses — there is no point at which psychologic trauma and stress can safely be ignored. Greater accuracy of both the scientific models for conceptualizing these relationships and the data that permit understanding them will be important.

With increasing sophistication of psychosomatic medicine, a sharp conceptual distinction has been made between *conversion symptoms,* which literally (albeit unconsciously) translate an impulse or wish into a physical effect, and *psychophysiologic reactions,* in which stress elicits autonomic and neuroendocrine responses adapative for fight or flight, but maladaptive in other ways (see, for example, Seiden, 1978*b*). In the case of pregnancy, one might particularly look for ways in which the hypothalamic-pituitary-adrenocortical-sympathetic nervous system responses to stress might adversely affect either the maternal physiology of pregnancy or the developing fetus. For example, a number of studies have shown that catecholamines can produce varied effects, including uterine hyperactivity and vasoconstriction, changes in fetal neuroendocrine growth and development, and variations in the timing and quality of labor.

TABLE 11–1　Use and Abuse of Psychosomatic Concepts in Obstetrics

Uses

1. Psychosocial stress plays a role in the most common and serious obstetric high-risk situations. Hope of decreasing rates of prematurity, preeclampsia, and dysfunctional labor through prevention or early treatment of stress syndromes could be a major frontier for improving obstetric outcomes.
2. More specific awareness of mechanisms by which stress impairs obstetric outcomes permits targeted interventions, which are more likely to be effective.
3. General sensitivity to the psychosocial side of the obstetric patient's experience is supportive and therefore stress-reducing in itself.

Abuses

1. A medical condition may be wrongly attributed to psychosocial causes or to a personality deficit.
2. The effects of psychosocial stress may be wrongly attributed to a personality deficit.

Results of Such Abuses

1. Misdiagnosis leading to ineffective or harmful treatment and/or omission of effective treatment.
2. Labeling and blaming the victim for personality deficit leading to impaired self-esteem, secondary depression, further demoralization, impaired self-confidence and coping abilities, impaired ability to enjoy pregnancy and manage it well, impaired ability to bond with and rear child.
3. Impaired medical and obstetric care. The physician untrained in psychiatry or psychologic management often feels inadequate to help patient, responds with "fight or flight," both of which impede the giving of not only appropriate psychiatric care but also of good regular obstetric care. Impaired communication may further affect care by causing patient to fail to report, or physician to not believe, early symptoms of serious complications.
4. The patient who is perceived as crock, crazy, or complainer may be overmedicated either to quiet her, or in the belief that she needs it, with consequent risks to the baby.

Several of the many animal studies showing effects on the fetus of maternal stress, presumably catecholamine-mediated, have been recently reviewed (Morishima et al., 1978). However, the applicability of such studies to human clinical situations has been limited by both species differences and the problem of nonphysiologic doses of catecholamines. Retrospective human clinical studies have generally suffered from possible confounding of variables and biased sample selection. Until recently the more direct measurement of stress effects on the human fetus was not possible: the absence of noninvasive techniques for evaluating possibly subtle effects on the fetus prevented much active research in this area. Recently, Wilds (1978) has reviewed ultrasound studies showing effects of maternal glucose levels, drug use, motor activity, and other variables on fetal activity, breathing movements, and heart rate.

Currently a number of new conceptual and methodologic advances are opening up the field of human maternal-fetal psychophysiology for active study.

A society for prenatal psychology has been formed and has held five international conferences; not surprisingly, a variety of approaches, from the mystical to the strongly physiologic, were represented.

Within the next decade major clarifications of effects, mechanisms, and possible modifiers of effects can be expected. This review will attempt to summarize present knowledge, point to some expected areas of forthcoming knowledge, and indicate particularly some cautions and clinical concerns that appear to be warranted from the present state of knowledge.

RELATIONSHIPS OF PHYSICAL AND PSYCHOLOGIC TRAUMA DURING PREGNANCY

It is important to remember that almost any kind of physical trauma to the mother during pregnancy is accompanied by psychologic responses. Indeed, psychologic trauma may be far more clinically significant than the original tissue trauma, as when an automobile accident causes minor scratches but serious and persisting anxiety or depression with insomnia or anorexia, or both.

Physically traumatic events precipitate both organic and functional behavioral responses. For example, cerebral functioning can be disrupted organically by trauma itself or by the disturbed physiology that results. Obvious examples include *direct head injury,* with intracranial hemorrhage or microhemorrhage, subsequent swelling, and increased intracranial pressure. Less directly, injuries with blood loss can impair cerebral functioning as a result of *hypovolemia. Hypoxia* can result from hypoperfusion, lung injury (puncture, smoke inhalation, and so forth), or carbon monoxide poisoning. *Electrolyte imbalance* can occur as an indirect result of either the injury (particularly in burns) or its treatment (improperly monitored intravenous therapy). *Hypoglycemia* can impair cerebral functioning in the patient whose injury and its sequelae unduly delay feeding. Brain hypoperfusion can result from the *supine hypotensive syndrome,* particularly late in pregnancy when the pressure of the gravid uterus on the inferior vena cava impairs venous return; if this possibility is not kept in mind, the comatose patient left lying on her back for radiologic studies or routine care may have added temporary damage to her cerebral functioning, while the fetus may suffer potentially serious longer lasting damage to the brain. Indeed, several studies indicate that there is a real risk of serious hypoperfusion to the fetus from maternal hypovolemia even before the maternal compensatory mechanisms fail in sustaining her blood pressure within normal levels (Buchsbaum, 1968).

Temporary organic brain syndromes of varying degrees of severity may be caused iatrogenically, by drugs administered for relief of pain, anxiety, or depression; it is important to keep in mind the fact that usual doses of such drugs can have synergistic and unusually strong effects in the presence of any of the other sources of compromised cerebral functioning. Functionally, *pain* is an almost inevitable response to physical trauma in the awake patient. *Anxiety* about the extent of the injury, its outcome for mother and fetus, and its effect on others involved in the situation is quite likely. *Depression* may be related to grief over losses — losses of loved ones if they were killed or injured in the same accident, loss of the idealized view of the loved one if he/she inflicted the injury or carelessly caused the accident; loss of self-esteem if the patient feels she contributed to the occurrence of the accident or injury. More complex and often more intractable depressions may be related to guilt: if the patient feels she caused or contributed to the traumatic event by her own behavior or negligence, guilt may be considerable. The clinician needs to be alert to the fact that patients may blame themselves for situations which were actually quite beyond their control; moreover, they may not verbalize this unless asked.

All of the above affects may be considerably amplified if the patient's physical injuries or need for medical care severely restrain her activities. Biologically, the organism in pain or anxiety, and to a lesser extent depression, prepares for "fight or flight." If the physical positioning of the patient (restraints, siderails, etc.), or the perceived need for medical treatment, effectively restrain the patient from either fight or flight, the reaction itself may be escalated. The patient with an organic brain syndrome is especially sensitive to environmental overstimulation and to misperception of unfamiliar places and objects.

Furthermore, interventions designed to treat physical trauma during pregnancy may cause or increase psychologic trauma. For example, hospitalization following a car accident during pregnancy may subject the pregnant woman to such psychologic traumas as *isolation* from familiar persons and places, *overstimulation* in an overcrowded accident ward, *insomnia* resulting from excessive noise and unfamiliar sleep surroundings, *pain* resulting from the injury or from medical procedures, and *fear, anxiety,* or *rage* as secondary affects which themselves are stressful. Similarly, medications given to decrease maternal anxiety, depression, pain, or insomnia may have physical effects on the fetus.

In addition, in our society psychologic stress is quite commonly handled by a variety of chemical and physical means, which are to varying degrees safe for the ordinary person, but may be damaging to the fetus if used in pregnancy. Alcohol, sedatives, tranquilizers, even aspirin are examples of commonly used drugs that may be hazardous to the fetus at doses that are generally safe in the nonpregnant adult. Even such a non-pharmacologic means of achieving relaxation as the sauna bath has been recently implicated in teratogenesis, as a result of maternal hyperthermia! Cigarette smoking, which may have remote consequences dangerous to the health of the smoker, may have more immediate consequences for the health of the fetus (see, for example, Yerushalmy, 1964).

Either anxiety or depression may be manifested in the pregnant patient, as in the nonpregnant one, by sleep disturbances, loss of appetite with poor nutrition, and failure of mother and fetus to gain weight. The consequences in the pregnant patient can be severe, because of the strong association between low birth weight and many other obstetric hazards.

Thus, all of the kinds of trauma described in other sections of this book are ipso facto accompanied by or in themselves psychologic trauma. Similarly, studies showing fetal or infant outcomes of physical trauma during pregnancy are all inadvertently studies of the outcome of psychologic trauma; some of the outcome may result more directly from psychologic responses than from the original insult.

No sharp differentiation, therefore, can be made between physical and psychologic trauma in pregnancy. To repeat, all physical traumas have psychologic concomitants and results, and all psychologic traumas have physiologic results, the study of which forms a major part of psychophysiologic medicine and obstetrics.

Clearly there are hazards to mother and fetus from both physical and psychologic stress and trauma, as well as from treatment methods used to try to mitigate them. Accordingly, some cultures have organized themselves to provide maximum protection of the pregnant woman from predictable sources of trauma. Our society is not one of these; on the contrary, the pregnant woman is susceptible to all the usual causes of physical and psychologic trauma, and in addition there are specific sources of psychologic trauma related to the pregnancy itself.

A word about nomenclature is in order here. Psychologic trauma may be acute and overwhelming, or chronic and persistent. In the case of the chronic, persistent type, it is probably somewhat more common to speak of stress than trauma (Wolff, 1958). The former is a more neutral term, the latter a more clinical one: a stressor may be a positive or negative event, a challenge that is met and mastered or which overwhelms. Trauma, by contrast, refers more often to a single external event that is seen as intrinsically damaging. Since major trauma sets in motion secondary stresses, we will in this paper use both terms heuristically and sometimes almost interchangeably. However, it is clear that both acute trauma and chronic stress, however conceptualized, have definite physiologic effects. Hinkle (1973) has recently provided an important review and critique of the concept of "stress." He points out that it has been used to refer to the apparently nonspecific responses of animals to a variety of physical and social environmental changes. He views the "stress concept" as an oversimplified model, drawn originally from eighteenth and nineteenth century physics and engineering, and brought into biology and medicine in an attempt to explain the apparent paradox that many manifestations of disease are produced by host reaction rather than a direct result of external damaging agents. He points out that this apparent paradox is no longer paradoxic when one recognizes that, in social animals, "the animal in a social group behaves in a manner such as to maintain its role relationships, even at the expense of its health and life." This important observation anticipates some of the thinking which has been more recently organized in the emerging field of sociobiology (Wilson, 1975). While some concepts along this line may be highly pertinent to the understanding of psychophysiologic aspects of pregnancy, birth, bonding and lactation, they lie somewhat outside the scope of this paper.

POSSIBLE SOURCES OF PSYCHOLOGIC TRAUMA IN PREGNANCY

There are three major groups of psychologic trauma: those stemming from the pregnancy itself, those related to the situation in which the pregnancy occurs, and those that are coincidental to the pregnancy. In turn, the pre-existing personality and coping style of the mother, and the characteristics of her social support system, will interact with the trauma, amplifying or modifying her psychologic and physiologic responses to stressors. Also, the health care system within which the woman receives prenatal and perinatal care or treatment for physical trauma can be either an added part of her social support system or a source of new stressors (and most typically is both).

Sources of Trauma Related to the Pregnancy Itself

It is obvious that *the circumstances of conception in themselves may be traumatic to the pregnant woman.* Pregnancy may occur as a result of rape, incest, or a casual liaison which was not expected to generate a pregnancy. Pregnancy may occur within an established union, but unexpectedly, either because of contraceptive failure or lack of planning, or because a previous infertility unexpectedly corrected itself. The woman may have become pregnant with the expectation of cementing a union with the baby's father — only to find that the opposite occurred.

Undoubtedly, unexpected and unwanted pregnancies have always been traumatic; but there are added problems in today's world. The very expectation that every gestation should be planned and wanted makes it more complicated to adjust to the all too frequent exceptions. The woman may have to deal with not only the pregnancy itself, but a sometimes severe blow to her self-esteem. She and/or her partner and significant others may regard the fact of the pregnancy as proving that she was immoral, careless, naive, inconsiderate, or otherwise failing to meet her own internal or imposed standards. Although pregnancy was once regarded as proof of biologic maturity at least — one of the major ways that a young woman could prove she was adult, and an older woman could prove she was still young — today it may be re-

TABLE 11–2 Organic Sources of Psychologic Trauma in Pregnancy

Trauma
>   Head injury: concussion, hemorrhage (extradural, subdural)
>   Indirect head injury: whiplash (multiple cerebral microhemorrhage)
>   Hypoperfusion: blood loss with hypotension, vascular occlusion
>   Hypoxia: Pulmonary trauma, smoke inhalation
>   Electrolyte imbalances and/or shifts between intracellular and extracellular fluid spaces

Iatrogenic Organic Brain Syndromes
>   Drugs: sedative, hypotensive, psychotomimetic
>   Supine hypotensive syndrome: especially in comatose patient late in gestation
>   Sensory deprivation or overload: intensive care unit syndrome

Endocrine Disorders
>   Thyroid disease
>   Diabetes, hypoglycemic syndrome
>   Adrenocortical insufficiency or excess

Characteristics of Organic Brain Syndrome Causing Further Psychologic Trauma
>   1. Cognitive disorganization and disorientation:
>   Impaired cooperation
>   Markedly decreased usual coping skills and defense mechanisms
>   Anxiety provoked more easily and less well managed
>   Assessment and judgment of situation markedly impaired
>   2. Environmental sensitivity:
>   Need for structure and familiarity to permit cognitive restructuring
>   Need for familiar trusted persons
>   3. Affective discontrol:
>   Increased manifest affect: anxiety, guilt, depression, rage
>   Inappropriate affect, which may or may not be related to misjudgment of situation
>   Affective lability, irritability
>   Decreased or increased pain threshold
>   Apparent severe pain, which may be largely due to anxiety
>   4. Vegetative disturbances:
>   Sleep disturbance
>   Diminished or distorted appetite
>   Impaired thirst and thermal mechanisms
>   Secondary electrolyte imbalances may result

garded more as proof of *immaturity* in terms of the person's being able to orchestrate sexual activity with contraceptive effectiveness.

Although methods of abortion and regulating fertility have been known since antiquity, it is only recently that we have come to expect them to be universally available, medically safe, and ethically acceptable. In practice we have not reached that ideal, nor is it in principle entirely attainable, because it rests on the assumption that wanting a pregnancy is an either-or proposition. In fact, no matter how much the pregnancy is wanted, the mother who is at all realistic must have some appreciation of the costs it will bring, enough to yield some second thoughts. And no matter how much the pregnancy is unwanted, no matter how much its termination will bring relief, there is likely to be some degree of identification with, or fantasy attachment to, the fetus who could have become a baby.

But besides all the ancient sources of ambivalence about a pregnancy, in today's world the woman who becomes pregnant is likely to herself feel, and to be so assigned by others, a degree of *responsibility* and *choice* in conceiving and maintaining the pregnancy, which was not true in the past. With responsibility comes the possibility of enhanced guilt, self-blame, blame by others, and loss of self-esteem. There is likely to be less sympathy for the unhappily pregnant woman. Once viewed at least partly as the victim of one of life's saddest existential tragedies, today she is often likely to be viewed as merely stupid or careless. If unmarried, she is not likely to be seen as merely one who was carried away by passion or was the victim of a seducer; she is also one who did not avail herself of contraception or the morning-after pill, and one who may not choose to have an abortion. Even if married she may be subject to criticism by herself or others for having become pregnant at an inopportune time with respect to career, either hers or her husband's, the needs of her other children, or even the logic of zero population growth. The pregnancy itself may be a real embarrassment, and in some ways more strongly so now than in the past.

Furthermore, the availability of abortion means that the unexpectedly pregnant woman has to deal with not only adaptation to a pregnancy but also the need to make a decision, often in a very short time span: will she continue the pregnancy or end it? Before deciding, she may have complex social and biologic data to assimilate and weigh. Today she has potential access to new sources of data about the biologic course of the pregnancy itself. Depending on her age and medical and family history, she may have an amniocentesis before deciding whether to continue the pregnancy. If she elects this route, she will have a fairly long and often anxious period of time before results are available. Socially, in today's world, her expectations of her partner and her social network may be uncertain, confused, or at variance with theirs. Social pressures on a partner to automatically share responsibility cannot clearly be relied on. Even if they exist, his response to them is by no means certain. As she contemplates the possibility of bearing and rearing a child, she has more complex decisions than ever before, about whether to count on him for material support, or to invest her effort in preparing to support herself and the child. The cues that indicate which choice is better may be vague and unreliable, and the effort of assessing them may be considerable. More remote decisions about her ultimate plans for integrating work and child-rearing (whether in or out of the home) may also be sources of stress. Her fantasied adequacy or inadequacy for doing this may cause persistent and marked anxieties.

To reiterate, the existence of contraceptive methods, however imperfect or unavailable to a particular woman, makes our society feel that every conception represents a conscious or unconscious choice. And the existence of safe abortion methods, however unacceptable or unavailable to a particular woman, makes many people in our society feel that the maintenance of a pregnancy once begun likewise is an act of choice. Whereas choices that are freely exercised have many constructive possibilities for increasing the woman's sense of mastery, choices also can carry a heavy burden of increased sense of responsibility — including responsibility which other aspects of a woman's social system do not fully support her carrying out. She may even be pressured into exercising a "choice" that is not hers —for example, pregnant adolescents who idealistically reject abortion may be pressured into it to save their families embarrassment. Young married women who deeply want a child may be pressured to have an abortion in order not to interrupt either their or their husbands' schooling. Other women may be pressured into choosing to continue an unwanted pregnancy because someone else morally objects to an abortion or makes it economically unavailable or medically unsafe. When these pressures — in either direction — are strong and come from individuals whose opinion matters to the woman, it can at times be difficult for her to decide what her own choice is. The very knowledge of availability of a choice, for some women, may usher in a period of painfully obsessive decision-making, which is itself a psychologic stress, whichever decision she ultimately makes.

Psychologic implications of even a wanted pregnancy may be stressful. The bodily changes of pregnancy may make the woman feel either more attractive sexually, or less so; the partner's response may be the same as hers or different. As her abdomen enlarges, her pelvic vasculature increases: she may develop increased capacity for sexual arousal and release just at a time when she may regard herself as less attractive sexually (Masters and Johnson, 1966). Not all women react favorably to the body image changes that occur with pregnancy. The cult of slenderness and girlishness may make her unable to feel pride in her pregnant shape; many women in fact regard themselves as ugly or unattractive when pregnant. Normal symptoms of early pregnancy, such as fatigue and some degree of nausea, may make her feel sick rather than healthy. Old memories associated with the pregnant state may be re-evoked — memories associated with a previous pregnancy that was problematic, or memories associated with a pregnancy of her own mother's that led to difficulties for the mother or estrangement from her. If these memories are only dimly recalled or not well worked through, surprisingly strong feelings of anxiety, depression, or guilt can be mobilized. The fact that the source of these feelings is obscure, and the contrast between such negative affects and a conscious positive wish for a child, can be surprisingly terrifying. Sophisticated women who have read of "maternal rejection" can become obsessively concerned with the possibility that even mild negative affect means deep unconscious conflict portending ultimate bonding failure.

Sources of Trauma Related to Situation

The relationship to *the child's father* is a major potential source of stress and trauma. It is simplistic to relate this only to whether or not they are married, though of course that is a major situational variable. Married fathers-to-be as well as unmarried ones may react in unpredicted ways to the fact of the woman's pregnancy (Fein, 1976; Wente and Crockenberg, 1976; Coley and James, 1976). Some men regress, become childish either from sibling rivalry with the prospective baby or from seeing the wife more as a mother. Because they see her as "mother," some become unable to function sexually with the pregnant woman since having sex with her would violate an incest taboo. Others become jealous of her evident proof of adult femininity and feel the need to make similar proofs of their own masculinity, either by having affairs with other women or buying expensive "masculine" toys, such as new cars, with money that is needed for the baby. Others become overanxious about the financial aspects of responsibility for a family, and overinvest time and energy in work just when their wives most need them to spend more time and energy on being together. Although the medical team will ordinarily know when the woman in prenatal care is unmarried, often the members will not know when the married woman is experiencing significant psychologic situational stress, because she may not say so or make it obvious. She may be embarrassed or feel guilty and blame herself; if her husband is known to the doctor, she may be concerned about impairing his image.

Indeed, male discomfort with the wife's pregnancy is sufficiently common and severe that research on wife-battering has found pregnancy to be a time of increased risk. Specific trauma to the pregnant abdomen (beating, kicking, gunshot wounds) is frequent (Roy, 1977). Even in a well functioning marriage, sexual intercourse can be inhibited by taboos or medical advice (sometimes warranted, sometimes not); this is likely to place added strains on a marriage (Bing and Colman, 1977).

Other major relationships may be sources of situational trauma as well. Primitive envy of the pregnant woman is surprisingly widespread and may be quite blatant in its expression; when this comes comes from persons whom the woman had previously experienced as support figures, the loss can be devastating. Thus, the woman's own mother or sister may be more envious than supportive, particularly if their own childbearing years are over.

The employed woman or student may find that her boss or academic mentor, previously a highly encouraging person, now acts in hostile or unpredictable ways. Their motivations for doing so may be complex. They may fear that her pregnancy and later the child will interfere with career commitments, and if they sympathize with the child also, feel guilty about wanting the mother to maintain an undiminished career commitment. They may fear minor inconveniences to themselves. In a primitive way, they may have conscious or unconscious fantasies that she will give birth in the office itself and they will be somehow responsible. If the relationship is a close one, they may be troubled by the unconscious fantasy that the child is really theirs and that their unexpressed attraction to the mother — a guilty secret — is now to be betrayed by the evolving pregnancy. Surprisingly often, male bosses or co-workers of pregnant women have dreams involving the woman's pregnancy which may be disturbing to them, and which of course they may feel unprepared to discuss with her. Male peers may feel distinctly inadequate, if they see the pregnant co-worker doing the same job they do and preparing to cope with a pregnancy and baby as well. Female co-workers may have the same feeling, coupled with envy of the pregnancy, or possibly fear that they may soon face the same issues. Female co-workers who have had children themselves are somewhat more likely to be supportive, unless they have had major unresolved difficulties in coping with their own children and the job. Some women may be harshly critical of the pregnant woman's plans for child care. Accurately or inaccurately, the woman herself may view the coming child as interfering with both her work performance or ambitions and her relationships with other women and men at work and in her community.

In today's world, when many women have serious career commitments and the majority of women expect paid employment during most of their lifetimes, major conflicts may seem to arise between plans for work and commitment in the labor market and work and commitment in the home. Some of these conflicts are intrinsic, but some are quite arbitrary results of social customs and traditional expectations. For many women, the arbitrary conflicts may be more troublesome than the intrinsic ones.

Work-mothering conflicts may be grouped as absolute, relative, and social or customary. Absolute conflicts are few but real. For example, active labor and the immediate postpartum hours are incompatible with the performance of almost all jobs, including the care and supervision of other children. Work of a critical nature which could not be postponed — such as airline pilot — would therefore not be possible at a time when a woman was either in labor or likely to go into labor before landing. Relative conflict exists when performance of the job is substantially hampered by the mothering tasks, or mothering is substantially hampered on the job. Thus, work requiring high energy levels might be impaired by the fatigue of first trimester pregnancy. The pregnancy might be endangered by work in a chemical factory involving potential exposure to teratogenic chemicals (see chapter 9).

It is the socially based conflicts, however, that give the most trouble. Although many jobs are physically compatible with pregnancy and with on-the-job care of a nursing infant, there are often taboos and constraints which irrationally limit this. In primitive societies the new mother typically carries her nursling with her as she goes about her work, but in our society the work image may be seen as incompatible with a mother image. Many women unnecessarily feel they have to choose between giving up working or giving up breast-feeding, and they may feel guilty either way, as well as anxiously obsessive about the decision (Saloman et al., 1976) well in advance of the birth.

Indeed, there may be significant anxiety and conflict about employment regardless of how the mother plans to feed the baby. Maternal employment outside the home has been widely regarded as harmful to children, or as hazardous to the child's attachment to the mother. Anxiety related to this belief may be quite strong, despite the fact that systematic reviews of the available scientific literature do not support it (Hoffman and Nye, 1974; Howell, 1973).

The woman's other children may be sources of situational trauma, particularly in the case of a second pregnancy when things have gone very well with the first child until now. Depending on the first child's age and personality, and the mother's capacity for empathy with the child under stress, there may be unexpected major disruptions in a hitherto highly gratifying relationship. Often the very highly gratifying nature of the relationship with a first child is part of the motivation for having a second, but as the woman becomes involved in the second pregnancy, the first child may sense a withdrawal of interest. If the child handles this by regression to more babyish ways of relating just when the mother expected her/him to act like a mature older sibling, there may be a crushing collapse of a cherished closeness. This can give rise to overpowering guilt in the mother, regrets about the second pregnancy, anger and irritability at the first child at the very time when that child needs extra empathy. In extreme (but all too common) cases the relationship to the older child may deteriorate into a vicious circle of excessive punishment or frank abuse. The ability of the father and/or others in the mother's social network to give emotional support to the child and the mother at this time can be critical.

Economic aspects of the situation surrounding pregnancy can be obvious sources of stress and trauma. Most young people today have their children at a time in the life cycle when they are not well established economically. The costs of obstetric care itself are escalating rapidly, and health insurance often does not cover these adequately, yet the extended family often feels less responsibility to help out than in the past. Many couples have established their lifestyles on the basis of combined earnings; loss of the woman's income, if she does not return to work shortly after delivery, may make more difference than anticipated. Plans she had to continue working may collapse if it appears to entail inadequate child care, or if there are unanticipated complications of pregnancy.

Women bearing and rearing children alone can anticipate even more difficult economic situations. Welfare and child support do not ordinarily begin until after the child is born, yet medical complications of pregnancy or even the time required for prenatal care in clinics may interfere materially with her ability to continue working.

Sources of Trauma that are Coincidental to the Pregnancy

Nothing about pregnancy itself, obviously, prevents the occurrence of other sources of psychologic trauma, which could occur to anyone. Parents or spouses may die, or depart, or fall ill. Accidents or illnesses may occur, to the woman herself or those close to her. Job situations may deteriorate, expected promotions may not be made, the economy may deteriorate, wars may break out, environmental stresses impinge.

Nevertheless, these usual hazards of life are likely to have special impact on the pregnant woman, both practically and psychologically. Requirements for prenatal care and nutrition make economic reverses harder to handle. Expectations of receiving special support during the pregnancy may make it harder to deal with reality if less support than usual is received. Stresses which are unpleasant but tolerable to the woman herself may have lasting effect on the fetus, as has apparently been demonstrated for crowding in mice (Keeley, 1962) and noise in humans (Jones, 1978).

POSSIBLE EFFECTS OF PSYCHOLOGIC TRAUMA IN PREGNANCY

In principle, psychologic trauma during pregnancy can exert its effects in a number of different times and places. It may affect the woman's sense of well-being, appetite, diet, and management of the pregnancy. It may affect the quality or duration of the pregnancy, contributing to premature or delayed onset of labor or to prolonged or dysfunctional labor. It may affect the

**TABLE 11–3 Psychosocial Sources of
Psychologic Trauma in Pregnancy**

Sources Related to the Pregnancy Itself
1. Circumstances of conception (rape, incest, seduction-abandonment, ambivalence)
2. Decision whether to maintain or terminate pregnancy as a source of stress and obsessional crisis
3. Continued ambivalence about pregnancy itself:
   Negative reaction to body image changes
   Anxiety or frustration provoked by changes in sexual interest
   Fear of pregnancy impact on other relationships
   Fear of implications of ambivalence

Sources Related to the Situation in which Pregnancy Occurs
1. Relationship to baby's father:
   Overt or latent conflict
   Complicated marital or extramarital situations
   Disappointments in his reaction to pregnancy
2. Relationships to other adults: family, work, school situations
3. Relationships to other children
4. Economic factors

Sources Coincidental to the Pregnancy Itself
1. All usual sources of trauma can occur in pregnancy
2. Effect may be greater than similar trauma occurring at other times:
   Increased economic needs of pregnancy and childrearing
   Increased need for intact effective social network to provide care to mother and support in childrearing role
   Increased vulnerability to changes in relationships and psychosocial support systems

Preexisting Psychiatric Illness or Personality Disorder or Deficit
1. An often overrated source of difficulty, due to insufficient attention to social environmental factors. Serious psychiatric illness occurs in roughly 10 per cent of population, while psychosocial stress is virtually ubiquitous and endemic to contemporary situations of childbearing and childrearing.
2. Preexisting illness may be enhanced, occasionally resolved, or more often temporarily improved by pregnancy, depending on circumstances.
3. The patient who rigidly denies *any* difficulties may be at risk of sudden collapse of denial, leading to emergence of overt serious illness during pregnancy or postpartum period.
4. Neither the diagnosis of preexisting illness nor that of situational response during pregnancy excludes the other as a possible or *the* possible modifiable source of current difficulties.

character of labor itself, or the woman's capacity to handle pain; thus, it may affect the amount of medication she requests or requires, leading in turn to further effects on the quality of labor. Dysfunctional or heavily medicated labor and delivery may affect the infant's status at birth. Finally, psychologic factors may materially affect the quality of the mother-infant attachment process at birth and in the immediate and remote postpartum periods. Besides all of these effects of trauma on the mother, the baby, and the pregnancy itself, there may be indirect effects which result from attempts to *manage* psychologic trauma and its sequelae: psychotropic medication or psychiatric hospitalization may have direct effects on the baby or indirect effects mediated by their effects on the mother's ability to mother.

During pregnancy, stress to the mother can be transmitted to the fetus, causing transient or permanent effects on the development and functioning of the fetal neuroendocrine systems, and perhaps other organs and systems as well. Both anatomic and behavioral teratogenesis can result from drugs given to the mother as part of treatment of physical or psychologic aspects of trauma and stress.

Among the most disturbing findings of human and animal research, to be reviewed later in this chapter, is the extent of the risk of causing serious iatrogenic damage from approaches currently in common use. The lessons of the thalidomide and diethylstilbestrol tragedies, and the recently accumulating evidence for the fetal alcohol syndrome, unfortunately seem so far to have been learned too specifically for those drugs alone. Pregnant women continue to take large numbers of drugs, both before and after learning that they are pregnant, and both on their own initiative and by prescription. Moreover, the physician consulting standard sources of prescribing information such as *Physician's Desk Reference* typically finds vague warnings such as "the safe use of [drug X] in pregnancy and lactation has not been established; therefore, its use in pregnancy, in nursing mothers, or in women of childbearing potential requires that the possible benefits of the drug be weighted against the potential hazards."

In assessing these kinds of effects in detail, and evaluating the quality of evidence for them, we need to pay careful attention to possible mechanisms capable of mediating them. Only through knowledge of the mechanisms and of their possible variations across species and at different times of gestation will we be able to plan rational and safe interventions.

MECHANISMS OF PSYCHOLOGIC TRAUMA IN PREGNANCY

Abortion or Premature Induction of Labor

The possibility that either stress or trauma could induce abortion has been invoked since ancient times in order to account for the disparity between sometimes apparently minor maternal injury and major effects on the fetus. Buchsbaum (1968) has reviewed some of the literature on this topic and the possible mechanisms involved. The issues are complicated. It is, of course, clear that the relationship is not invariant, or all stressful pregnancies would end without the need for induced abortion! Possible mechanisms remain controversial, and it is likely that more than one may be operative. Earlier writers suggested that direct myometrial stimulation via the autonomic nervous system could initiate premature labor. Stress-induced adrenal secretion of epinephrine could have oxytocic effects on the uterus, but these effects appear to be both dose-related and modified by other factors, many of them unknown. Kaiser and Harris (1950) concluded that only higher doses of epinephrine, high enough to elicit severe systemic effects, were oxytocic. Indeed, in the lower doses, which would be more likely to be associated with clinical levels of anxiety, epinephrine had an inhibitory effect on the myometrium. A number of studies have shown that clinical maternal anxiety is related to a variety of obstetric complications (McDonald et al., 1963; Davids and DeVault, 1962;

TABLE 11–4   Mechanisms and Effects of Maternal-Fetal Transmission of Stress and Trauma

Virtually all mechanisms in Column 1 have been associated, alone or synergistically, with virtually all effects in Column 2. The strength of the relationship, or the evidence for its importance, varies with species, and with dose or strength of the stress, and its timing in gestation.

Column 1. Mechanisms	*Column 2. Effects*
1. Direct effect on fetal behavior (loud noises)	1. Ovulation, sperm transport, implantation, corpus luteum formation
2. Maternal neural transmission	2. Uterine motility
Autonomic nervous system (uterine contraction or inhibition; uterine vasoconstriction)	3. Uterine vasoconstriction or dilatation
Voluntary nervous system (voluntary modification of breathing affecting oxygenation; abdominal pressure modification in labor)	4. Fetal behavior in utero
	5. Fetal growth and development – general
3. Maternal humoral transmission	6. Fetal growth and development – neuro-endocrine systems
Catecholamines	7. Fetal growth and development – other systems, specifically those capable of becoming target organs for psychosomatic illness
Hormones (thyroid, steroid, sex hormones, insulin, others)	
4. Iatrogenic	8. Onset, timing, and quality of labor
Direct effects of drugs and procedures	9. Quality and intensity of maternal-infant attachment in postpartum minutes and hours
Self-medication with drugs and other agents; dietary changes	
Environmental factors in treatment settings	10. Late effects on child's emotional, intellectual, psychosomatic behavior:
Anxiety (hence catecholamine release) provoked by unfamiliar *physical environment*, loss of control, pain	Mental retardation
Human environment	General emotionality
Frightening or rage-engendering behavior by staff	Hyperactivity
Isolation and/or separation from familiar persons	Vulnerability to psychiatric illness
	Vulnerability to psychosomatic illness

Blau et al., 1963; Stott and Latchford, 1976; Nuckolls et al., Gorsuch and Key, 1974). In none of these studies was any specificity of relationship demonstrated between anxiety and prematurity as compared with other complications. Indeed, McDonald and co-workers found both the length of labor and the weight of the infant to be *positively* correlated with maternal anxiety levels.

Stress effects causing termination of very early pregnancies were shown in mice by Weir and DeFries (1963) as well as by Bruce and Parrot (1960), Eleftheriou and co-workers (1962), and Runner (1959). In these studies, stress in early gestation (up to the first seven days) was produced through a variety of stressors, such as forced swimming, loud noises, and forced exposure to a brightly lit open field. Earlier studies reviewed by these authors had shown that other environmental stimuli such as the odor of strange males, handling by humans, and changes in the physical environment inhibited implantation and corpus luteum for motion.

Neuroendocrine Mechanisms *Not* Causing Abortion but Affecting Fetal Growth and Development

The existence of an interaction between the maternal and fetal adreno-cortical systems was well established by the 1950's. A good review of prior work is provided by Christiansen and Jones (1957), who attempted to pin down the specificity of these results. Earlier work had established that the fetal adrenal gland does not normally appear to secrete hormones but does enlarge after adrenalectomy of the mother. Fetuses of adrenalectomized mothers had enlarged adrenals but did not appear to produce adrenal hormones beneficial to the mother. The fetal adrenal enlargement appeared to be due to activity of the fetal pituitary.

A series of studies in the 1960's investigated what might be called behavioral teratogenesis, although that term was not used at the time (Ader and Belfer, 1962; Thompson and Goldenberg, 1962; Thompson et al., 1962; Thompson et al., 1963). The research question asked was whether stress applied to the mother during pregnancy could affect fetal development, as manifested in behavioral change, demonstrable in later periods of life. Sufficient replications have been accomplished in different laboratories to present compelling evidence that rodent behaviors generally used as models of "emotionality" can be affected by a variety of forms of direct stress or "conditioned anxiety" to the mother or by injection of catecholamines during gestation. In general both changed adrenal weight in offspring and increased "emotionality" of offspring tested at varying ages were found. There appeared to be differential effect in the case of epinephrine injection, depending, as one might expect, both on dose and on timing during gestation. Another series of studies indicate that different strains of rats and mice are differentially susceptible to these effects (Thompson and Olian, 1961; Defries, 1964; Weir and Defries, 1964; Defries et al., 1967). A replication of Morra (1965) used an avoidance learning paradigm in both early and late pregnancy at three levels of stress, and found that lower fertility and viability were associated with the higher stress, and that the latter half of pregnancy seemed to be more sensitive to these treatments. Interestingly, the surviving offspring of prenatally stressed mothers showed greater levels of conditioned stress themselves (as tested in a water T-maze) but also faster swimming time and greater accuracy in maze learning. In contrast, Joffe (1965) found impaired maze learning but no difference in emotionality as measured in open field tests in the offspring of mothers who had undergone a prolonged approach-avoidance conflict sufficiently stressful to cause gastric ulcers. An ingenious study by Bell and co-workers (1965) showed that offspring stressed by maternal epinephrine injection at the time during which the fetal gut is developing had a greater frequency of ulcers when stressed in adulthood than did controls whose mothers had received similar injections at other times in gestation.

Young (1964) found the effects of norepinephrine injection during the second trimester on open field behavior of offspring to be similar to that of epinephrine injection at the same time. Joffe (1963) emphasizes the need for testing the offspring at different ages.

Human studies relating stress and trauma during pregnancy to later outcome for the child are necessarily less precise. A number of studies show that both obstetric complications and later adverse effects, such as mental retardation and behavior disorders, including hyperactivity, neurosis, character disorders, and autistic or psychotic disorders in childhood and adult life, are more prevalent among pregnancies complicated by increased anxiety, physical illnesses, trauma, and stressful life events (Stott, 1973; Stott and Latchford, 1976; Ottinger and Simmons, 1963, 1964; Ferreira, 1965; Joffe, 1969, Pasamanick et al., 1956; Zitrin et al., 1964; Sontag, 1941; Montagu, 1962; Davids et al., 1963; Gorsuch and Key, 1974). Pyloric stenosis in the infant has been related to third trimester stress, presumably mediated by a neurohumor, perhaps gastrin (Dodge, 1972). Huttunen and Niskanen (1978) showed that the apparent effects of a prenatal stress (death of father) on adult schizophrenia and criminality were *not* accompanied by higher incidence of overt obstetric complications. Rather, they appeared to be associated with effects of maternal stress responses on the developing fetal brain — particularly hypothalamic organization occurring during the third to fifth months of gestation.

Sontag (1966), as part of longitudinal studies at the Fels Institute, was able to collect reports of eight incidents in which severe and sudden emotional trauma during late pregnancy was associated with measurable (over tenfold) increases in fetal activity. These children showed no gross anatomic congenital defects but tended to be irritable and hyperactive in childhood.

The problem with all such human studies, of course, is the difficulty in identifying possibly significant etiologic variables. Women who are of lower socioeconomic status tend to have poorer nutrition and more life stress and trauma, and to raise their children under more adverse circumstances. Thus pre- and postnatal psychologic effects are difficult to separate from each other and from physical effects of these events on the developing fetal nervous system. It has been possible to demonstrate experimentally transient effects of mild maternal stress (e.g., cold pressor test, noise or voluntary hyperventilation) on fetal heart rate (see, for example, Fotheringham and Doust, 1963). For obvious ethical reasons, more severe and prolonged stresses would not be produced intentionally, and it is hard to know therefore to what extent they exert cumulative effects as opposed to causing adaptation.

As a further complication, there is every reason to believe that these effects interact with each other. Thus, the infant whose prenatal stress caused changes in development of, for example, nonadrenergic pathways in the limbic system, might be born with a greater susceptibility to postnatal stresses.

Even though maternal stress can produce permanent effects on the fetus, it nevertheless cannot always be avoided. As noted above, the pregnant woman may have to endure a variety of avoidable and unavoidable stresses. The obstetric team responsible for her care would ideally like to reduce stress or, failing that, minimize its consequences for mother and child alike. Since psychoactive drugs are generally used to decrease stress responses, for women even more commonly than men, the safety and efficacy of such drugs during pregnancy becomes a critical clinical issue.

The issue becomes more complex when one recognizes that immediate and long-range effects may differ. Thus, Morishima and colleagues (1978) found that immediate stress effects in rhesus monkeys could be mitigated by sedation. However, the evidence for long-range effects on the child are disturbing, both for self-administered drugs like alcohol and opiates and for typically prescribed ataraxic drugs.

Effects of Maternal Psychoactive Medication on the Fetus

A paper by Kornetsky (1970) reviews the effects of psychoactive drugs on the immature organism, including the fetus, and incorporates a few studies of preconceptional drug administration to the mother. Both increases in prematurity and associated complications, as well as withdrawal symptoms, are reported for infants born to opiate-addicted mothers, and a few reports of alcohol withdrawal syndrome are described.

Animal studies which were reviewed suggested the possibility of permanent alterations in development of the infant cerebral cortex from meprobamate administration to the mother. Similar deficits were not seen in offspring whose mothers had been given tranquilizing agents (reserpine and chlorpromazine), which act subcortically rather than cortically.

Earlier reviews by Werboff and Gottlieb (1963) and Young (1967) provide additional references on other classes of drugs. Several cases of severe limb malformations have been reported in women taking haloperidol during the first trimester, a result similar to that produced by the same drug in rodents and rabbits, and similar to effects produced by thalidomide in rodents, rabbits, and humans (Kopelman et al., 1975).

Kris (1965) clinically followed 52 children born to mothers on phenothiazine during gestation but found no adverse effects. However, Levy and Wisniewski (1974) reported and reviewed a number of cases of extrapyramidal effects, sometimes severe, and persisting for days to months, in infants born to mothers taking phenothiazines. Adverse effects on motor activity and audiogenic seizure susceptibility have been shown in rats (Jewett and Norton, 1966).

Lithium carbonate, originally considered safe if proper precautions were followed (Goldfield and Weinstein, 1971, Weinstein and Goldfield, 1975) now appears liable to cause an increased incidence of cardiovascular malformation (Weinstein and Goldfield, 1975). Teratogenic effects of tricyclic antidepressants have been suggested but not established (Bourke, 1974).

Minor tranquilizers (Athinarayan et al., 1976) and tricyclic antidepressants (Webster, 1973) have been associated with withdrawal symptoms in the neonate, on occasion lasting through the first postnatal month. More recently, a series of papers have documented the potential severity of the fetal alcohol syndrome, including effects such as gross teratogenesis, mental retardation, and behavior disorders in offspring of women using alcohol in pregnancy (see review by Breese et al., 1978). The extent to which alcohol alone, as opposed to nutritional deficiencies frequently associated with heavy alcohol use, is responsible for these effects has not yet been entirely clarified.

Of obvious concern to obstetricians are studies indicating persistent effects of drugs given during labor and delivery. These have been reviewed by Kornetsky (1970), Brackbill (1970), Aleksandrowicz (1974), and Haire (1973). The conclusions of these studies are disturbing. A variety of agents are capable of delaying onset of respiration and of causing persistent changes in infants' spontaneous and elicited behavior, including those that are of potential importance in the establishment of bonding and nursing (Kron et al., 1966; Brazelton, 1970). Aleksandrowicz concludes: "Summing up we may say that there is enough evidence to date that obstetric analgesia and anesthesia in any form involves an element of calculated risk to the infant. Without denying the great beneficial possibilities of analgesia and anesthesia one should consider carefully the alternative of natural childbirth by means of hypnosis or one of the various relaxation techniques whenever the physical and emotional condition of the mother allows it."

Effects of Stress and Trauma on the Course of Labor

Labor has been regarded as intrinsically traumatic in the past; indeed, attempts to manage it by means of anesthesia and analgesia have been based on this concept. However, in modern obstetrics it has become clear that much of the trauma and stress to the laboring woman is the result of pain augmented by anxiety, lack of knowledge about what is happening to her, unfamiliar persons and surroundings, and a situation which generally compromises her sense of mastery (Seiden 1977, 1978). Prenatal psychologic adaptation has also been shown to affect the amount of medication received during labor (Brown et al., 1972):

In the past, of course, the very real fear of obstetric catastrophe and even death in childbirth made anxiety hard to avoid for many women. Today, the knowledge that good obstetric care can handle most intrinsic risks is a potential source of confidence. The problem is how to make that care unobtrusively available, so that the mother's sense of mastery is not undermined by the very care which ought to enhance it.

Psychologically, a normal birth is better conceptualized as an athletic event than a medical one — a situation in which, if no unexpected trauma occurs, one expects pain but expects to experience the thrill of mastering it in attaining a valued goal. Educated and sophisticated couples today increasingly expect to master pain and avoid trauma by educational and psychophysiologic approaches, with husband participation in the events of labor and birth, with or without the use of specific Lamaze techniques.

Much customary obstetric ritual has traumatic potential which has not been shown to confer commensurate benefits: procedures such as routine enemas, perineal shaving, and confining the patient to bed during labor can all compromise the patient's mastery of well-advanced labor, making analgesia necessary where it might not have been otherwise. Surprisingly, however, several studies have shown that in psychologically prepared women, those who are also given analgesia do not report less pain (Klopfer et al., 1975, Davenport-Slack and Boylan, 1974, Henneborn and Cogan, 1975), and that in fact even regional as well as general anesthesia can impair a positive sense of mastery (Doering and Entwisle, 1975).

Indeed the experience of "having the birth taken away from me" by medication or an authoritarian attitude on the part of medical personnel has been bitterly traumatic for many women, and has undoubtedly contributed both to liability to litigation processes and the current increased interest in giving birth in nonmedical settings (Arms, 1975; Shaw, 1974; Ward et al., 1976, Hazell, 1976).

Factors Affecting the Psychology of Attachment Behavior

In many mammals besides humans, there is clear evidence of a critical period for maternal-infant attachment during the immediate postpartum period. Mothers who are prevented from touching the infant, licking and grooming it, and nursing it, carrying out the generally species-specific initial contact behaviors during the first postpartum minutes or hour, may not do so later. Even the presence of strangers, unfamiliar sounds, bright lights, or other disrupting events can break up the smooth patterning of the attachment or bonding process. These behaviors are particularly strong in those mammals that typically bear one infant at a time, and are necessarily truncated in those species that bear litters (including domestic pets).

TABLE 11–5 Psychophysiologic Management of Stress and Trauma in Pregnancy and Birth

The Apparently Normal Pregnancy
1. Assessment of overall psychosocial situation
2. Assessment of wish to continue pregnancy, degree of ambivalence, support vs. pressure from key figures in psychosocial environment
3. Continuity of care—obstetrician or midwife who will attend birth should become familiar to patient during prenatal care.
4. Matching of patient to obstetrician (or midwife) who can relate to her in a mutually satisfying way psychologically. Referral or consultation if personality clash occurs during prenatal care.
5. Prenatal education with informational, technical, psychosocial components:
   Effective nutritional education
   Effective learning of psychologic techniques for pain management
   Understanding of pharmacologic techniques for pain management, with enough information about hazards to give informed consent
   Familiarity with environments in which birth will take place, either if uneventful or if unanticipated complications develop
   Inclusion of at least one key family member or substitute throughout process—generally the husband, but in particular situations someone else may be more appropriate.

The Obviously Psychosocially Stressful Pregnancy
1. All factors applying to apparently normal pregnancy apply here even more strongly. Many severely stressful pregnancies will have presented as "apparently normal" because of woman's denial or reluctance to discuss sources of stress, or because members of the medical staff have not asked her.
2. Risk of poor nutrition will be greater if there are economic factors, time pressures interfering with food preparation, depression interfering with appetite.
3. Use of prescription, over-the-counter, and recreational drugs may be greater because of attempts to deal with stress and its consequences.
4. Temptation to use more medication/intervention during labor may be greater because of stress effects, emotionality, anxiety, and impaired cooperation, but should be resisted because the risk to the already compromised fetus, who is more susceptible to drug effects, is greater. Psychologic techniques of pain management are both more important and more difficult to achieve.
5. Need for psychosocial support of familiar persons and environment is both more important and often more difficult to achieve.

A fast expanding research area establishes that at least some of these effects occur in humans also. In births with minimal intervention, the human attachment process proceeds with the particularly salient events being skin-to-skin contact, eye contact, and nursing in the minutes immediately after birth. Eye contact is a particularly important variable in that the human infant in the hour or so after birth is able to make focussed eye contact in a way which it will not be able to again for some 6 weeks (Klaus and Kennel, 1976). Previous research had established that for many women, feelings of maternal attachment do not occur until eye contact is made (Robson and Moss, 1970).

PSYCHOPHYSIOLOGIC MANAGEMENT OF STRESS AND TRAUMA IN PREGNANCY AND BIRTH

The Apparently Normal Pregnancy

Initial assessment of the pregnant woman, whether she presents for prenatal care or for termination of pregnancy, should be unhurried enough to permit

TABLE 11–5 Psychophysiologic Management of Stress and Trauma in Pregnancy and Birth *Continued*

The Obviously Psychosocially Stressful Pregnancy (Continued)

6. Because of all the above factors, risk of all kinds of obstetric complications is greater. The obstetrician's dilemma is how to be more reassuring in the face of objectively greater risk.
7. Both the effects of preexisting stress and the frequency of greater obstetric complications and intervention make risk of bonding failure greater—and of more ominous prognosis—since childrearing in the stressful environment carries with it greater risks for child abuse if not mitigated by strong attachment.

Psychologic Management of Obstetrically Complicated Situations

1. Psychologic techniques of pain management (Lamaze or equivalent). These are preferably taught in advance, but good labor coach can do a great deal in active labor if rationale is explained to patient.
2. Single team member should be assigned, who has no other responsibility but psychological management.
3. Avoid increasing stress by use of language which patient does not understand, or by adverse remarks about patient or outcome, regardless of apparent level of consciousness.
4. Where feasible provide honest and concrete reassurance about safety of baby—visual and tactile contact after birth, hearing heart tones before birth.

Where Baby is Born Alive but Compromised

1. Maintain contact; if necessary, transport both mother and baby in same ambulance if at all possible.
2. Maintain mother's ability to give personal care to as great a degree as is consistent with survival of both.
3. Permit continued presence of significant others for mother.
4. Encourage breast feeding or at least pumping and use of mother's own milk.

Where Death or Persistent Gross Damage Occurs to Mother and/or Infant

1. Support healthy mourning process in survivors. Permit time for saying goodbyes, contact with the body if at all desired, use of other persons such as family, religious counselors, medical and social work staff.
2. Mother of dead infant in most circumstances should not be put in obstetric ward with other, happy mothers—bed in gynecology section may be preferable.
3. Psychosocial follow-up for other family members is essential, either by obstetric staff or social worker.

both a careful assessment of her situation and the opportunity for her to talk about her concerns freely. She may or may not have considered alternatives; her decision may represent a hasty response to stresses associated with the pregnancy or other factors. The physician may or may not be the best person to make this initial assessment. Barriers of age, ethnicity, language, and social class may impede communication and can sometimes be overcome by collaborative use of other members of the obstetric team. However, if she is going to continue the pregnancy, it is important that she should meet the obstetrician or midwife who will attend the birth as early and as often as possible in prenatal care. The greater the psychologic complications or risks, the more important is the principle of continuity of care. Unfortunately, our systems of delivery of obstetric care often make it most difficult for those patients who need it most to obtain the psychosocial support of personal familiarity with the person who will attend the birth. However, as the importance of these factors becomes more known, they will be regarded as an intrinsic part of obstetric care. Providing them competently yields not only better outcomes for the patient, but considerable gratification for obstetric personnel. Training programs can be adapted to recognize these needs, as they have been to meet other important needs. Aseptic technique, when first introduced into obstetrics, seemed to pose intolerable difficulties; members of the obstetric team adjusted to it as its importance became better known. Some obstetricians have a particular gift for relating to certain types of patients who may be difficult for others, such as adolescents, those with manifest psychologic problems, patients of particular ethnicity, patients who want to take an active role in the birth process or who value birth customs unfamiliar to the staff. The doctor who cannot respect and empathize with a particular patient should not attend her in labor and birth. Obviously, such a potential clash should be detected early enough in the prenatal course to permit changing the birth attendant, or receiving consultation to modify attitudes and enhance empathy. Particularly early in training, the doctor's anxiety can lead to rigidity and a need to control the patient's birth experience. More experienced obstetric staff can serve as role models and consultants to help the trainee develop an attitude of flexibility and respect for *every* patient, even those initially found difficult.

Such preparation allays anxiety by giving information about pregnancy and birth as well as specific coping techniques for labor. The efficacy of psychoprophylaxis in reducing anxiety and need for medication in labor has now been demonstrated in controlled studies (Enkin et al., 1972). Group support and actual practice of these techniques are important, so that even the patient who is medically sophisticated should be encouraged to participate. Co-participation with the person who will share the labor and birth experience is important, whether this is the husband, another relative or friend, or a staff member.

Another source of anxiety can be giving birth in an environment which is unfamiliar to the patient, perceived as someone else's territory, full of strange equipment with frightening implications. This source of anxiety can be much decreased by architectural innovations such as the homelike labor-delivery room, and by giving the pregnant woman opportunities to tour the environment and ask questions about any puzzling aspects of equipment and routine well before the expected date of delivery.

The Overtly Psychosocially Stressful Pregnancy

Patients who are not happy about the pregnancy, who are fearful of delivery, or who maintain active ambivalence or frank rejection of the expected baby pose special problems in both pregnancy and birth. There is a temptation to handle them by authoritative overly "medical" approaches, often making use of excessive instrumentation, heavy medication, even general anesthesia at the time of birth. This may seem particularly tempting when there is a firm plan for adoption of the baby. However, it is almost always unwise. The troubled pregnancy, if the mother elects to keep the baby, is at particularly high risk of later attachment failure and even frank child abuse. There is little advantage to delivering an intact baby only to have it return to the emergency room within a few weeks or months with a fractured skull. In addition, the mother who is going to give up the child has a particular need to have a positive experience of the birth. These difficult situations require especially good prenatal preparation, and it may be particularly difficult to provide it. A mature and experienced childbirth educator, who has dealt with similar situations in the past, can be enormously helpful.

Unfortunately there is often a tendency to include the husband or male partner when things are going well, but to omit him from prenatal education and the birth if the relationship has conflicts or if he is ambivalent or immature. Probably it is in these situations of marginal attachment that his participation may be more important to his future relationship to mother and baby. If he is shaky or there is doubt about his reliability, it may be wise to have a member of the nursing staff assigned to provide support for him and some supervision, rather than automatically exclude him. However, it is important to respect the mother's wishes in these matters. There are situations in which her own mother, sister, or friend may be a more appropriate personal support figure than the husband or partner, and the latter may of course not be available. Generally, the younger adolescent should attend childbirth preparation classes with the one who is likely to be with her during labor and birth, such as her mother, sister, or an older friend.

Prenatal classes in preparation for childbirth have often been omitted in these troubled pregnancies — a paradox because they are of greatest importance here. The psychologic high-risk pregnancy is most likely to be also the obstetric high-risk pregnancy, but a large proportion of the variance in outcome is accounted for by nutritional variables. Anxiety and depression are frequently associated with loss of appetite or distorted appetites. The economically deprived patient may have difficulty affording high quality protein. The adolescent may have special nutritional deficits because of her own recent or still existing growth spurt and because of adolescent food fads or lack of access to a kitchen where she can prepare foods for herself. Assuring a proper prenatal diet may be the single most important controllable factor in her ultimate obstetric outcome, but it is not easily achieved. Simple dietary prescription by obstetric personnel is *not* enough, and may even backfire. For example, a well-balanced diet prescribed in an attempt to provide good nutrition while restricting weight gain can cause iatrogenic malnutrition if there is only partial compliance. The patient who is unable to resist favorite high-calorie foods may attempt to compensate by reducing her intake of needed protein. General emotional support and specific peer group support in modifying dietary habits is especially important for the adolescent patient, whose otherwise poor diet is often a peer group phenomenon.

Patients who initially mistrust medical personnel may resist attempts to have them join prenatal groups, but these have potentially the most to gain. Providing an opportunity to ventilate concerns with others of similar attitudes may be the only way to prevent having an otherwise terrified, recalcitrant, even combative patient reach the stage of active labor.

Psychologic Management of Obstetrically Complicated Situations

Unfortunately, circumstances may make it impossible for many of the patients who might most need the kind of psychologically sophisticated prenatal care which has just been outlined to receive it. They may arrive in active labor, with no prenatal care, at term or very prematurely. They may have suffered a gunshot wound to the abdomen, severe trauma from automobile accidents or domestic quarrels, or any of the other intrinsic or extrinsic complications of pregnancy. There may be no time at all to establish a relationship; immediate care may be necessary on an emergency basis. In these situations, needless to say, one does the best one can.

If the patient is conscious, some member of the team must be prepared to assume responsibility for psychologic management, talking to her to relieve her anxiety, explaining what procedures are being done and what their purpose is. Psychologic approaches to management of anxiety and pain may be particularly important in that the patient's condition may make her a poor anesthesia risk. Short-term pain is often bearable to the patient in emergency situations, who tends to dissociate herself from it; and much of what looks like response to pain may in fact be response to anxiety. This is a particularly important consideration when there is risk of shock or hypovolemia from blood loss, in that anesthetic or analgesic agents that cause further hypotension can pose real hazards to mother or infant. Additionally, there is some evidence that the administration of obstetric drugs, always a calculated risk, has special hazards for the already compromised infant.

The patient who appears to be unconscious cannot be assumed to be unreceptive just because she is unresponsive; we have far too many anecdotal accounts of "unconscious" patients later repeating comments of medical personnel which they overheard and understood or misunderstood. Adverse remarks about the patient or the probable outcome to herself and to the baby must not be made in her presence, even if she appears to be unconscious. After the immediate stabilization of the conditions of mother and infant, if both survive, a number of issues arise in planning for their further care. Some of the same issues, and some different ones, will arise if either or both do not survive, or survive in a severely compromised condition. These will be discussed separately.

If the emergency has been resolved with the pregnancy intact, but there is need for further medical or obstetric care for the mother, we can anticipate anxiety on her part for the baby's well-being. She may or may not voice these concerns, and a simple one-time reassurance may well not be enough. She may not believe such reassurances, and in many situations of course they cannot be given with full honesty. Situations which have involved significant maternal hypotension, for example, may or may not have damaged the baby. It is not wise to give overly simplistic reassurance, particularly when it cannot be honestly given. The mother is likely to perceive the doctor's anxiety or reservations in the process of giving false reassurance. It is much better to give an honest discussion of what is known, with some emphasis on the positive possibilities, but no blanket statements that all is certainly well when this is unwarranted. Concrete evidence may be more reassuring than a number of words: for example, as soon as possible let the mother feel fetal heart tones, and review other evidence that the fetus is alive.

When the crisis has been resolved with delivery of a compromised baby at term or prematurely, or an infant who requires precautionary observation in a high-risk setting, a variety of other problems arise. Recent data provide quite compelling evidence for the higher risk of attachment failure where mother and infant are separated after birth (Klaus and Kennell, 1976). This must be countered in every possible way, with the following goals kept in mind:

1. The mother must have as much opportunity for contact with the baby as is consistent with the life-support needs of both.

2. The mother must have as much opportunity to provide personal care to the baby as is consistent with the life-support needs of both.

3. The sense of helplessness and inadequacy which the mother tends to have in these circumstances must be countered as vigorously as possible.

4. Those other family members who will be important in the care of the baby and the support of the mother must be as maximally involved as possible.

In practical terms, these goals have the following implications:

1. If the baby must be transferred to a high-risk perinatal center for further care, every possible effort must be made to transport the mother to the same center and if at all possible in the same vehicle. Opportunities to see, touch, hold, or nurse the baby must be given if at all possible, and however fleetingly; the memory of these moments helps the mother keep the reality of the baby in mind during periods of later separation if these are inevitable. Literally only seconds of contact in this period may make more lasting difference in attachment than hours together later. Even in situations of very grave risk, brief moments of contact may be possible and their importance cannot be overemphasized. This is particularly important in situations of risk in which the baby may die, in that the mother's ability to complete the mourning process and form unimpaired attachments to later children may be materially affected. Women often carry for a lifetime a sense of incompleteness about having never held the baby during its abbreviated moments of life. Being able to hold and if necessary "say goodbye" to a possibly dying infant may be important in order to complete mourning, reduce stress levels in subsequent pregnancies, and bond to later children as other individuals rather than as a substitute for the infant who died.

2. If there are significant others who are supportive to the woman — husband, male partner, her own mother, or others — the presence of one or more of them during critical transitions is extremely important. Now that we have

generally come to recognize how important this is during a normal birth, it is even more essential to recognize its importance when the birth is not normal or the outcome is uncertain. It is, of course, especially critical when the emergency circumstances of birth result in the delivery being attended by personnel who are strangers to the mother. A wide variety of rationalizations have been recently used to exclude husbands from presence at a cesarean section. Some of these are similar to the rationalizations that were formerly used to exclude fathers from the delivery room; they should be recognized for what they are. It becomes especially important if the mother will be unconscious at the time of birth, since allowing her "significant other" to hold the baby immediately after birth, and describe that experience to her later, may permit some vicarious participation.

3. Nursing the baby is likely to be especially important to the mother who has had an impaired birth experience in that it provides a restitutive opportunity to feel that things are following a normal course later on. Breast pumps should be used to initiate and maintain lactation if the infant is in too compromised a condition to suckle. The milk should be used if possible to feed the mother's own baby. If she has an abundant supply, use of the excess as donor milk for other premature or high-risk infants can help maintain her sense of self-worth.

In recent years, the attachment and bonding experience has been emphasized and brought to the attention of personnel in high-risk infant nurseries. The data indicate that infants who are separated from their mothers at birth are at higher risk of bonding failure and of subsequently being victims of child abuse, facts which have already had an impact on practice in many centers. Unfortunately, the following situation is all too common: the baby has some condition at birth that requires temporary observation in the high-risk nursery, followed by transfer after 12 or 24 hours to the regular nursery. The mother finds personnel in the high-risk nursery sensitive to attachment and bonding needs but is dismayed to find that this philosophy is not likewise followed in the regular nursery.

Situations in Which the Mother Survives, but the Baby Dies

The loss of an infant around the time of birth requires a psychologic experience of mourning that is in many ways even more complicated than that required by the loss of an older person. The tragedy may seem greater in that this child never had a chance to live at all. Depending on the circumstances under which death occurred, the opportunities for the mother to blame herself may be very great indeed. Paradoxically, she may even try to blame herself as a form of reassurance, so as to ensure success of a subsequent pregnancy by avoiding whatever she feels she may have done wrong with this one. If there was an accident or illness, she or other members of the family may blame herself or each other in an attempt to reassert mastery over the tragedy. The death of an unwanted infant may cause especially strong guilt. Many of these events may be outside the obstetrician's immediate purview, but it is well to be aware of them for ensuring that comprehensive care is given. Some inquiry into this area should be made at the time of postpartum check-ups, with psychologic follow-up by other personnel if the obstetrician does not feel competent to do so.

Again, the mother should be offered an opportunity to see and touch the baby soon after its death if she wishes; this opportunity should be extended to other family members if she does not. It may be an important part of the mourning process, which we invariably recognize in funerals of adults, but often do not in the case of infant death. In the case of a very premature infant, the decision whether to treat it psychologically as a miscarriage, or as a death with funeral ceremony may be one which the mother wishes to ponder. The psychologic definition of death of a "person" may be different for the family than the medicolegal definition of miscarriage vs. death (which generally depends on the presence or absence of air in the infant's lungs). In some cases, the mother will want the physician to make that decision for her; in other cases, she will need time to discuss the issue with other family members and/or religious counselors.

Situations in Which the Baby Survives, but the Mother Dies

Fortunately far rarer today than formerly, this event still occasionally occurs, particularly in cases of trauma in late pregnancy. The car accident en route to the hospital for what would otherwise have been an uneventful birth is a particularly tragic example. Obstetric and medical attention in such desperate emergencies will naturally be directed at attempts to save the lives of both mother and baby; the needs of the father and other family members can easily be shunted aside in the upheaval. Opportunity for the father to hold the baby immediately after birth and make eye contact before instillation of eye drops — indeed, all the actions that are important in the bonding process in any normal birth — may be especially critical when the mother has died. A father who may be raising a child under such difficult circumstances will need all the help he can get in forming an attachment. Someone from nursing or social service should be assigned on an emergency basis to the family members, to stay with them until the situation has stabilized, and to follow it up; the obstetrician will obviously not have the usual opportunity at 6 weeks' postpartum to pick up difficulties which may have emerged. A visiting nurse familiar with postpartum issues may be an appropriate person to provide psychosocial follow-up; another possible agent is the leader of childbirth preparation classes which the couple may have attended.

Situations in Which Neither Mother nor Baby Survives

This is the situation that is most likely to escape needed psychosocial follow-up, because there may be no member of the family who seems to require immediate medical attention. Assignment of someone from social services for follow-up interviews or care during the first week and again at 6 weeks is extremely important. Some family members who may never come to obstetric attention, such as the woman's other children, may be particularly at risk. The author has treated a woman who is in her sixties and was still suffering effects of the death of her pregnant mother when she was 8 years old. The death, which occurred from pneumonia, may not have been preventable in those days, but the child's trauma could have been lessened. Unfortunately the little girl had come home from school with a cold which her mother had caught, and her unavoidable grief had been vastly compounded by a tragic sense of responsibility, which impaired the whole course of her life and her own childbearing experience.

EPILOGUE

It becomes clear that the general principles of treatment and prevention of psychologic trauma in pregnancy are extensions of general principles of good medical practice. Some aspects of understanding of possible mechanisms involve highly sophisticated psychophysiologic investigation. Most aspects of treatment involve meticulous attention to the general principles of comprehensive care, and appropriate use of the whole obstetric and social service team. Present-day health planning makes a valid distinction between levels of care, but it is important to realize that the highly sophisticated perinatal care that may be provided at a tertiary care center for mother and/or infant requires close attention to primary care concepts where their psychologic well-being and often that of other family members is concerned.

REFERENCES

Ader R, Belfer ML: Prenatal maternal anxiety and offspring emotionality in the rat. Psychol Rep *10*:711, 1962.

Aleksandrowicz MK: The effect of pain relieving drugs administered during labor and delivery on the behavior of the newborn: A review. Merrill-Palmer Quarterly of Behavior and Development *20*(2), April 1974.

Arms S: Immaculate Deception: A New Look at Women and Childbirth in America. Boston, Houghton Mifflin, 1975.

Athinarayan P, et al: Chlordiazepoxide withdrawal in the neonate. Am J Obstet Gynecol *124*:212, 1976.

Bell RW, Drucker RR, Woodruff AB: The effects of prenatal injections of adrenalin chloride and d-amphetamine sulfate on subsequent emotionality and ulcer-proneness of offspring. Psychonomic Sci *2*:260, 1965.

Bing E, Colman L: Making Love During Pregnancy. New York, Bantam Books, 1977.

Blau A, et al: The psychogenic etiology of premature births: A preliminary report. Psychosom Med *25*:201, 1963.

Bourke, GM: Antidepressant teratogenicity? Lancet *1*:98, 1974.

Brackbill Y: Obstetrical medication and infant outcome: A review of the literature. Monographs of the Society for Research in Child Development, Serial 137, *35*:1, 1970.

Brazelton, TB: Effect of prenatal drugs on the behavior of the neonate. Am J Psychiat *126*:95, 1970.

Breese, GR, et al: Developmental neuropsychopharmacology. *In* Lipton, MA, DiMascio A, Killam F (eds): Psychopharmacology: A Generation of Progress. New York, Raven Press, 1978, pp 609–620.

Brown WA, et al: The relationship of antenatal and perinatal psychologic variables to the use of drugs in labor. Psychosom Med *34*:119, 1972.

Bruce, HM: A block to pregnancy in the mouse caused by proximity of strange males. J Reprod Fertil *1*:96, 1960.

Bruce HM, Parrott DMV: Role of olfactory sense in pregnancy block by strange males. Science *131*:1526, 1960.

Buchsbaum HJ: Accidental injury complicating pregnancy. Am Obstet Gynecol *102*:752, 1968.

Christianson M, Jones IC: The interrelationships of the adrenal glands of mother and foetus in the rat. J Endocrinol *15*:17, 1957.

Coley SB Jr, James, BE: Delivery: A trauma for fathers? Family Coordinator, pp 359–363, October 1976.

Conway E, Brackbill Y: Delivery medication and infant outcome: An empirical study. Monographs of the Society for Research in Child Development, Serial 137, *35*:24, 1970.

Davenport-Slack B, Boylan CH: Psychological correlates of childbirth pain. Psychosom Med *36*:215, 1974.

Davids A, DeVault S. Maternal anxiety during pregnancy and childbirth abnormalities. Psychosom Med *24*:464, 1962.

Davids A, et al: Maternal anxiety during pregnancy and adequacy of mother and child adjustment eight months following childbirth. Child Dev *34*:993, 1963.

DeFries JC: Prenatal maternal stress in mice. J Hered *55*:289, 1964.

DeFries JC, Weir MW, Hegmann JP: Differential effects of prenatal maternal stress on offspring behavior in mice as a function of genotype and stress. J Comp Physiol Psychol *63*(Suppl):332, 1967.

Deutsch H: The Psychology of Women. Vol. II, Motherhood. New York, Grune & Stratton, 1945.

Dodge JA: Psychosomatic aspects of infantile pyloric stenosis. J Psychosom Res *16*:1, 1972.

Doering S, Entwisle DR: Preparation during pregnancy and ability to cope with labor and delivery. Am J Orthopsychiatry *45*:825, 1975.

Eleftheriou BE, et al: Interaction of olfactory and other environmental stimuli on implantation in the deer mouse. Science *137*:764, 1962.

Enkin M, et al: An adequately controlled study of the effectiveness of POM training. *In* Psychosomatic Medicine in Obstetrics and Gynecology. Proceedings of the 3rd International Congress of Psychosomatic Medicine in Obstetrics and Gynecology, London, March 29–April 2, 1971. Basel, S Karger, 1972.

Erhardt A: Behavioral sequelae of prenatal hormonal exposure in animals and man. *In* Lipton et al (eds): Psychopharmacology: A Generation of Progress. New York, Raven Press, 1978, pp 531–540.

Fein RA: Men's entrance to parenthood. Family Coordinator, pp 341–348, October 1976.

Ferreira AJ: Emotional factors in prenatal environment: A review. J Nerv Ment Dis *141*:108, 1965.

Fotheringham JB, Doust JWL: The effects of maternal stress on the fetal heart rate. Wortis (ed): Recent Advances in Biological Psychiatry. Vol V. New York, Plenum Press, 1963, pp 13–23.

Goldberg, HL, DiMascio A: Psychotropic drugs in pregnancy. *In* Lipton et al (eds): Psychopharmacology: A Generation of Progress. New York, Raven Press, 1978, 1047–1055.

Goldfield M, Weinstein MR: Lithium in pregnancy: A review with recommendations. Am J Psychiatry *127*:64, 1971.

Goldfield MD, Weinstein MR: Lithium carbonate in obstetrics: Guidelines for clinical use. Am J Obstet Gynecol *116*:15, 1973.

Gorsuch RL, Key MK: Abnormalities of pregnancy as a function of anxiety and life stress. Psychosom Med *36*:352, 1974.

Haire D: The cultural warping of childbirth. (A special report on U.S. Obstetrics prepared for the International Childbirth Education Association, 1972, 1976.) Environmental Child Health *19*:171, 1973.

Hazell LD: Commonsense Childbirth. New York. Berkeley, 1969. Revised edition, 1976.

Henneborn WJ, Cogan R: The effect of husband participation on reported pain and probability of medication during labor and birth. J Psychosom Res *19*:215, 1975.

Hinkle LE Jr: The concept of "stress" in the biological and social sciences. Science, Medicine and Man *1*:31, 1973. (Also published in Inter J Psychiatry Med *5*:335, 1974.)

Hoffman LW, Nye FI (eds): Working Mothers: An Evaluated Review of the Consequences for Wife, Husband, and Child. San Francisco, Jossey-Bass Publishers, 1974.

Howell MC: Employed mothers and their families. Pediatrics *52*:252, 1973.

Huttunen MO, Niskanen P: Prenatal loss of father and psychiatric disorders. Arch Gen Psychiatry *35*:429, 1978.

Jewett RE, Norton S: Effect of tranquilizing drugs on postnatal behavior. Exp Neurol *14*:33, 1966.

Joffe JM: Note on "emotional behavior in the rat as a function of maternal emotionality." Psychol Rep *13*:734, 1963.

Joffe JM: Emotionality and intelligence of offspring in relation to prenatal maternal conflict in albino rats. J Gen Psychol *73*:1, 1965.

Joffe JM: Prenatal Determinants of Behavior. New York, Pergamon Press, 1969.

Jones FN: Residents under an airport landing pattern as a factor in teratism. Unpublished report; cited in Med. World News *19*:7, Apr. 1978.)

Kaiser IH, Harris, JS: Effect of adrenalin on pregnant human uterus. Am J Obstet Gynecol 59:775, 1950.

Keeley K: Prenatal influence on behavior of offspring of crowded mice. Science 135:44, 1962.

Kelly JV: Effect of fear upon uterine motility. Am J Obstet Gynecol 83:476, 1962.

Klaus MH, Kennell J: Maternal-Infant Bonding: The Impact of Early Separation or Loss on Family Development. St. Louis, CV Mosby, 1976.

Klopfer FJ, et al: Second stage medical intervention and pain during childbirth. J Psychosom Res 19:289, 1975.

Kopelman AE, et al: Limb malformations following maternal use of haloperidol. JAMA 231:1, 1975.

Kornetsky C: Psychoactive drugs in the immature organism. Psychopharmacologia 17:105, 1970.

Kris EB: Children of mothers maintained on pharmacotherapy during pregnancy and postpartum. Curr Ther Res 7:785, 1965.

Kron RE, et al: Newborn suckling behavior affected by obstetric sedation. Pediatrics 37:1012, 1966.

Lennane KJ, Lennane RJ: Alleged psychogenic disorders in women — a possible manifestation of sexual prejudice. N Engl J Med 288:288, 1973.

Levy W, Wisniewski K: Chlorpromazine causing extrapyramidal dysfunction in newborn infant of psychotic mother. NY State J Med 74:684, 1974.

Looney JG, et al: A new method of classification for psychophysiologic disorders. Am J Psychiatry 135:304, 1978.

Masters W, Johnson V: Human Sexual Response. Boston, Little, Brown and Company, 1966.

McDonald RL, et al: Relations between maternal anxiety and obstetric complications. Psychosom Med 25:357, 1963.

Mead M, Newton N: Cultural patterning of perinatal behavior. In Richardson, SA, Guttmacher, A (eds): Childbearing — Its Social and Psychological Aspects. New York, Williams & Wilkins, 1967, pp 142–244.

Monckeberg F: The effect of malnutrition on physical growth and brain development. In Prescott J, Read M, Coursin D (eds): Brain Function and Malnutrition: Neuropsychological Methods of Assessment. New York, John Wiley, 1975, pp 15–40.

Montagu MFA: Prenatal Influences. Springfield, Illinois, Charles C Thomas, 1962.

Morishima HO, et al: The influence of maternal psychological stress on the fetus. Am J Obstet Gynecol 13:286, 1978.

Morra M: Level of maternal stress during two pregnancy periods on rat offspring behaviors. Psychonomic Sci 3:7, 1965.

Nuckolls KB, et al: Psychosocial assets, life crisis and the prognosis of pregnancy. Am J Epidemiol 95:431, 1972.

Ottinger DR, Simmons JE: Maternal anxiety during gestation and neonate behavior. In Wortis, J (ed): Vol V, Recent Advances in Biological Psychiatry. New York, Plenum Press, 1963, pp 7–12.

Ottinger DR, et al: Maternal emotionality, multiple mothering, and emotionality in maturity. J Comp Physiol Psychol 56:313, 1963.

Ottinger DR, Simmons JE: Behavior of human neonates and prenatal maternal anxiety. Psychol Rep 14:391, 1964.

Pasamanick B, et al: Pregnancy experience and the development of behavior disorder in children. Am J Psychiatry 112:613, 1956.

Robson K, Moss HA: Patterns and determinants of maternal attachment. Pediatrics 77:976, 1970.

Rothman D, et al: Psychosomatic infertility. Am J Obstet Gynecol 83:373, 1962.

Roy M: A current survey of 150 cases. In Roy M (ed): Battered Women: A Psychosociological Study of Domestic Violence. New York, Van Nostrand Reinhold, 1977.

Runner MN: Embryocidal effect of handling pregnant mice and its prevention with progesterone. Anat Rec 133:330, 1959 (abstract).

Salomon M, et al: Breastfeeding, "Natural Mothering" and Working Outside the Home. In Stewart D (ed): Twenty-First Century Obstetrics Now. Chapel Hill, North Carolina, NAPSAC Publications, 1976.

Seiden A: The sense of mastery in the childbirth experience. In Nadelson C, Notman M (eds): Women in Context: Development and Stress. Vol III, The Woman as Patient, New York, Plenum, 1978a.

Seiden, A: Psychophysiological illness. In Franks V, Gomberg E (eds): Gender and Disordered Behavior, New York, Brunner/Mazel, Inc., 1978b.

Shaw NS: Forced Labor: Maternity Care in the United States. Elmsford, New York, Pergamon Press, 1974.

Sontag LW: The significance of fetal environmental differences. Am J Obstet Gynecol 42:996, 1941.

Sontag LW: War and fetal relationship. Marriage and Family Living *6*:1, 1944.

Sontag LW: Implications of fetal behavior and environment for adult personalities. Ann N Y Acad Sci *134*:782, 1966.

Spencer RF: Embryology and obstetrics in preindustrial societies. *In* Landy D (ed): Culture, Disease, and Healing: Studies in Medical Anthropology. New York, Macmillan, 1977, pp 289–299.

Steinschneider A: Obstetrical medication and infant outcome: Some summary considerations. Monographs of the Society for Research in Child Development, Serial 137, *35*:35, 1970.

Stott DH: Follow-up study from birth of the effects of prenatal stresses. Develop Med Child Neurol *15*:770, 1973.

Stott DH, Latchford SA: Prenatal antecedents of child health, development, and behavior. J Am Acad Child Psychiatry *15*:161, 1976.

Thompson WR: Influence of prenatal maternal anxiety on emotionality in young rats. Science *125*:698, 1957.

Thompson WR, Olian S: Some effects on offspring behavior of maternal adrenalin injection during pregnancy in three inbred mouse strains. Psychol Rep *8*:87, 1961.

Thompson WR et al: The effects of prenatal maternal stress on offspring behavior in rats. Psychological Monographs: General and Applied *76*:1, 1962.

Thompson WR, Goldenberg L: Some physiological effects of maternal adrenalin injection during pregnancy in rat offspring. Psychol Rep *10*:759, 1962.

Thompson WR, et al: Behavioral effects of maternal adrenalin injection during pregnancy in rat offspring. Psychol Rep *12*:279, 1963.

Ward C et al: The Home Birth Book. Washington DC, Inscape Publishers, 1976.

Webster PAC: Withdrawal symptoms in neonates associated with maternal antidepressant therapy. Lancet *2*:318, 1973.

Weinstein MR, Goldfield MD: Cardiovascular malformations with lithium use during pregnancy. Am J Psychiatry *132*:529, 1975.

Weir MW, DeFries JC: Blocking of pregnancy in mice as a function of stress. Psychol Rep *13*:1963.

Weir MW, DeFries JC: Prenatal maternal influence on behavior in mice: Evidence of a genetic basis. J Comp Physiol Psychol *58*:412, 1964.

Wente AS, Crockenberg SB: Transition to fatherhood: Lamaze preparation, adjustment difficulty and the husband-wife relationship. Family Coordinator, pp 351–357, October 1976.

Werboff, J, Gottlieb JS: Drugs in pregnancy: Behavioral teratology. Obstet Gynecol Surv *18*:420, 1963.

Wilds PL: Observations of intrauterine fetal breathing movements — a review. Am J Obstet Gynecol *131*:315, 1978.

Wilson EO: Sociobiology: The New Synthesis. Cambridge, Harvard University Press, 1975.

Winick M, Rosso P: Malnutrition and central nervous system development. *In* Prescott JW, et al (eds): Brain Function and Malnutrition: Neuropsychological Methods of Assessment. New York, John Wiley & Sons, 1975, pp 41–52.

Wolff HG: *In* Wolf S, Goodell H (eds): Stress and Disease. 2nd Ed. Springfield, Illinois, Charles C Thomas, 1968.

Yerushalmy J: Mother's cigarette smoking and survival of infant. Am J Obstet Gynecol *88*:505, 1964.

Young RD: Effect of prenatal drugs and neonatal stimulation on later behavior. J Comp Physiol Psychol *58*:309, 1964.

Young RD: Developmental psychopharmacology: A beginning. Psychol Bull *67*:73, 1967.

Zitrin A, et al: Pre- and paranatal factors in mental disorders of children. J Nerv Ment Dis *139*:357, 1964.

Chapter 12

POSTMORTEM CESAREAN SECTION

*Herbert J. Buchsbaum
and Dwight P. Cruikshank*

Cesarean section, one of the oldest surgical procedures, was *first* performed on the dead woman, and later on the dying woman, in an attempt to save the unborn infant. The origins of removing the unborn infant from the dead mother date back to antiquity.

With changes in society, the pregnant woman has been exposed to the hazards of accidental injury and death in the home, in the working environment (Chap. 9) and on the highway (Chap. 6). With improved transport and life sustaining equipment, the critically injured, moribund patient can now be brought to a medical facility, where the physician must decide whether to institute resuscitative measures and perform a cesarean section on the dead or dying mother.

MYTHOLOGY

References to postmortem cesarean section can be found in Greek and Roman mythology. Bacchus, the Roman god of wine, and Dionysus, son of Zeus, both allegedly were born by postmortem cesarean section. Aesculapius, the renowned healer, was delivered by Apollo from the womb of the dead Coronis on her funeral pyre. Whether Aesculapius was originally a god or a man is still unsettled. Nevertheless, temples were built in his honor and he became so renowned in the art of healing that he was worshiped as a god; ". . . for hundreds of years after his death the sick and maim, and the blind, came for healing to his temple" (Hamilton, 1942). Aesculapius (god or man), born by postmortem cesarean section, is still referred to in the Hippocratic oath, and his staff and coiled serpent are the universal symbols of the healing arts.

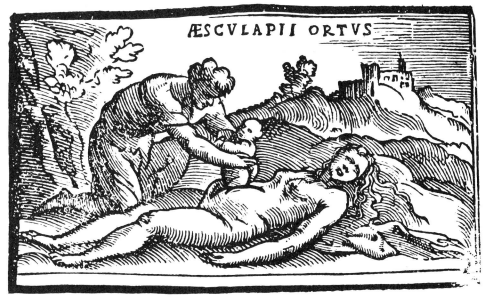

Figure 12-1   The delivery of Aesculapius by postmortem cesarean section. Woodcut from the 1549 edition of Alessandro Benedetti's *De re medica*. (P. Gall, L'econografia del taglio cesareo, 1936.)

HISTORY

The ancient Hebrews and Egyptians routinely removed the unborn child prior to burial of the mother. References to the rights of children born by postmortem cesarean section can be found in the Mishayoth, the earliest written collection of Hebrew legal traditions, compiled by Rabbi Judah at the close of the 7th Century AD. The practice of removing the infant after death of the mother was practiced in the Orient by the worshipers of Buddha. The ancient Hindus removed the unborn infant from the dead mother if fetal movements were detected. A Roman decree of 715 BC required that the fruits of pregnancy be removed before a dead woman could be placed in a sepulcher. This decree eventually became part of the *Lex Caesare* (Emperor's Law) from which the modern term "cesarean" derives. Scipio Africanus, the first Caesar, was born by postmortem cesarean section, according to Pliny the Elder.

Only Islam, among the world's major religions, forbade delivery of an unborn fetus from a dead mother. Any child so born was to be put to death, since it was felt to be the reincarnation of the devil. In Christian society, in contrast, concern about baptism and salvation required that the unborn child be removed from the mother's womb immediately after her death. In 1280, the Catholic Church at the Council of Cologne decreed that postmortem cesarean section must be done before a dead woman could be buried, to allow the child to be baptized. The Church played a leading role in stressing postmortem cesarean section; numerous references to the procedure can be found in Church writings and canon law.

Nearly 500 years after the Council of Cologne, King Charles of Sicily sentenced a physician to death for failing to perform the procedure on a dead woman. In 1757 a secular Austrian law made it compulsory for a physician to perform a cesarean section when maternal death occurred after the sixth month of gestation. Similar laws and decrees came into effect in Central Europe: in Wurtemberg, 1775; Frankfurt, 1786; the Duchy of Kurhessen in 1767 and 1787; the Grand Duchy in Bavaria, 1816; and the Grand Duchy of Baden in 1827.

The delivery of a living infant from the womb of a dead woman caught the public's fancy during the Middle Ages. Two royal British personages were rumored to have been born by postmortem cesarean section; Robert II, King of Scotland, in the fourteenth century, and Edward VI, son of Henry VIII and Jane Seymour, in 1537. However, Young (1944) finds little evidence to support the contention that either of these men was born by postmortem cesarean section.

William Shakespeare (1564–1616), reflecting the popular medical and social climate of the period, makes reference to postmortem cesarean section in two works: in *Cymbeline,* and in his more famous *Macbeth.* In the climactic scene (Act V, Scene 7) Macduff confronts Macbeth:

> MACBETH. . . . I bear a charmed life, which must not yield to one of woman born.
>
> MACDUFF. . . . Macduff was from his mother's womb untimely ripped.

The reference to "ripped" suggests abdominal delivery, and Young (1944) cites authorities who feel that "untimely" refers to postmortem cesarean section. Cesarean section, during Shakespare's time, was performed only on dead women.

Ambroise Paré (1510–1590), the renowned French surgeon and the father of trauma surgery, recognized that the interval from maternal death to postmortem cesarean section was critical for fetal survival: "If all signs of death appear in the woman that hath been in travail, and cannot be delivered, there must be a surgeon ready at hand which may open her body as soon as she is dead, whereby the infant may be preserved in safety. . . . It is far better to open her body as soon as she is dead . . ." (Paré, 1678).

Paré's pupil, Jacques Guillemeau (1550–1613), commented on the importance of maintaining an airway during the mother's agonal period to improve fetal oxygenation. His method of neonatal resuscitation was not as enlightened. Bystanders were advised to take "a little wine in their mouth and to spit it into the child's nose, ears, and mouth" (Young, 1944).

Schwarz (1862), the Recorder of Vital Statistics in the Duchy of Kurhessen, reported 107 postmortem cesarean sections without a surviving infant among 336,941 births in the Duchy between 1836 and 1848. By the late 19th Century, isolated cases, and later series, of successful postmortem cesarean sections were being reported.

Accidental Cesarean Section

In addition to surgical postmortem cesarean section, the historical medical literature contains numerous references, some factual and some fanciful, to fatal accidental maternal injury resulting in *unplanned* cesarean section. Maternal injury from blunt or penetrating trauma may result in the delivery of a live infant through the abdominal wall while causing the death of the mother.

Gould and Pyle (1897) cite the case of a pregnant woman going to draw water at a stream, who was cut in half by a cannon ball. The intact amniotic sac was removed from the water by a soldier, who delivered a living infant. Maternal injuries resulting from goring have been recorded since the time of Moses. In some cases a live infant was born through a laceration in the abdominal wall and uterine wall, whereas the mother died as a result of the injury. The mechanisms of fatal maternal injury have changed with the mechanization of our society. In a recent case (Griep, 1971), a woman nine months pregnant was thrown from an automobile as it left the highway and overturned. She sustained a laceration of the abdominal wall and a vertical rent in the anterior wall of the uterus, from which the child was expelled. The mother died at the scene of the accident; the infant, found on the ground, survived without evidence of injury.

Recent Cases

A review of recently reported cases would suggest that the causes of maternal death in which postmortem cesarean section was successful are changing. In Ritter's series (1961) of 120 successful cases, eclampsia and tuberculosis were the leading causes of maternal death; accidental death was not listed among the contributing causes. One of two cases reported by Vitsky (1964) followed fatal maternal injury in an automobile accident. The medical literature was again reviewed by Breen and Peraglie (1966), and they reported 142 successful cases, in six of which maternal death resulted from accidental injury. Weber (1971) lists traumatic accidents as the cause of death in five patients among his series of 153 successful postmortem cesarean sections. Two additional cases have been reported since Weber's review, in which maternal death can be classified as accidental; an electrocution and an automobile accident.

We have now come full circle with respect to cesarean section. First performed on the dead mother, the operation during this century has become a safe and widely performed procedure for maternal and fetal indications in the living woman. Now because of the increased likelihood of accidental injury and death during pregnancy, we must again consider cesarean section in the dead or dying woman.

Although the incidence of postmortem cesarean section is probably far greater than the reported cases would indicate, it nevertheless is an infrequently performed procedure. A busy obstetrician may never encounter this type of situation in his professional lifetime; an emergency physician is likely to.

CLINICAL SITUATIONS

A physician may be faced with the decision of whether to perform a cesarean section in two situations. In the truly emergent case, the physician is confronted with a gravida who has recently died — either at the scene of the accident or in the emergency room. In the second situation the criteria of cerebral death may be fulfilled (Table 12–1), but the maternal vital life functions are continued with ventilatory or cardiovascular support, or both. In such cases, there is time to obtain obstetric and pediatric assistance, and the procedure can be delayed to evaluate the status of the infant.

TABLE 12–1   Criteria for Cerebral Death

1. No sedative, hypnotic, or paralytic drugs have been administered to the patient for at least 24 hours.
2. Two electroencephalograms, 24 hours apart, showing electrocortical silence (must be interpreted by qualified electroencephalographer).
3. No spontaneous movement in 24 hours. No movement in response to painful or other stimuli except those based on spinal cord reflexes.
4. No respiratory effort for at least 24 hours. No spontaneous respiratory effort during 2 min of apnea (respirator disconnected).
5. No cough with carinal stimulation.
6. No brainstem reflexes:
   a. Eyes fixed forward.
   b. No eye movement on turning of head.
   c. No corneal reflex.
   d. Pupils dilated 3 mm or more, and unreactive to light.
   e. No jaw jerk, jaws loose.
   f. No snout reflex.
   g. No gag reflex.
7. Rectal temperature 90° F (32.2° C) or less.

The likelihood of successful outcome in postmortem cesarean section is related to several factors: (1) the duration of gestation; (2) the time interval between maternal death and delivery; (3) the cause of maternal death; (4) resuscitative efforts instituted in the interim; and (5) the status of the fetus, compromised as the result of maternal trauma. We define successful postmortem cesarean section as the delivery of a live infant surviving without physical or mental sequelae.

Duration of Gestation

Postmortem cesarean section is futile when the gestation has not progressed far enough for the infant to survive. With intensive intrapartum and neonatal care, survival rates of 23 per cent are attainable for infants weighing 501 to 1000 gm. However, under the emergency conditions surrounding a postmortem cesarean section, survival of infants weighing less than 1000 gm is extremely unlikely. With optimal care, 69 per cent of infants weighing 1000 to 1500 gm at birth can be expected to survive and develop normally (Stewart and Reynolds, 1974). Even under less than optimal conditions, survival of infants of this size is likely enough to justify performance of a postmortem cesarean section. A fetal weight of 1000 gm corresponds roughly to a gestational age of 28 weeks. In the emergent situation, the physician must decide solely on the basis of a rapid physical examination whether the fetus has reached 28 weeks or 1000 gm.

The duration of gestation can be best determined by such information as the date of the last menstrual period, size of the uterus at initial prenatal examination, date of quickening, and date fetal heart tones were first heard. Unfortunately, when the patient is moribund, this information may not be available.

Estimation of fetal weight by palpation of the fetus through the maternal abdomen requires considerable experience and frequent practice. However, after the twentieth week the height of the uterine fundus, in centimeters above the symphysis pubis, corresponds roughly to weeks of gestation. Thus, a 28 cm fundus corresponds approximately to a gestational age of 28 weeks. Similarly, at 28 weeks the uterine fundus is usually halfway between the umbilicus and the costal margin (see Fig. 2–2). These rules do not apply in situations such as intrauterine growth retardation or multiple gestation. However, when confronted with a dead gravida, the physician is justified in performing postmortem cesarean section if the fundal height is 28 cm or more, or if the uterus is halfway (or more) between the umbilicus and the costal margin.

Interval Between Maternal Death and Delivery

Many obstetricians of the last century, including Scanzoni, believed that the conceptus, like the maternal organs, died at the death of the mother. Duer (1879) cites reports of 21 infants born alive 1 to 5 min postmortem, and 13 born alive within 15 min of maternal death. There are fanciful reports in the literature of fetal survival among infants born 24 and even 36 hours after maternal death.

A critical review of the literature suggests that there are no authenticated cases of fetal survival when cesarean section was performed over 20 min following maternal death. Weber (1971) rated the chances of fetal survival against elapsed time as follows:

Less than 5 min — excellent
5 to 10 min — good
10 to 15 min — fair
15 to 20 min — poor
20 to 25 min — unlikely

Recent clinical reports would support this conclusion. Toongsuwan (1972) reported survival of an infant delivered 15 min after the death of the mother by electrocution at 38 weeks' gestation. The infant's condition was poor for the first 45 min, but improved after active resuscitation. The child was reported to be normal at 8 years of age. Smith (1973) reported a postmortem cesarean section performed on a mother killed at term in an automobile accident. While the mother was being transported to the hospital, cardiac massage was performed. After an interval of 25 min a 2650 gm infant with a heart beat but no respirations was delivered. The infant started breathing spontaneously after 30 min of aggressive resuscitation. During the time of resuscitation the infant experienced several convulsions. At 9 months the infant was found to have extensive brain damage with spastic quadriplegia. Autopsy on the mother revealed an aortic laceration involving five sixths of its circumference. The cardiac massage was unsuccessful in maintaining fetal oxygenation in this case, because extensive hemorrhage compromised placental circulation.

As these two cases illustrate, the elapsed time is crucial, not only for survival but also for the quality of subsequent life. The fact that survival of the infant may be possible if delivery occurs 25 min after maternal death should not be interpreted as allowing time for procrastination or consultation. With every passing minute after maternal death, the chance of permanent neurologic damage to the infant increases, and to insure optimal growth and development, delivery should occur *within* 5 min of maternal death.

Cause of Maternal Death

Postmortem cesarean section is more likely to result in the birth of a healthy infant when maternal death follows an acute insult in a previously healthy woman than when death follows a long chronic illness marked by hypoxia, acidosis, and undernutrition. The birth of a healthy infant by postmortem cesarean section is more likely to follow head trauma or electrocution than an injury with hemorrhage, hypotension, and shock. With maternal hemorrhagic shock, uterine blood flow is disproportionately reduced. The mother acts to maintain her own homeostasis. Postmortem delivery of an infant following maternal death by drowning or smoke inhalation is not likely to result in the delivery of a normal infant, since in these situations fetal oxygenation is markedly reduced secondary to the maternal insult.

The cause of maternal death as a prognostic factor in fetal outcome has long been recognized. As early as 1772, a physician noted: "In case the mother dies of a long, slow, and wasting disease, the infant dies with her always; therefore the operation [postmortem cesarean section] is useless. . . . If she dies suddenly, the child may yet be saved. . . " (Duer, 1879).

Interim Resuscitative Measures

Fetal salvage is more likely if appropriate resuscitative and supportive efforts are maintained for the mother until delivery. All efforts directed toward improving chances of maternal survival improve the chances of fetal survival. The fetus has biochemical and circulatory buffers to combat maternal hypotension and hypoxia, but these are limited and dependent on restitution of maternal blood pressure and respiration.

Maternal circulatory function must be maintained, blood volume replaced, and gas exchange supported. An adequate airway must be maintained. Maternal ventilation should be accomplished by mouth-to-mouth resuscitation, with bag and mask ventilation, or optimally, by an endotracheal tube. Open chest wounds should be sealed to assure effective respiratory exchange. In the absence of adequate heart rate and blood pressure, closed chest cardiac massage should be instituted. Circulating volume should be supported with infusions of lactated Ringer's solution or whole blood, or both. One ampule (50 mEq) of sodium bicarbonate should be administered intravenously every 5 min. Even when it is apparent that maternal resuscitative efforts have failed, ventilation, cardiac massage, and bicarbonate therapy should be continued until postmortem cesarean section is accomplished and the fetus delivered.

Status of the Fetus

In the emergent situation, there is no time for elaborate methods of fetal surveillance. Auscultation of the fetal heart tones is recommended, since postmortem cesarean section is futile if fetal cardiac activity has ceased. A Doppler unit, if available, can help to amplify fetal heart tones. A fetal heart rate of 120/min to 180/min is reassuring, but postmortem cesarean section is justified if any fetal heart activity is present, regardless of rate.

THE EMERGENT SITUATION

Operative Technique

In the truly emergent situation, only a blade is needed to perform a postmortem cesarean section. Clamps and retractors will facilitate performing the procedure but are not essential. One or two assistants are helpful in gaining exposure by retraction, in diminishing the likelihood of trauma to the infant, and in resuscitation of the newborn, but they are not essential.

The abdomen need not be prepared. A vertical midline incision which extends from the symphysis pubis through the umbilicus into the epigastrium should be utilized. The incision should be carried through all layers of the abdominal wall until the peritoneum is entered. A vertical incision should then be made into the anterior wall of the uterus, extending from the fundus to the bladder reflection. Because of the thick, well vascularized myometrium, extensive bleeding can be anticipated. If membranes are intact they should be incised. An anterior placenta, encountered after the myometrial incision, should be ignored and the incision carried through the placenta. This long "classic" incision facilitates the rapid removal of the fetus with minimal trauma. After delivery, the infant's head is held lower than the body to facilitate drainage from the nasopharnyx, but the infant should not be held vertically by the ankles. After delivery, the umbilical cord should be doubly clamped promptly and divided.

Resuscitation of the Newborn

The infant's mouth and nose should be suctioned with a bulb syringe, with the infant in a head-down position. All neonates, especially premature ones, have limited ability to maintain body temperature; therefore, efforts must be made immediately to prevent cooling. The infant should be placed in an environment where the ambient temperature is 37° C to 37.5° C, such as a radiant heat infant warmer or incubator. The infant's entire body should be dried with a towel to prevent evaporative heat loss. If the infant is crying and has sustained respirations, an oxygen-enriched environment should be provided by a mask delivering 5L/min of oxygen held loosely over the infant's nose and mouth. If, however, the infant is apneic, or has labored, slow, or gasping respirations, assisted ventilation should begin immediately. Before mechanical respirators are available, the resuscitator can place a tube delivering oxygen in the corner of his own mouth and perform mouth-to-mouth resuscitation on the infant. This should be done at a rate of 40 to 60 respirations per minute, and the pressure delivered should be just the amount required to cause excursions of the neonate's chest wall. If a small oral airway is available it should be in place during mouth-to-mouth ventilation, and the infant's head should be extended. Immediate ventilation can also be accomplished by an oral airway and a reservoir ventilation bag (Ambu bag) and mask, provided that an infant face mask and a

TABLE 12–2   Emergency Equipment for Newborn Resuscitation

Rubber bulb syringe

Plastic oral airway, newborn size

DeLee suction catheter with mucus trap

Reservoir ventilation bag, 500–1000 ml size, with newborn face mask

Laryngoscope with size 0 Miller blade

Endotracheal tubes with metal stylet
   #15 French, internal diameter 3.5 mm (for term infants)
   #13 French, internal diameter 3.0 mm
   #10 French, internal diameter 2.5 mm (for prematures)

Stethoscope

Source of oxygen

---

newborn bag is available. Reservoir ventilation bags designed for adults should *not* be used, as they may generate pressure sufficiently high to cause pneumothorax in the newborn. Table 12–2 lists the equipment which should be available for newborn resuscitation.

At 1 min after delivery the infant should be assigned an Apgar score (see Table 12–3). A 1 min Apgar score of 3 or less indicates a severely depressed and asphyxiated newborn who needs vigorous resuscitative efforts. These infants should have immediate laryngoscopy with suctioning of mucus and meconium and placement of a neonatal (size, #10 to #15 French) oral endotracheal tube. Through this the infant should be ventilated 40 to 60 times per minute, either by mouth-to-tube or with a neonatal ventilation bag (see above). The infant's heart rate should be monitored during this time. If the heart rate falls below 50 and does not respond to adequate ventilation, external cardiac massage should be instituted. This is accomplished by compressing the infant's sternum with the operator's thumb two times per second or 120 times per minute. In severely asphyxiated infants the first spontaneous gasping respirations will usually occur after 3 to 5 min of therapy, but assisted ventilation of up to 30 min may be necessary (Evans and Glass, 1976). If the infant remains flaccid, bradycardic, and apneic after 5 min of these vigorous resuscitative efforts, sodium bicarbonate (3 mEq/kg) should be administered through a catheter placed in the umbilical

TABLE 12–3   Apgar Score

Sign	0	1	2
Heart rate	None	Below 100	Over 100
Respiratory effort	None	Slow, irregular	Good, crying
Muscle tone	Flaccid	Some flexion of extremities	Active motion
Reflex irritability	No response to stimulus	Weak cry	Vigorous cry
Color	Blue or pale	Body pink; extremities blue	Completely pink

artery. This technique requires considerable experience and expertise, however, and should only be attempted by qualified obstetric or pediatric personnel.

Endotracheal intubation of a flaccid newborn is generally easily accomplished. However, it is imperative that auscultation of the chest and abdomen be done to ascertain that the tube is in the trachea and not the esophagus. Furthermore, observation of the chest wall will confirm placement of the tube, as the chest wall will move with respiration if the tube is in the trachea. If endotracheal intubation cannot be performed promptly, attempts should cease and ventilation by mouth-to-mouth or bag and mask should be resumed.

Infants with 1 min Apgar scores of 4 to 6 are moderately depressed. Usually they will respond to adequate ventilation with bag and mask or mouth-to-mouth, and tactile stimulation (drying with a towel, lightly slapping the soles of the feet). Vigorous slapping of the infant's buttocks and immersion in cold water should be avoided as resuscitative techniques.

At 5 min after birth the infant should be assigned another Apgar score. The 5 min Apgar score is prognostically significant in identifying those infants who may have neurologic damage at 1 year of age (Dranges and Berendes, 1966). If the resuscitative efforts have been appropriate and if the infant has not already suffered a marked insult, the 5 min Apgar should be 7 or more.

NONEMERGENT SITUATION

In the nonemergent situation, the physician is confronted with a moribund patient in whom biological life functions are being maintained by respirators and other life support systems. In these situations there is adequate time for deliberation regarding postmortem cesarean section, to obtain obstetric and pediatric consultation, and to evaluate the fetus.

The first decision which must be made is whether the patient is dead. Our institution uses the criteria listed in Table 12–1 to establish that cerebral death has occurred. When these criteria are satisfied, postmortem cesarean section is indicated. The necessary support of maternal respiratory and cardiovascular function should be maintained until delivery is accomplished.

In the nonemergent situation a number of techniques are available to help the physician determine fetal maturity.

An estimation of fetal size and gestational age can be obtained by ultrasound examination with determination of the fetal biparietal diameter. As can be seen in Table 12–4, the range of error increases as gestation progresses. However, as a general rule, a fetus with a biparietal diameter of 75 mm is usually of at least 28 weeks' gestational age, and a biparietal diameter of 95 mm or more indicates a term gestation. Caution must be exercised in assigning gestational age on the basis of biparietal diameter, however, for (1) the examination must be performed by someone skilled in obstetric ultrasound, and (2) average fetal size at any gestational age will vary, depending on the patient population and the geographic area.

Amniocentesis can also be used to determine fetal maturity (Table 12–5). The lecithin to sphingomyelin (L/S) ratio in the amniotic fluid is an indicator of the amount of pulmonary surfactant present in the fetal lungs. Surfactant is

TABLE 12–4   Fetal Biparietal Diameter as an Indicator of Gestational Age

Biparietal Diameter (mm)	Mean Gestational Age (weeks)	Range of Gestational Age (weeks)
45	19.4	18.5–20.0
50	20.9	20.1–21.7
55	22.5	21.7–23.6
60	24.1	23.3–25.0
65	25.7	25.0–26.7
70	27.2	26.6–28.4
75	28.9	28.2–30.3
80	31.1	29.8–32.8
85	33.7	32.1–35.3
90	36.4	34.7–38.1
95	40.5	38.3–43.1

necessary in the lungs to lower surface tension and prevent alveolar collapse during expiration. Its absence from the lungs of premature infants is a cause of the respiratory distress syndrome (RDS), the predominant cause of mortality among prematures. Lecithin, a phospholipid, is a major component of surfactant, and as the fetal lung matures, the proportion of lecithin relative to sphingomyelin increases. If the L/S ratio is 2/1 or greater, the fetus is producing surfactant and should not develop RDS.

Amniotic fluid creatinine concentration is a useful index of fetal muscle mass and renal maturity, and a concentration of 2.0 mg per 100 ml or more usually indicates a mature fetus, provided that the maternal serum creatinine level is normal. Amniotic fluid also contains desquamated fetal cells, and in the mature fetus these become filled with lipid. When the sediment of centrifuged amniotic fluid is stained with Nile blue stain, these cells become orange ("orange cells"). If 20 per cent or more of the cells in amniotic fluid stain orange with this technique the fetus is probably mature.

All of these tests can be performed on 20 ml of amniotic fluid. If the laboratory is familiar with the tests, results should be available in 1 hour (creatinine, Nile blue stain) to 3 hours (L/S ratio). Information obtained by amniocentesis should not be the deciding factor in whether or not to perform a postmortem cesarean section, however, for not all premature infants develop the respiratory distress syndrome, and of those who do develop the syndrome 40 to 70 per cent survive (Evans and Glass, 1976). In the nonemergent situation, if there is evi-

TABLE 12–5   Amniotic Fluid Fetal Maturity Studies

Test	Measures	Mature Value
Lecithin to sphingomyelin ratio (L/S ratio)	Pulmonary surfactant; pulmonary maturity	≥ 2
Creatinine concentration	Fetal muscle mass; renal maturity	≥ 2 mg/100 ml
Nile blue stain ("orange cells")	Lipid in desquamated fetal cells	$\geq 20\%$

dence from the history, physical examination of the abdomen, or ultrasound examination that the fetus has reached 28 weeks of gestation or a weight of 1000 gm or more, postmortem cesarean section should be performed.

There is considerable evidence accumulating from animal and human studies that administration of parenteral betamethasone to the mother will accelerate lung maturation in the premature fetus. Liggins and Howie (1972, 1974) have demonstrated that two intramuscular doses of 12 mg betamethasone given to the mother 24 hours apart will markedly reduce the incidence of the respiratory distress syndrome prior to 34 weeks' gestation (treated group, 11 per cent with RDS; controls, 40 per cent with RDS), provided delivery can be delayed for at least 48 hours after betamethasone therapy. However, the side effects and long-term effects of this therapy are unknown, and it should still be regarded as highly experimental. This therapy must never be used after 34 weeks' gestation, when it does not alter the incidence of RDS, or in hypertensive or toxemic patients, in whom it *increases* the perinatal mortality for reasons as yet unclear.

Assessment of Fetal Health

There is little that can be done at present in terms of fetal assessment to determine which infants are damaged beyond salvage. Electronic fetal heart rate monitoring may demonstrate patterns believed by some to represent an agonal fetus (Fig. 12–2). However, infants with severe, irreversible hypoxic central nervous system damage may have completely normal heart rate patterns. Like-

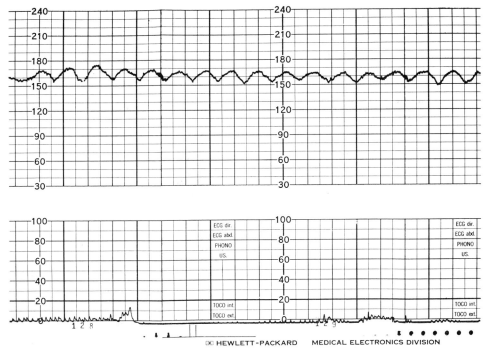

Figure 12–2 External fetal monitor tracing showing "sinusoidal" fetal heart pattern, thought to be a sign of fetal hypoxia (Baskett and Koh, 1974). This fetus was severely anemic secondary to trauma.

wise, the presence of meconium in the amniotic fluid may indicate a recent hypoxic stress upon the fetus, but most infants with meconium-stained fluid are normal, and conversely, a severely compromised fetus may have perfectly clear amniotic fluid. As in the emergent situation, postmortem cesarean section should be performed if there is any fetal heart beat present, provided the fetus meets the 28 weeks/1000 gm criterion.

Technique of Operation and
Resuscitation of Newborn

In the nonemergent situation the operation will be performed by an obstetrician with a pediatrician in attendance.

LEGAL ASPECTS

There is considerable historical, religious, and, some would agree, moral support for the performance of cesarean section on a dead mother. However, the current concern regarding medical liability may cause misgivings on the part of the physician about possible civil and criminal liability.

Every effort should be made to obtain consent for postmortem cesarean section from the patient's next of kin. This consent addresses itself to the rights of the dead mother, but who is to speak for the rights of the unborn infant in this situation? Since 1943, Oklahoma has had a law giving legal right to the physician to perform postmortem cesarean section *with* the consent of the next of kin (Vitsky, 1964). But what about the situation in which consent cannot be obtained?

Absence of informed consent for a surgical procedure may constitute a tort (battery). But *implied* consent exists in emergency situations (life-threatening situations requiring immediate medical intervention), where, due to unconsciousness or incapacity, expressed consent cannot be obtained. Under the conditions of postmortem cesarean section the rights of the child become paramount, and no jeopardy or risk is incurred by the dead mother. The greatest legal threat to the physician therefore, might be a charge of violation (mutilation) of a corpse. Ritter (1961) notes that no physician has ever been successfully prosecuted in the United States for performance of a postmortem cesárean section, even when accomplished *against* the expressed wishes of the next of kin. Thus, the rights of the child demand that precious time not be wasted in obtaining consent if it is not immediately available, or even if it is refused.

Other legal considerations are discussed in detail in Chapter 13.

REFERENCES

Baskett TF, Koh KS: Sinusoidal fetal heart pattern, a sign of fetal hypoxia. Obstet Gynecol *44*:379, 1974.

Breen JL, Peraglie RR: Postmortem cesarean section. Report of a case. Pacif Med Surg *74*:102, 1966.

Dranges JS, Berendes A: Apgar scores and outcome of the newborn. Pediatr Clin North Am *13*:635, 1966.

Duer EL: Postmortem delivery. Am J Obstet Gynecol *12*:1, 1879.

Evans HF, Glass L: Perinatal Medicine. Hagerstown, Md, Harper & Row, 1976.

Gould GM, Pyle WM: Anomalies and Curiosities of Medicine. Philadelphia, W. B. Saunders Company, 1897.

Griep EA: Traumatic live birth of a normal infant. JAMA *217*:477, 1971.

Hamilton E: Mythology. Boston, Little, Brown, 1942.

Liggins GC, Howie RN: A controlled trial of antepartum glucocorticoid treatment for prevention of the respiratory distress syndrome in premature infants. Pediatrics *50*:515, 1972.

Liggins GC, Howie RN: The prevention of RDS by maternal steroid therapy. *In* Gluck L: Modern Perinatal Medicine. Chicago, Year Book Medical Publishers, 1974.

Paré A: Cited in Young JH: The History of Cesarean Section. London, HK Lewis, 1944, p 224.

Ritter J: Postmortem cesarean section. JAMA *175*:715, 1961.

Schwarz J: Monats f Geburtsh *18*(Suppl.):121, 1862.

Smith GE: Postmortem cesarean section. A case report. J Obstet Gynaecol Br Commonw *80*:181, 1973.

Stewart AC, Reynolds EOR: Improved prognosis for infants of very low birth weight. Pediatrics *54*:724, 1974.

Toongsuwan S: Postmortem cesarean section following death by electrocution. Aust NZ J Obstet Gynaecol *12*:265, 1972.

Vitsky M: Cesarean section on the dead and critically ill. Am J Obstet Gynecol *90*:17, 1964.

Weber CE: Postmortem cesarean section: Review of the literature and case reports. Am J Obstet Gynecol *110*:158, 1971.

Young JH: The History of Cesarean Section. London, HK Lewis, 1944.

Chapter 13

CIVIL LIABILITY FOR THE INFLICTION OF PRENATAL HARM

*David Kader**

INTRODUCTION

This chapter attempts to essay a comprehensive and critical history[1] of the noncriminal legal treatment in the United States[2] of injuries wrongfully inflicted on the unborn in cases of maternal traumatic experience.[3] This particular legal dimension on trauma in pregnancy will be presented in two general parts. First, the current state of the law concerning civil liability for the wrongful infliction of prenatal harm will be summarized. This presentation will include a discussion of the historical evolution of the doctrine[4] and the primary criteria — viability and live birth — upon which judicial decisions were founded. The criteria assessment reveals both the intimate relationship between the progress in medical understanding of prenatal injuries and the law's doctrinal development, and the substantial conceptual difficulties attending the adoption of medical models for resolving social issues legally framed.[5] Second, this chapter will provide a more in-depth analysis of the current law by reviewing the judicial decisional history within three frameworks: (1) prenatal harm resulting in birth and later life with injuries; (2) prenatal harm resulting in death before birth; and (3) prenatal harm resulting in death after birth. This fact-oriented categorization is responsive to the judicially employed dominant criteria of live birth.

THE CURRENT STATE OF THE LAW — HISTORY AND CRITERIA FOR DECISION

Summary of Current State of the Law

All jurisdictions that have ruled on the issue allow a child who survives birth to recover compensation for injuries sustained before birth.[6] Although only a

*Grateful acknowledgment is given for substantial assistance in writing this chapter to Gary Dietsch, J. D., 1977, University of Iowa; member of the Ohio Bar.

few jurisdictions have permitted recovery by live infants for injuries sustained before they reach viability, no state has recently denied an infant the right to recover compensation on the ground that it had not reached viability when the injury was sustained.[7] No jurisdiction denies compensation for the wrongful death of infants who survive birth,[8] and at least two jurisdictions have allowed such recoveries when the injuries were inflicted prior to the stage at which the fetus was viable.[9] Once the child is born alive the courts show no hesitation in recognizing the child's independent legal existence at the time of the injury and tend to focus on the issue of causation in personal injury and wrongful death cases alike.[10]

The major area of contemporary conflict exists in the context of recovery sought for the wrongful death of the stillborn.[11] The principal debate here involves the adoption of appropriate criteria by which to define the legal status with regard to personhood of the unborn fetus ultimately stillborn. Twelve jurisdictions at present hold that the fetus does not achieve "personhood" within the meaning of their respective wrongful death statutes.[12] Twenty-four jurisdictions hold that the fetus need not survive birth to qualify as a "person" for the purposes of their wrongful death acts.[13] The vast majority of these decisions involved the stillbirth of a fetus which was viable at the time of infliction of harm.[14] Only one jurisdiction has upheld a suit for the stillbirth of a fetus that had not reached viability.[15] Thus, the wrongful death of the stillborn fetus constitutes the last major situation of prenatal harm infliction for which, as yet, the majority of jurisdictions in the United States decline to permit recovery of compensation.

Historical Development

The first case in the United States to decide the issue of whether the unborn could hold a wrongdoer liable for inflicting harm prior to birth was *Dietrich v. Northampton,* decided in 1884 by the Supreme Judicial Court of Massachusetts.[16] In *Dietrich,* a woman between four and five months pregnant slipped on a defect in a street in the town of Northampton and fell. Her fall resulted in the premature birth of her child, who survived birth for ten or fifteen minutes.[17] The administrator of the deceased child's estate commenced an action against the town for the wrongful death of the child pursuant to the Massachusetts wrongful death statute.[18]

Justice Oliver Wendell Holmes wrote the opinion of the court denying recovery. Holmes reasoned that no judicial precedent warranted such recovery and that no previous case had even recognized the right of the child itself to seek compensation for injuries inflicted prenatally. In addition, Holmes adopted without examination the premise popular in those times that the unborn child is a part of its mother and thus could not be granted any legal existence independent of the mother. Therefore, such a child was not deemed to be a "person" within the meaning of the statute, for the loss of whose life a lawsuit may be brought.

Although all states that have addressed the question[19] now reject the reasoning and ruling in *Dietrich,* Holmes' decision greatly influenced the law of prenatal harm for at least the ensuing sixty years. Indeed, much of the ideological basis of the present laws on prenatal harm is traceable to the logic of *Dietrich*. The nexus between Holmes' premise and current legal views is the issue of viability, whose adoption was a partial response to and rejection of Holmes' premise.[20]

The judicial origin of the viability rule can be traced to the now famous dissent of Justic Boggs in *Allaire v. St. Luke's Hospital*[21] in 1900. In *Allaire*, the majority, relying on Holmes' opinion in *Dietrich*,[22] denied a child born alive the right to maintain an action for prenatal injuries. Boggs in dissent argued for legal recognition of the independent existence of the fetus once it reaches viability, stating:

> Medical science and skill and experience have demonstrated that at a period of gestation in advance of the period of parturition the foetus is capable of independent and separate life. . . .[23]

With the continued judicial reliance on evidence made available by progress in medical science, the law on prenatal harm in time underwent rapid change.

Forty-six years after *Allaire* — and over sixty years after *Dietrich* — the United States District Court for the District of Columbia, in *Bonbrest v. Kotz*,[24] rejected Justice Holmes' decision in *Dietrich* and reasoned, like Justice Boggs, that an unborn viable fetus is capable of living outside its mother's womb, and should therefore be recognized as an independent legal being.[25] In *Bonbrest*, the court recognized the legal right of a child to commence a civil action for damages for injuries caused by the negligence of the doctor and hospital during his delivery. Thus began what the American Law Institute has called "the most spectacular complete reversal of a well-settled rule in the history of the Law of Torts" until the cases on products liability arose.[26]

While many commentators correctly cite *Bonbrest* as the case which started the doctrinal rebellion against *Dietrich*,[27] *Bonbrest* was not in fact the first decision by an American court to reject the holding and reasoning of *Dietrich*. At least four cases can be located which anticipated modern thought.[28]

Shortly after the *Bonbrest* decision, the Minnesota Supreme Court heard a case that was the first reported United States decision to recognize the independent legal existence of the unborn child that fails to survive birth.[29] In *Verkennes v. Corniea*, the court upheld an action brought for the wrongful death of an unborn child which had reached viability, quoting Justice Boggs with approval and concluding:

> It seems too plain for argument that where independent existence is possible and life is destroyed through a wrongful act a cause of action arises under the statutes cited.[30]

The *Bonbrest* and *Verkennes* decisions reversed the previous trend, which had adhered to *Dietrich*. They provided the necessary impetus and authority for courts that had not yet ruled on the question to escape the restraining influence of *Dietrich*. The body of precedent that rapidly formed, coupled with a growing judicial recognition of advancing medical understanding of fetal life, gradually induced those jurisdictions that had adopted Holmes' reasoning prior to *Bonbrest* and *Verkennes* to reverse themselves and join the trend of the majority of jurisdictions.

Criteria for Decision

The Viability Rule

Fetal viability has been relied upon as a ground for recognizing existence independent from the mother prior to birth[31] and thus the existence of personhood sufficient in law to permit recovery for wrongfully inflicted prenatal harm. In cases of live birth, the modern trend has been to move away completely from considerations of viability. However, those courts that recognize a right to recovery for the wrongful death of a stillborn fetus rely on viability as the point at which the fetus achieved personhood within the meaning of the statutes[32] authorizing the cause of action. Because of the continued importance of viability criteria in this area, an enumeration of the various definitions of viability that the courts have advanced would be useful. Almost all of the definitions of viability are phrased in terms of the fetus's capability of independent existence separate from its mother.[33] The various judicial formulations have included the following: capable of living outside the uterus or womb;[34] capable of independent existence, not part of the mother;[35] capable of separate existence apart from the mother;[36] capable of independent life;[37] capable of remaining alive after birth independent of the mother;[38] when destruction of the mother's life would not necessarily mean its death, and when, if separated from the mother, it would be mature enough to live and grow;[39] when it is at such a stage of development as to permit continued existence, under normal conditions, outside the womb.[40]

The definition formulations themselves suggest that no exact temporal measure of viability exists. The decisions generally do agree, however, that viability is usually attained between the sixth and the eighth months of pregnancy.[41] As for fetuses less than six months old who are *eventually stillborn,* the decisions illustrate a significant amount of variance in their viability analysis and conclusion. Some, such as *Carroll v. Skloff,*[42] made no reference to viability and relied exclusively on the live-birth distinction to deny recovery. Two other courts[43] have, on the other hand, looked to the physical condition of the fetus itself at the time of its stillbirth, finding viability from the fact that it was fully or perfectly formed at birth.

In *In re Logan's Estate,*[44] which involved a suit in New York for the wrongful death of a five and one-half month old stillborn fetus that was injured in its third month of development, the parties approached the case as if the fetus were viable at the time of birth. Yet, in *Occhipinti v. Rheem Manufacturing Company,*[45] which involved a mother's suit for personal injuries and mental distress stemming from an automobile accident which caused the stillbirth of her five and one-half month old fetus, the parties treated the case as if the fetus were not viable.

The cases of *Peterson v. Nationwide Mutual Insurance Company*[46] and *Torigian v. Watertown News Co.*[47] also illustrate the confusion in this area. In *Peterson,* the Ohio Supreme Court decided that a child who was injured in its twenty-second week of prenatal development, who was born two weeks later, and who died twenty-one hours after birth was a "person" within the meaning of a liability insurance contract providing death benefits for a "person" killed as a result of a motor vehicle accident.[48] The court held that the situation fell within the ambit of the holding of a previous case, which upheld liability for prenatal injuries suffered "by a viable child delivered alive."[49] Thus, the court treated the twenty-four week old fetus as viable, relying on the fact that it lived for twenty-one hours after birth and on the issuance of the certificate of live birth as proof of the child's capability of independent existence.[50] Yet, in *Torigian,* which upheld a suit for the wrongful death of a child who was injured when its mother was three and one-half months pregnant, born eight and one-half weeks later, and who died approximately two and one-half hours after birth, the Supreme Judicial Court of Massachusetts analyzed the case under the assumption that the child was not viable, without referring to the child's ability to survive birth as evidence of its viability.[51] These two cases raise a potential issue which those cases adhering to the viability rule have not discussed; namely, whether viability is to be determined at the moment of injury infliction or death. Most of the decisions, like *Torigian,* characterize the fetus as viable or previable in relation to its development at the time of the injury.[52] However, certain cases, such as *Peterson,* apparently have looked to the child's development at the time of birth in order to ascertain whether it was viable.[53] In any event, in those jurisdictions that reject the live-birth requirement and adhere to the viability requirement,[54] this issue of the relevant time at which to ascertain the fetus' viability will undoubtedly arise.

In light of these various interpretations and uses of viability criteria it is not surprising that a number of decisions have criticized the viability rule. Some of these criticisms have been made by courts which favored the live-birth distinction,[55] while others were made in the context of suits where the child had been born alive after being injured before it had reached viability.[56]

One of the major objections advanced against the viability rule is that it is "impossible of practical application" because of difficulties of proof[57] and medical uncertainty.[58] The rule has also been criticized as being irrelevant[59] and arbitrary.[60] The cases have stated, for example, that the viability of the fetus is irrelevant: to the purpose of protecting the child's "right to begin life with a sound mind and body;"[61] in view of medical knowledge;[62] to the purposes of justice;[63] for the purposes of duty, because the separate existence of a live-born child is recognized at conception;[64] because with a stillborn child, damages are too speculative to allow a recovery of compensation.[65]

Outright rejection of viability as a criterion was made in *Smith v. Brennan.*[66] In this ruling the New Jersey Supreme Court stated that the viability criterion was an historical anomaly and no longer necessary in light of the law's repudiation of the *Dietrich* rationale of the unity of identity of the unborn fetus and its mother. The court stated that the rule was first advanced in Justice Bogg's dissent in *Allaire v. St. Luke's Hospital* as an attempt to refute the *Dietrich* premise, and in view of the repudiation of *Dietrich,* has outlived its relevance. Consistent with this view, at least in the context of the child's suit for its own prenatal injuries, the cases have stated that causation is the issue, not viability, and that lack of viability does not necessarily render the problem of proving causation insurmountable.[67]

In the context of the wrongful death suit for the death of a stillborn fetus, the courts that favor the live-birth distinction reject the viability rule for its impossibility in practical application and argue that it is no less arbitrary than the live-birth distinction.[68] Finally, in *Presley v. Newport Hospital,*[69] a plurality opinion of the Rhode Island Supreme Court posited it as absurd to rely on the viability of a fetus in order to uphold an action for its wrongful death, while other decisions in Rhode Island have held that the viability of a fetus is irrelevant for the purposes of the live-born child's right to sue for injuries inflicted prior to reaching viability.

The viability rule and its application in the different contexts of suits for injuries and wrongful death actions for live-born and stillborn infants will be discussed further in separate sections of the chapter.[70]

The Live-Birth Requirement

The previous discussion has shown that some courts limit the law's protection of the unborn fetus from wrongful injury by requiring survival to live birth.[71] Twelve jurisdictions flatly hold that the stillborn child is not included within the coverage of their wrongful death statutes and adhere to live birth as the decisive criterion.[72] Once the child is born alive — even if it is able to survive only a few minutes[73] — most courts relate the child's independent legal existence back to the moment of conception;[74] but if it is unable to survive birth, it receives no legal protection at all. The primary judicial criticisms[75] of the live-birth requirement are that it is unjust, arbitrary, absurd, and even unconstitutional. Judicial defenses[76] of the live-birth requirement rest on the relative certainty of the event of birth, making it an unambiguous requirement for determining presence or absence of legal protection for wrongful infliction of injury. Reference is made to the medical uncertainty as to the moment of viability as a reason for adopting live birth as the test. However, the premise that a line must be drawn at all is not examined, neither is the general judicial assumption that there is medical agreement on the meaning of live birth or on its apparent ease of proof.[77]

Those jurisdictions that adhere to the live-birth requirement face the responsibility and necessity of selecting, from among a number of available "life signs,"[78] those deemed most appropriate in defining the live-birth requirement.

LIFE WITH INJURIES

Introduction and History

No jurisdiction currently denies a child the right to sue for injuries wrongfully inflicted prior to birth.[79] Since the historical development to this current state of the law was a process of rejecting the reasons for denying the child's lawsuit, it would be useful in understanding the modern law to first briefly discuss the now rejected early rationales advanced to oppose such suits.

A number of reasons were given in the case law for denying the injured child's lawsuit. In addition to the *Dietrich* premise that the injured unborn child is a part of its mother,[80] courts also denied relief on the ground that proof of a causal relationship between the injury and the alleged tortious conduct was so difficult as to invite speculative awards and fraudulent claims.[81] Furthermore, those participating in these decisions felt compelled by the doctrine of *stare decisis* to persist in denying a cause of action because of the lack of precedent favorable to a contrary view.[82] As a result of the absence of progressive precedent, some courts felt that any recognition of a right to sue should await legislative action.[83] Finally, of major concern to some courts was the prospect that an infant would later be able to sue its own mother for injuries caused by her negligent conduct during pregnancy.[84]

Beginning with *Bonbrest,* however, the *stare decisis* argument was undercut and the path paved for the ensuing wholesale abandonment of the *Dietrich* decision. Although Judge McGuire purported to factually distinguish *Dietrich* from the situation involved in *Bonbrest,* he directly criticized Holmes' premise in *Dietrich* that the unborn child is a part of its mother as a long-outmoded legal fiction[85] which could no longer be allowed to leave unremedied the obvious harm to the child without being inconsistent with notions of natural justice. Judge McGuire cited medical sources on fetal development in support of his claim that even a nonviable fetus is not a part of its mother.[86] Judge McGuire rested his decision, however, on the fact that the Bonbrest child was viable at the time of the injury and capable of living independently of its mother.[87] Judge McGuire found precedent for his decision in the civil law and in Canadian law, and also by analogy to property and criminal law.[88] Finally, he refused to allow the threat of false claims and difficult problems of proof to bar recovery of compensation, expressing confidence in the law's ability to recognize and utilize the progress of medical sciences in the area of fetal development.[89]

Other courts rapidly accepted the reasoning of Judge McGuire and began to echo his arguments.[90] Many cases analogized this to the protection of various interests of the unborn child in property and criminal law to support the argument that tort law should recognize and protect the right of an unborn child to begin life unimpaired by physical or mental defects caused by the wrongful conduct of others.[91] The decisions also harmonized the change in the law with the principles of *stare decisis* by noting that contemporary medical knowledge had advanced since *Dietrich* and arguing that, to remain meaningful, the law had to change to keep pace with these developments in the medical sciences.[92] Finally, as more and more decisions recognized the cause of action for prenatal injuries, the "lack of precedent" argument was found simply to no longer apply.[93]

Like *Bonbrest,* most of the early decisions which upheld the child's damage suit for prenatal injuries relied on the fact that the fetus was viable at the time of the injury — the courts still feeling constrained to overcome Holmes' premise by reference to the physical fact of the viable fetus's capability of existing independently of its mother.[94] Illustrative is *Woods v. Lancet,*[95] in which the New York Court of Appeals overruled its earlier decision barring the child's recovery of compensation for prenatal injuries and upheld a suit by a child for injuries inflicted when it was in its ninth month of development. In *Woods,* Judge Desmond rejected the earlier precedent, stating that to deny the independent existence of a viable fetus is "to deny a simple and easily demonstrable fact."[96] Having thus recognized the legal right of the unborn child to begin life free of negligence-caused physical and mental impairment, Judge Desmond also held that the mere uncertainty or difficulty of proof was not an acceptable ground for totally denying the right.[97]

As the pace of the acceptance of *Bonbrest* quickened, some courts ceased relying on the child's physical independence and ability to survive outside the mother and began to relate the independent legal existence of the injured child to stages of fetal development prior to viability, eventually to the moment of conception.

In 1953, New York became the first state to recognize a cause of action on behalf of a child for injuries sustained before reaching viability. In *Kelley v. Gregory*,[98] the Appellate Division allowed the child to sue for injuries sustained in an automobile accident which occurred when the child's mother was three months pregnant. The court relied partially upon property law, which treats a posthumous child as an independent being from the moment of conception, to reject the requirement of viability.[99] The court asserted that the fetus is a separate organism from the moment of conception and that its dependence on its mother for nourishment and protection does not destroy that separability but simply describes the conditions under which its life will not continue.[100] To date, ten other states have followed New York and have upheld suits for injuries without regard to the stage of fetal development at the time of the injury, and at least one state has stated in dictum that it did not base its decision to uphold recovery on the ground that the child was viable at the time of the injury.[101] The real issue in these cases of live birth is proof of a causal connection between the tortious conduct and the child's injuries rather than the ability of the child to survive independently of its mother at the time of the injury.[102]

A number of decisions have stated that to deny relief would be unjust as the child is no less hampered by the injuries inflicted in its fourth month of development than it would be if it had been injured in the eighth month.[103] Indeed, the injustice would be peculiarly severe in light of medical evidence that the fetus is most susceptible to harm in its first trimester of development; thus, in the period in which the fetus has its greatest physical vulnerability, the law provides the least protection.[104]

Perhaps the strongest testimony of how far the law has developed in the ninety-three years since *Dietrich* is in the two recent cases[105] that held that a child can hold another liable even for harm-causing wrongful conduct that occurred prior to the child's conception. In both cases the courts judged that the only bar to recovery would be the inability to prove a causal connection between the conduct and the injury, stating that the duty to the as yet nonexistent child stemmed from the foreseeability that the mother would one day become pregnant, and noting that the child was no longer nonexistent when the effects of the conduct were finally felt.[106]

The Modern Question: Causation, Not Viability

No state court that has in modern times addressed the question refuses to recognize the child's right to compensation for injuries tortiously inflicted prior to birth.[107] The modern judicial analysis has moved away from viability as the relevant criterion to the question of the causal relationship between the alleged wrong and the harm suffered. This move by the judiciary to a new focus of inquiry will be considered by evaluating cases of injury infliction occurring both after[108] and before[109] fetal viability.

After the *Bonbrest v. Kotz* decision set into motion the wave of reversals of early decisions that denied recognition of a cause of action on behalf of the child for prenatal injuries,[110] those courts that joined the new trend toward such recognition had the least trouble with the cases involving a child's suit for injuries sustained after it had reached viability. Many of the cases involving this factual circumstance in the past twenty years assume the child's right to recover compensation and instead focus on the issues of causation, negligence, and damages.[111]

The advancement of medical knowledge, or perhaps simply the law's willingness to acknowledge it, was in part responsible for removing some of the earlier perceived obstacles to recognition of a cause of action in this area. Medical evidence of the viable fetus's ability to survive independently of its mother allowed courts to avoid the *Dietrich* premise that the unborn child was a part of its mother.[112] Increased medical knowledge of fetal development also gave courts more confidence in the ability to establish a causal connection between injury and negligent conduct, thereby alleviating the old fear of fictitious claims and speculative proof.[113] Finally, those jurisdictions that had previously decided not to recognize a cause of action on behalf of the child incorporated strong references to advances in medical knowledge and the law's need to keep pace with such advances in order to harmonize their change with the principles of *stare decisis.*[114]

These advances in medical science, especially those that enhanced the ability to prove causation of prenatal injuries, also invited judicial recognition of a right to recover for injuries inflicted prior to the fetus's viability.[115] Acknowledging that the proof of harm is no less simple because the injury occurred before viability, a sense of justice moved the courts to extend the protection of tort law to include that stage.[116] In one of the early decisions to extend the protection to stages prior to viability, *Hornbuckle v. Plantation Pipe Line Company,*[117] the concurring and dissenting members of the court would have limited the extension to the stage at which the child was "quick," or "able to stir in the mother's womb."[118] However, the majority held that the stage of prenatal development at the time of the injury was irrelevant so long as causation is shown.[119]

The causation questions have become central to the modern cases and the answers given have not in all cases escaped criticism. In *Sinkler v. Kneale,*[120] the Pennsylvania Supreme Court faced a complaint on behalf of a child afflicted with Down's syndrome (mongolism) against a person who was involved in an automobile accident with the child's mother when she was one month pregnant. The complaint sought to establish a causal connection between the child's condition and a nutritional imbalance caused by the accident, and the court held that recovery would be upheld if the causal connection were proved. The American Law Institute sharply criticized the court for "being taken in by [this] wild theory" of causation[121] and while rejecting the viability test cautions that

> [Under the] present state of medical knowledge of embryology, as we approach the beginning of pregnancy medical testimony in proof of a causal connection becomes increasingly speculative, unreliable and unsatisfactory, and tends to become mere conjecture. For that reason a court may properly require more in the way of convincing evidence of causation when the injury is claimed to have occurred during the early weeks of pregnancy than when it comes later. This is not a matter of viability, nor is there any fixed and definite line to be drawn at any particular state of development of the fetus.[122]

Recently, a Florida Court of Appeals cited this cautionary note of the Institute in a decision which upheld a child's suit for injuries allegedly caused by an automobile accident in which the mother was involved when she was in her sixth week of pregnancy. In *Day v. Nationwide Mutual Insurance Co.*,[123] the court held that viability at the time of the injury is irrelevant when the child was born alive, both in view of the child's separate existence from the moment of conception and for the purposes of achieving justice. The court refused to allow either the fear of false claims or the difficulty of proof of causation to preclude recovery, expressing confidence that advances in medical science and the judicious use of a higher standard of proof of causation for injuries allegedly inflicted in the early stages of pregnancy would minimize these dangers.

DEATH AFTER BIRTH

No state currently refuses to recognize the right of the proper party to commence a wrongful death or survival action for the death of a child injured before birth who survives birth.[124] The decisional history of the law related to the wrongful death of children born alive parallels the development of the law regarding suits by the child itself for prenatal injuries.[125] This parallelism resulted in part from the fact that many courts have held that the test of recovery under their state's survival statute is whether the child could have brought an action for injuries on its own behalf had it not died. Consequently, as more states recognized the child's right to sue in its own right, those states which applied this test automatically recognized the right to commence the survival action provided by statute.[126] Most of these statutes are phrased in terms of the death of a "person," and the courts readily held that the child demonstrated its "personhood" within the meaning of the statute by surviving birth. Later in this chapter (page 261) the law regarding actions brought for the death of the stillborn will be discussed, and it will be noted that in some states the child's ability to survive birth is decisive on the issue of whether a suit will be allowed.[127] The discussion immediately following indicates that, in suits involving the wrongful death of children who survived birth, the primary question is whether the courts will allow a cause of action regardless of the stage of fetal development at the time of the alleged injury.[128] The few cases that have involved injuries to previable fetuses which eventually resulted in the child's death after birth answer affirmatively.[129]

Cooper v. Blanck,[130] decided by a Louisiana Court of Appeals in 1923, was the first reported American case to uphold an action for the wrongful death of a child who survived birth, yet died because of harm inflicted prior to birth. However, *Cooper* did not serve as authority for national change of the law, an historical role performed twenty-three years later by the *Bonbrest* decision.[131] Indeed, the *Verkennes v. Corniea*[132] decision, which recognized the right to sue for the wrongful death of a stillborn fetus, antedated the first decision rendered after *Bonbrest* to uphold a cause of action for the wrongful death of a child who survived birth. Consequently, it was somewhat anticlimactic when, in 1950, the Ohio Supreme Court decided in *Jasinsky v. Potts*[133] to uphold the suit for the wrongful death of a child who survived for three months after birth before succumbing to injuries suffered in an automobile accident which occurred after it had reached viability. The court relied primarily on its decision of the previous year, *Williams v. Marion Rapid Transit, Inc.,*[134] which upheld an infant's suit for prenatal injuries, concluding that an unborn viable child is a "person" within the meaning of both the Ohio Constitution and the Ohio Wrongful Death statute.[135] The court found it would be absurd to impute a legislative intent to reward the wrongdoer who inflicts the ultimate harm of death, by allowing recovery for injuries if the child lives yet refusing to recognize a cause of action when the child dies.[136] The states quickly fell in line with the *Jasinsky* result and analysis.[137]

However, while the courts recognized a cause of action for injuries inflicted prior to viability as early as 1953,[138] and for the wrongful death of a stillborn child injured prior to viability — yet after "quickening" — in 1955,[139] the first decision to uphold a suit for the wrongful death of a child injured prior to viability who died after surviving birth was not rendered until the 1967 decision of *Torigian v. Watertown News Co.*[140] In *Torigian,* the child's mother, when three and one-half months pregnant, was involved in an automobile accident which caused the premature birth of her child eight and one-half weeks later. The child lived for only about two and one-half hours and the administrator of the child's estate brought a survival action for the injuries to and death of the child. The court cited the many cases that had involved injuries to previable fetuses who were stillborn or who survived birth with injuries, as well as the perceived unanimity of the commentators, in holding that the nonviability of a fetus should not bar recovery.[141] The cited cases defeated the traditional lack of precedent argument and the court expressed confidence that the advancement of medical science had removed the need for speculation and conjecture about causation and eliminated the danger of fraudulent claims.[142]

Subsequent cases involving this type of fact pattern have adopted this general reasoning and the reasoning of the cases that upheld suits for injuries inflicted prior to viability and have related the separate existence of the child born alive back to the moment of conception.[143] At least one case that involved a suit for the death of a stillborn fetus has also employed this reasoning, mentioning in dictum that viability should not be the determinative factor.[144] Given the similarities between the reasoning employed in these death after birth cases and those cases involving suits by living children for injuries, it is safe to say that future cases for the wrongful death of children who survive birth, but later die, will be less concerned with the child's stage of fetal development at the time of the injury than with the ability to prove a causal connection between the tortious conduct and the injury and death.

The only potential bar to such suits rests on the ground that the pecuniary loss caused by such death is too speculative. While this view has barred recovery in a number of lawsuits involving the stillborn,[145] only one decision, *Stetson v. Easterling,*[146] has employed this view to bar a suit for the death of a child who survived birth. The reasoning of *Stetson,* coupled with that of subsequent decisions in that jurisdiction, indicates that the decision was based on a defect in the complaint filed in the case rather than on a general principle that damages will always be too speculative in the situation involving the death of a child who survived birth.

In *Stetson v. Easterling,* the court denied recovery under its wrongful death statute for the death of a five month old child who suffered brain damage during its delivery on the grounds that the complaint contained no allegations sufficient to provide a basis for assessing the pecuniary loss caused by the child's death. The analysis contained in two subsequent cases decided by intermediate courts of appeal — *Yow v. Nance,* 29 N.C.App. 419, 224 S.E.2d 292 (1976); and *Cardwell v. Welch,* 25 N.C.App. 390, 213 S.E.2d 382 (1975), cert. denied, 287 N.C. 464, 215 S.E.2d 623 (1975) — suggests that *Stetson* does not bar all suits for the wrongful death of children who are born alive and later die from injuries incurred before birth. Each case involved a suit for the wrongful death of a stillborn and in denying the cause of action the reasoning of each case implicitly recognized that, had the child survived birth, recovery would have been possible if appropriate allegations of pecuniary loss had been demonstrated.

DEATH BEFORE BIRTH

Introduction

Though the current state of the law reveals unanimity on the issue of the right of the child born alive to claim damages for injuries or wrongful death by tortious acts, the courts are in substantial disagreement on the issue of the right to sue where the injured unborn dies before birth. The courts seemingly agree that once the child is born alive the issues are one of negligence, causation, and extent of damages. However, in the area of the stillborn most courts continue to raise the threshold issue of the legal status of the unborn. Various criteria for resolution have been put forward in the cases in this area. Some cases require the live birth,[147] others assess the child's stage of prenatal development at the time of the injury,[148] and still others view the child as an independent being from the moment of conception and focus on the issue of causation instead.[149] In order to facilitate analysis of these different positions and the reasoning advanced for each, those cases that require live birth as a prerequisite to recovery and those that do not view live birth as the crucial event will be discussed separately.

Stillbirths Precluded from Recovery

A number of decisions in twelve jurisdictions have held that no wrongful death or survival action can be recognized for the death of a child injured prior to birth unless the child survives birth.[150] These decisions have held that the stillborn, which fails to survive birth, is not a "person," "child," or "minor child" within the meaning of the wrongful death or survival statutes that authorize lawsuits on behalf of those allegedly killed by wrongdoing. By so interpreting the personhood language of the authorizing statutes, these courts require adherence to the live-birth requirement. The following list summarizes reasons frequently advanced for accepting live birth as a prerequisite with subsequent elaboration of a number of the more frequently offered reasons: (1) by reason of legislative intent;[151] (2) by analogy to property law;[152] (3) by analogy to abortion laws and other criminal laws;[153] (4) because a line must be drawn at some point and using viability is too imprecise;[154] (5) the damages attributable to birth of a stillborn are too speculative to be awarded justly;[155] (6) the loss due to the stillbirth is recoverable as an element of the mother's damage award thereby permitting the danger of a double recovery;[156] and (7) the fear that allowing such suits would enable the child to sue its mother.[157]

Legislative intent is perhaps the reason most frequently advanced against the recognition of a wrongful death action for a stillborn fetus. As the previous discussion indicated, since the wrongful death action is exclusively statutory, the crucial issue is whether the statute itself covers the situation of the stillborn fetus. Many courts have argued, for various reasons, that the legislature could not have intended to include the stillborn fetus within the coverage of the statute. Some courts have looked to the circumstances surrounding the original enactment. Since most of these statutes were originally passed in the nineteenth century, before the case law recognized a cause of action for prenatal injuries, the courts conclude that the original statutes could not have contemplated inclusion of the stillborn fetus within its coverage. Noting that the statutes remain in substantially the same form as when originally passed, the courts have concluded that this legislative failure to amend the statutes to extend its coverage signified a legislative intent to exclude coverage of the stillborn fetus.[158] Thus, any extension of the acts' coverage beyond that which existed at the time of original passage must await future legislative action.[159] Where the statutes have received judicial construction barring the stillborn fetus a cause of action, the courts have subsequently argued that the legislature's failure to amend the statute to overrule such a judicial interpretation indicates the legislature's assent to the previous construction.[160]

Many courts have also concluded that the use in statutes other than the wrongful death act of similar terms (such as "person" or "child") indicates that the legislature must have contemplated only live-born children when it used that terminology.[161] Illustrative is the California Court of Appeals decision in *Justus v. Atchison,*[162] in which the court held that the term "minor person," as used in the California wrongful death statute, could not include within its coverage a child which failed to survive birth because the computation statute for the period of minority of a "person" provided that the period of minority be calculated from the first minute of the day upon which the person is born.[163] Thus, the court reasoned, "the minority of a person begins only at birth," and the use of the word "minor" to modify the word "person" in the statute indicated the legislature's intent to cover the child only after its live birth.[164] Since the statute has now been amended to delete the term "minor" as a modifier of "person,"[165] it should be interesting to see if the California courts will construe the change as legislative action designed to include the stillborn child within the coverage of the statute.

It must be noted that the court in *Justus* also justified the live-birth requirement by reference to a general statutory provision which provided that an unborn child "is to be deemed an existing person, so far as may be necessary for its interests in the event of its subsequent birth."[166] Since this statute conditions general protection of the unborn child's potential interests upon survival of birth, it not only fails to protect the stillborn child, but also provides a basis for concluding by analogy that the wrongful death statute also fails to extend that protection.[167] The troubling aspect of this reasoning lies in the fact that the interest at stake — protection against tortious interference with the right to be born — is by its very nature one that is totally destroyed before the child is able to survive birth, and therefore it differs from the typical proprietary interests which the more general statute is designed to protect.[168]

The courts that have discarded the live-birth requirement have rejected these arguments of legislative intent on various grounds. Most of these courts simply state that the statute must be construed broadly to fulfill its remedial purposes.[169] Others have stated that the statutory wrongful death action is coextensive with the common law action for damages.[170] Both of these lines of argument avoid inquiry into "legislative intent," and instead look to changes in medical and biological conditions in order to keep the statute in tune with contemporary knowledge.[171]

Some judges have argued that the constitutional law of abortion as articulated in *Roe v. Wade*[172] requires the live-birth distinction.[173] For example, in *State ex rel. Hardin v. Sanders*,[174] the administrator of the estate of a child who was stillborn as a result of an automobile accident that occurred when the mother was eight months pregnant brought a wrongful death action for the death of the child. The defendant commenced a suit against the judge presiding over the wrongful death action to prohibit the proceeding on the ground that the statute did not apply to the death of stillborn fetuses. On appeal of the prohibition suit proceeding, the Missouri Supreme Court held that a fetus is not a "person" within the meaning of the wrongful death statute until it is born alive.[175] In addition to the arguments based on legislative intent, statutory construction, and the imprecision of the viability criterion, the court reasoned, on the basis of the United States Supreme Court decision in *Roe v. Wade,* that "the unborn have never been recognized in the law as persons in the whole sense" and that "the word 'person,' as used in the Fourteenth Amendment, does not include the unborn."[176] Justice Ryan also feared the potential conflicts of upholding an action for the wrongful death of a stillborn fetus while allowing abortion of the fetus at the request of the pregnant woman.[177] Other courts have flatly held that *Roe v. Wade* supports the viability rule for stillbirths rather than the live-birth distinction.[178]

An extensive analysis of the impact of the landmark United States Supreme Court abortion decision in *Roe v. Wade* upon the law of prenatal harm will not be undertaken here, since it exceeds the scope of this chapter.[179] This interface of abortion and tort law provides the seeming paradox of, on the one hand, permitting the imposition of liability for fetal death or injury when negligently caused but, on the other hand, of permitting immunity for harm intentionally caused and maternally desired. This apparent dilemma has spawned a number of state court decisions[180] that employ the Supreme Court abortion decision in a manner inconsistent with one another, thereby introducing new uncertainty in an area of law long plagued with ambiguity.

Certain states whose statutes limit the wrongful death recovery to the pecuniary loss of the statutory beneficiaries of the child's estate, have completely barred action for the wrongful death of the stillborn child on the ground that any estimate of such pecuniary loss would be totally speculative.[181] The cases reason that not only is there no basis for estimating the probable monetary contribution of the child to the household had it lived but in addition the possibility exists that the cost of raising and educating the child would exceed the estimate of its monetary contribution.[182] Several courts and commentators have attacked this reasoning — as well as the entire concept of limiting damages for wrongful death to pecuniary loss[183] — on the ground that it leaves an obvious loss (though possibly a quantitatively ambiguous one) totally uncompensated for.[184] However, some courts have responded to this challenge with the argument that the parental loss in the wrongful death of the stillborn child is recoverable by the parents in their own right as an aspect of the pain and suffering award to the mother and the father's loss of consortium action.[185] The North Carolina Supreme Court has precluded recovery in this situation on the ground that any damage award would be so entirely speculative as to amount, in effect, to be an award of punitive damages which the statute did not contemplate.[186]

Some courts have adopted the live-birth distinction partially because of their rejection of the viability rule.[187] Starting with the premise that "a line must be drawn somewhere," these courts perceive that the line between viability and nonviability is too imprecise and medically too difficult to draw, and thus settle on live birth, perceiving it to be much easier to identify. Of course, this reasoning is no more persuasive than its premises that a line must be drawn and that live birth is an easily identifiable event.[188]

A further rationale advanced in favor of drawing the line at live birth is that the need for compensation is more compelling in the situation involving a child who faces the prospect of living its entire life saddled with injuries than in the case of the stillborn, in which the parents (whose loss is viewed as less severe) can receive partial compensation in the form of the mother's action for her own pain and suffering.[189] This distinction has some merit, especially in states that limit the beneficiaries' damages to the pecuniary loss attributable to the death,[190] since it is difficult to quantify in pecuniary terms the injury or loss which accompanies the stillbirth of one's child. However, this position is difficult to reconcile with the unanimous recognition of the cause of action when a child is born alive, but dies after a very short period of life, even minutes.[191] It is difficult to imagine why the need for compensation to the beneficiaries is any more compelling — especially if the damage is limited to pecuniary loss — in the situation involving a child who survives birth by ten minutes before succumbing to its injuries than in the case of a child whose injuries are so severe as to cause its death before birth. The answer of the courts that require live birth is, again, simply that the line must be drawn at some point, and birth is no less arbitrary and easier to ascertain than viability or "quickening."[192]

Stillbirths Not Precluded from Recovery of Compensation, if Fetus is Viable

As noted previously,[193] a majority of the jurisdictions which have decided the issue have upheld the cause of action for the wrongful death of the stillborn child. The vast majority of the decisions permitting suit held that the fetus was a "person" within the meaning of the statute where the fetus was viable at the time of the stillbirth.[194] This section will analyze the reasoning of those decisions and the following section will discuss the few opinions that have argued for elimination of both the live-birth requirement and the viability distinction.

The decisions that have held that a viable unborn fetus is a "person" or a "minor child" within the meaning of the applicable wrongful death and survival statutes have relied on several different rationales. The most frequently advanced reason is based on medical or biologic evidence of the child's ability to exist independently of its mother. Under this reasoning, the unborn child attains separate legal existence as a "person" at the time it attains the capability of separate and independent physical existence.[195] Some courts have gone so far as to state that viability marks the point in time at which the fetus biologically becomes "a living human being."[196]

Support for the treatment of the viable unborn fetus as a "person" has also been drawn by analogy to the decision in *Roe v. Wade,* which extends the greatest amount of state protection to the fetus after it reaches viability, or in the third trimester of pregnancy.[197] The argument proceeds on the basis that the increased protection of the fetus's interest in being born after reaching viability justifies the protection of that interest by the liability provisions of tort law.[198]

These courts have rejected the arguments that legislative history and inaction preclude judicial recognition of coverage within the statute until affirmative legislative action, arguing that the inference of legislative intent is fictional and that changed medical and biological conditions,[199] as well as changes in the case law regarding suits for prenatal injuries, militate in favor of interpreting the statute to keep it abreast of the times.[200] These courts noted that the legislature is free to amend the statute in the event that it disagrees with the courts' interpretation.[201]

A number of courts have also rejected the argument that damages for the death of the stillborn child are so speculative as to bar the action totally. In some cases the rejection is based on the fact that the wrongful death or survival statute does not limit the damage award to the pecuniary loss attributable to the child's death, but rather allows the award to include loss of companionship, love, and affection of the stillborn child as an aspect of damages.[202] In this situation, the existence of a statutorily recognizable compensable loss is much more apparent than it is when the recognition of loss extends only to pecuniary matters. However, even in states that limit the recovery to the pecuniary loss some courts have held that it would be unjust to totally deny compensation simply because a specific measure of the amount of loss could not be calculated.[203] Finally, two decisions have stated that even if the loss attributable to the prenatal death of a child is so speculative as to amount to an award of punitive damages, this would not bar the action because it would be consistent with the purpose of the act to preserve human life and punish the person who interferes with that purpose by assessing the cost against the wrongdoer.[204]

In the course of upholding the cause of action for the stillbirth of a viable fetus these courts have criticized the live-birth requirement as a prerequisite to recovery. The most frequently raised criticism is that drawing the line at birth is absurd.[205] Some courts have attempted to illustrate the absurdity by citing a hypothetical situation in which twins are born and one has died before birth, while the other dies shortly after birth, arguing that to deny recovery for the death of the stillborn twin and allow recovery for the death of its sibling who outlived it by a few moments is absurd.[206] In this hypothetical case, the arbitrariness and absurdity of the distinction speak for themselves.

A more persuasive argument for the absurdity of the live-birth distinction is based on the fact that it results in the least amount of liability when the severity of the harm is the greatest;[207] namely, absolution in the face of having desolated. The infliction of death leaves the would-be defendant absolutely free from liability, while if the harm inflicted is short of death the defendant is liable for damages to the child.[208]

The courts have used these same arguments to criticize the live-birth distinction as being unjust.[209] Indeed, at least one litigant has argued that the distinction is so irrational as to deny the parents of the stillborn child their constitutional right under the Fourteenth Amendment to equal protection of the law. In *Justus v. Atchison*,[210] the California Court of Appeals employed rational basis scrutiny in rejecting the challenge, stating that the distinction was rationally related to the major purposes of the wrongful death statute. The court indicated that the distinction need not further all of the state purposes involved, and that it therefore was not invalid simply because it did not perfectly further the goal of deterring tortious interference with the unborn fetus's right to life. While it was not raised in the context of a challenge for equal protection, in *Eich v. Town of Gulf Shores*,[211] in which the Alabama Supreme Court upheld action for the wrongful prenatal death of an eight and one-half month old fetus, the court rejected the live-birth distinction because of its view that the distinction has no relevance to the statutory purpose to preserve human life by punishing the wrongdoer.

Additional criticisms of the live-birth distinction have been based on simple disagreement with the choice of birth as the moment that defines the beginning of human life. Thus, in *O'Neill v. Morse*,[212] the Michigan Supreme Court upheld a survival action brought on behalf of the estate of an eight month old fetus who was stillborn as a result of an automobile accident, stating in part:

> The phenomenon of birth is not the beginning of life; it is merely a change in the form of life. . . . One need not be alive in order to be born; as the delivery of stillborn babies demonstrates. Neither is it possible to be born alive unless he be living prior to the birth.[213]

The court also attacked the premise that the unborn child is a part of its mother until birth, citing Justice Boggs' dissent in *Allaire v. St. Lukes Hospital,* and then stating:

> If the mother can die and the fetus live, or the fetus die and the mother live, how can it be said that there is only one life?
> If tortious conduct can injure one and not the other, how can it be said that there is not a duty owing to each?[214]

An additional argument that objects to the live-birth distinction on grounds of injustice uses analogies to property law and asserts that it would be unjust to refuse to protect the unborn child's right to life, yet protect its property rights.[215]

In addition to the analogy drawn to the protection of the rights of the unborn child in property law, courts have analogized to criminal laws (including abortion statutes) that make or have made it an offense to cause the death of an unborn child. The decisions reason that since these laws recognize and protect the unborn child's right to life, it would be anomalous to withhold that protection in the wrongful death context.[216]

In *Eich v. Town of Gulf Shores*,[217] the Alabama Supreme Court argued that the abortion decision in *Roe v. Wade* also militated against making survival of birth a condition in granting cause of action (despite the United States Supreme Court's ruling that the unborn fetus is not a "person" within the meaning of the Fourteenth Amendment). The Alabama court argued that *Roe v. Wade* supports the proposition that, at least after the first trimester of fetal development has passed, the state has an interest and "general obligation" to protect prenatal life, so long as it does not unreasonably intrude on the prospective mother's right of privacy. Since in the wrongful death context the mother's privacy interest is not at issue, the state has a recognized interest, perhaps even a duty, in extending the statute's protection to the stillborn child.

Finally, in *Britt v. Sears*,[218] the Indiana Court of Appeals held in favor of recognizing the stillborn viable fetus's "personhood" within the meaning of the wrongful death statute by analogy, in part, to the treatment of the unborn fetus in the Public Health Code and the state Cemetery Act. The court noted that these laws, which defined the procedures for the filing of death certificates and for the disposal of the remains of deceased persons by burial, cremation, or donation pursuant to the Uniform Anatomical Gift Act, all treated the stillborn child's death and body identically to that of the child born alive. Indeed, the anatomical gift act's definition of "decedent" was framed to specifically include "a stillborn infant or fetus."[219] However, given the difference in the purposes furthered by these acts and the wrongful death act, the analogy is of limited validity. Indeed, the counterargument could be made that the legislature's specific inclusions of the stillborn child or fetus within the coverage of these acts and the absence of any such specific inclusion in the wrongful death act give rise to an inference of a legislative intent to exclude the stillborn child or fetus from the coverage of the wrongful death act unless specifically included.[220]

Stillbirths Not Precluded from Recovery Lawsuit, Irrespective of Fetal Viability

Finally, one court has upheld a suit for the wrongful stillbirth of a previable fetus and another court has stated in dictum that the stillborn fetus's lack of viability will not bar a suit for its wrongful death.

In *Porter v. Lassiter*,[221] an automobile accident injured a woman one and one-half months pregnant who three months later had a stillborn child. Evidence at trial showed that the stillbirth was caused by damage to the placenta suffered in the automobile accident. The Georgia Court of Appeals held that a wrongful death action would lie in the stillborn child's death because "a foetus becomes a child when it is 'quick' or capable of moving in its mother's womb," and the Georgia criminal law defines the killing of an unborn child which had reached the stage of quickening as murder.[222]

Presumably, the fetus or embryo might have been "quick" at the time of the accident, as most medical authorities state that quickening normally occurs in the very early stages of pregnancy, often long before the mother is even capable of feeling that movement. Whenever "quickening" commences, it is a previability phenomenon.

In a relatively recent decision, *Presley v. Newport Hospital*,[223] the Rhode Island Supreme Court by a vote of 3 to 2 upheld a suit for the wrongful death of a viable stillborn fetus which was allegedly caused by negligent care by the hospital and the attending physician during the mother's delivery. One justice voted to uphold the suit, but relied on the child's viability in reaching his conclusion, partially because of his view that *Roe v. Wade* supported the adoption of the viability requirement in the context of a suit for the wrongful death of a stillborn child.[224] Two justices, however, voted to uphold the action by rejecting the live-birth requirement as absurd and unjust, and expressly stating that they were not premising their decision on the fact that the child was viable.[225] Noting that a previous decision had held that the viability of the fetus at the time of injury was irrelevant to its right to recover for the injury after its birth, the justices also rejected the notion that a stillborn fetus had to be viable in order to be a "person" within the meaning of the wrongful death statute. The justices expressed the opinion that causation was the relevant inquiry in both the injuries and the stillbirth situation, and that the fetus's viability had no relevance to that issue in either situation.

NOTES

[1] Two articles taken together provide a rich look at the doctrinal evolution of liability for parental harm. See P.M. Winfield, "The Unborn Child," 4 *U. of Toronto L.J.* 279 (1942) (also published in 8 *Camb.L.J.* 76 [1942]); and D.A. Gordon, "The Unborn Plaintiff," 63 *Mich.L.Rev.* 579 (1965).

[2] For a recent review of the law on prenatal harm in other common law jurisdictions (including England, Canada, Ireland, Australia, New Zealand) see P.J. Pace, "Civil Liability for Pre-Natal Injuries," 40 *Modern L.Rev.* 141 (1977). See also P.A. Lovell and R.H. Griffiths-Jones, "'The Sins of the Fathers'—Tort Liability for Pre-Natal Injuries," 90 *Law Quarterly Rev.* 531 (1974).

[3] This chapters limits itself to the civil law's response to prenatal harm. Thus, no direct consideration is provided of the response of criminal law, nor of postnatal or preconception wrongs. The legal aspects of preconception wrong (typically involving failures in pregnancy or disease prevention) are undergoing rapid development. For discussion of this relatively new area of tort law, see *Note*, "Wrongful Birth in the Abortion Context—Critique of Existing Case Law and Proposal for Future Actions," 53 *Denver L.J.* 501 (1976).

[4] The principal historical discussion will occur in the text accompanying notes 16–30, *infra*. The text will also occasionally allude to historical matters relevant to the particular topic being discussed.

[5] See *Note*, "The Impact of Medical Knowledge on the Law Relating to Prenatal Injuries," 110 *U. of Pennsylvania L.Rev.* 554 (1962); and D.A. Gordon, "The Unborn Plaintiff," 63 *Mich.L.Rev.* 579, 603–628 (1965).

[6] See *Appendix* for the discussion of the cases involving this factual pattern, see notes 79–123, *infra*, and accompanying text.

[7] See *Appendix*. See notes 115–123, *infra*, and accompanying text. Two courts have held that a child may recover for injuries sustained before birth that were attributable to conduct that occurred before the child was conceived: *Renslow v. Mennonite Hospital*, 40 Ill.App.3d 234, 351 N.E.2d 870 (1976); and *Jorgensen v. Meade Johnson Laboratories, Inc.*, 483 F.2d 237 (10th Cir. 1973).

Rather than concerning themselves with the stage of prenatal development at the time of the injury, the *Renslow* and *Jorgensen* decisions relate the independent existence of the live-born child back to the moment of conception and focus on the issue of causation. See, for example, *Day v. Nationwide Mutual Insurance Co.*, 328 So.2d 560 (Fla.App. 1976); *Daley v. Meier*, 33 Ill.App. 2d 218, 178 N.E.2d 691 (1961); *Sinkler v. Kneale*, 401 Pa. 267, 164 A.2d 93 (1960); *Smith v. Brennan*, 31 N.J. 353, 157 A.2d 497 (1960); *Bennett v. Hymers*, 101 N.H. 483, 147 A.2d 108 (1958); *Hornbuckle v. Plantation Pipe Line Co.*, 212 Ga. 504, 93 S.E.2d 727 (1956); and *Kelley v. Gregory*,

282 App.Div. 542, 125 N.Y.S.2d 696, app. granted 283 App.Div.2d 914, 129 N.Y.S.2d 914 (1953).

[8]See *Appendix*. For the discussion of the cases involving this factual pattern, see notes 124–146, *infra*, and accompanying text.

[9]*Torigian v. Watertown News Co.*, 352 Mass. 446, N.E.2d 926 (1967); and *Wolfe v. Isbell*, 291 Ala. 327, 280 So.2d 758 (1973). *Cf. Justus v. Atchison*, 53 Cal. App.3d 556, 126 Cal. Rptr. 150 (1975) (dictum); *Jorgensen v. Meade Johnson Laboratories, Inc.*, 483 F.2d 237 (10th Cir. 1973) (implicit). In addition, one court has recognized a right to recover where the conduct which caused the death occurred prior to conception. *Jorgensen v. Meade Johnson Laboratories, Inc.*, 483 F.2d 237 (10th Cir. 1973).

[10]See, e.g., *Torigian v. Watertown News Co.*, 352 Mass. 446, 225 N.E.2d 926 (1967).

[11]For the discussion of the cases involving this factual pattern, see notes 147–225 and accompanying text, *infra*.

[12]*Kilmer v. Hicks*, 22 Ariz.App. 552, 529 P.2d 706 (1975); *Justus v. Atchison*, 53 Cal.App.3d 556, 126 Cal.Rptr. 150 (1975); *McKillop v. Zimmerman*, 191 N.W.2d 706 (Iowa 1971) (dictum); *State ex rel. Hardin v. Sanders*, 538 S.W.2d 336 (Mo. 1976); *Acton v. Shields*, 386 S.W.2d 363 (Mo. 1965); *Drabbels v. Skelly Oil Co.*, 155 Neb. 17, 50 N.W.2d 229 (1951); *Graf v. Taggert*, 43 N.J. 303, 204 A.2d 140 (1964); *Endresz v. Friedberg*, 24 N.Y.2d 478, 301 N.Y.S.2d 65, 248 N.E.2d 901 (1969); *Gay v. Thompson*, 266 N.C. 394, 146 S.E.2d 425, 15 A.L.R.3d 983 (1966); *Yow v. Nance*, 29 N.C.App. 419, 224 S.E.2d 292 (1976); *Cardwell v. Welch*, 25 N.C.App. 390, 213 S.E.2d 382 (1975) cert. denied 287 N.C. 464, 215 S.E.2d 623 (1975); *Marko v. Philadelphia Transportation Co.*, 420 Pa. 124, 216 A.2d 502 (1966); *Durrett v. Owens*, 212 Tenn. 614, 371 S.W.2d 433 (1963); *Nelson v. Peterson*, 542 P.2d 1075 (Utah, 1975); and *Lawrence v. Craven Tire Company*, 210 Va. 138, 169 (S.E.2d 440 (1969). *Cf. Stokes v. Liberty Mutual Insurance Co.*, 213 S.2d 695 (Fla. 1968) and *Hall v. Murphy*, 236 So.Car. 257, 113 S.E.2d 790 (1960).

[13]*Eich v. Town of Gulf Shores*, 293 Ala. 95, 300 So.2d 354 (1974); *Hatala v. Markiewicz*, 26 Conn.Sup. 358, 224 A.2d 406 (1966); *Porter v. Lassiter*, 91 Ga.App. 712, 87 S.E.2d 100 (1955); *Pleasant v. Certified Grocers of Illinois, Inc.*, 39 Ill.App.3d 83, 350 N.E.2d 65 (1976); *Maniates v. Grant Hospital*, 15 Ill.App.3d 903, 305 N.E.2d 422 (1973); *Chrisafogeorgis v. Brandenberg*, 55 Ill.2d 368, 304 N.E. 2d 88 (1973); *Britt v. Sears*, 150 Ind.App. 487, 277 N.E.2d 20 (1971); *Hale v. Manion*, 189 Kan. 142, 368 P.2d 1 (1962); *Rice v. Rizk*, 453 S.W.2d 732 (Ky. 1970); *Valence v. Louisiana Power & Light Co.*, 50 So.2d 847 (Louisiana App. 1951); *State use of Odham v. Sherman*, 234 Md.179, 198 A.2d 71 (1964); *O'Neill v. Morse*, 385 Mich. 130, 188 N.W.2d 785 (1971); *Pehrson v. Kistner*, 222 N.W.2d 334 (1974); *Rainey v. Horn*, 221 Miss. 269, 72 So.2d 434 (1954); *White v. Yup*, 85 Nev. 527, 458 P.2d 617 (1969); *Poliquin v. Macdonald*, 101 N.H. 104, 135 A.2d 249 (1957); *Stidam v. Ashmore*, 109 Ohio App. 431, 11 Ohio Op.2d 383, 167 N.E.2d 106 (1959); *Evans v. Olson*, 550 P.2d 924 (Okla. 1976); *Libbee v. Permanente Clinic*, 518 P.2d 636, (Ore. 1974); *Presley v. Newport Hospital*, 365 A.2d 748 (1976); *Fowler v. Woodward*, 244 S.Car. 608, 138 S.E.2d 42 (1964); *Moen v. Hanson*, 85 Wash.2d 597, 537 P.2d 266 (1975); *Baldwin v. Butcher*, 184 S.E.2d 428 (W.Va. 1971); *Kwaterski v. State Farm Mutual Automobile Insurance Co.*, 34 Wis.2d 14, 148 N.W.2d 107 (1967); and *Simmons v. Howard University*, 323 F.Supp. 529 (D.D.C. 1971). *Cf. Delaware: Worgan v. Greggo & Ferrara, Inc.*, 50 Del. 258, 128 A.2d 557 (1956) (dictum).

[14]Of the jurisdictions represented in note 13, *supra*, Illinois and Michigan have specifically denied recovery for a previable stillborn fetus: *Rapp v. Hiemenz*, 107 Ill.App.2d 382, 246 N.E.2d 77 (1969); *Toth v. Goree*, 65 Mich.App. 296, 237 N.W.2d 29 (1975). Alaska, in *Mace v. Jung*, 210 F.Supp. 706 (D.Alaska, 1962), denied recovery for the stillbirth of a previable fetus. However, it has not ruled on the right to recover for the stillbirth of a viable fetus. Two jurisdictions, in dictum, have stated that viability is the cut-off point for stillborn fetuses for wrongful death purposes. See *Poliquin v. Macdonald*, 101 N.H. 104, 135 A.2d 249 (1957) (dictum) and *Todd v. Sandidge Construction Co.*, 341 F.2d 75 (4th Cir. 1964) (dictum).

[15]Only Georgia has upheld a wrongful death action for a stillborn fetus which was not viable, and in that case the concurring and dissenting opinions would have limited the holding to fetuses that had passed the stage of "quickening." *Porter v. Lassiter*, 91 Ga.App. 712, 87 S.E.2d 100 (1955). Some decisions have, in dictum, indicated a predisposition to uphold recovery despite the absence of viability. *Presley v. Newport Hospital*, 365 A.2d 748 (1976) (dictum) (plurality opinion); *Valence v. Louisiana Power & Light Co.*, 50 So.2d 847 (Louisiana App., 1951) (dictum); and *Toth v. Goree*, 65 Mich.App. 296, 237 N.W.2d (1975) (dissent).

[16]*Dietrich v. Northampton*, 138 Mass. 14 (1884).

[17]*Id.* at 14–15. Interestingly, the conclusion that the child was born alive was based upon the observation of "motion in its limbs."

[18]Pub. Sts. C. 52, § 17; Mass. at 15. In common law death permitted no cause of action for personal torts as all claims, personal or for the decedent's estate, terminated with life's passing. Statutes have modified this absolute bar, though jurisdictions vary in the type of wrongful death and survival of action statutes authorizing the postdeath recovery. See W. L. Prosser, *Handbook of the*

Law of Torts (1971, 4th ed.), 898–914; and Speiser, *Recovery for Wrongful Death* (1975, 2d ed.). vol. 1, 35–36.

¹⁹See *Appendix.*

²⁰One court has criticized the viability distinction as an historical anomaly, urging that it is no longer necessary in light of the virtually unanimous repudiation of *Dietrich. Smith v. Brennan*, 31 N.J. 353, 157 A.2d 497 (1960). The viability rule is discussed in greater depth in the text accompanying notes 31–70, *infra.*

²¹184 Ill. 359, 368–74, 56 N.E. 638, 640–42 (1900) (Boggs, J., dissenting).

²²*Id.* at 365–68, 56 N.E. at 639–40.

²³*Id.* at 370, 56 N.E. at 641.

²⁴465 F.Supp. 138 (D.D.C. 1946).

²⁵*Id.* at 140–43.

²⁶*Restatement (Second) of Torts,* §869, Note to Institute at 174 (Tent. Draft No. 16, 1970).

²⁷See, for example, Comment, "Recovery for Prenatal Injuries: The Right of a Child Against His Mother," X *Suffolk U.L.Rev.* 582 at 586–587 (1976); Note, "The Unborn Child and the Constitutional Conception of Life," 56 *Iowa L.Rev.* 994 at 997 (1971); Note, "The Impact of Medical Knowledge on the Law Relating to Prenatal Injuries," 110 *U. of Pennsylvania L.Rev.* 554 at 556 (1962); D.A. Gordon, "The Unborn Plaintiff," 63 *Mich.L.Rev.* 579 (1965).

²⁸*Lipps v. Milwaukee Electric R. & Light Co.*, 164 Wis. 272, 159 N.W. 916 (1916) (the Wisconsin Supreme Court denied a child's suit for damages for injuries sustained before birth, but only for the stated reason that the child had not reached viability at the time of its injury. The court indicated in dictum that it would have recognized a right to recover if the child had been viable at the time of the injury). *Cooper v. Blanck*, 39 So.2d 352 (La.App. 1923) (a Louisiana Court of Appeals upheld the right of the parents of a deceased child to sue under the state's survival act for the pain and suffering experienced by the child prior to death. The court held that the eight month old fetus was a "child" within the meaning of the statute because it was viable. One explanation for *Cooper's* obscurity prior to *Bonbrest* is that it was not published until 1949. See *Toth v. Goree*, 65 *Mich.App.* 296, 237 N.W.2d 29 [1975] [Maher, J., dissenting]).

Kine v. Zuckerman, 4 Pa.D. & C. 227–231 (1924) (a Pennsylvania district court upheld a child's suit for damages for injuries suffered prior to the child's birth by relying, in part, on the advances in embryology which had demonstrated that the unborn child maintained a physiologic identity independent of its mother. The Pennsylvania Supreme Court ignored *Kine* in its first decision on this issue. *Berlin v. J.C. Penney Co.*, 339 Pa. 547, 16 A.2d 28 [1949]).

Scott v. McPheeters, 33 Cal.App.2d 629, 92 P.2d 678 (1939). A California Court of Appeals upheld a damage suit brought by an eleven year old child against a doctor who allegedly caused the child to sustain brain damage with resulting paralysis by his negligent use of forceps and metal clamps during the child's birth. The court relied heavily on a statute, 19 Cal. Stats. (Civil Code, §29), which provided:

A child conceived, but not yet born, is to be deemed an existing person, so far as may be necessary for its interests in the event of its subsequent birth.

The statute had previously been applied only to property rights, and the court held that the child's cause of action was a "property right" sufficient to trigger application of the statute. In dictum, the court discussed the viability distinction and expressed its view that a viable fetus—possessed of fully developed lungs and organs and capable of living if born—should be deemed a "human being" in actual existence.

²⁹*Verkennes v. Corniea*, 229 Minn. 365, 38 N.W.2d 838 (1949).

³⁰229 Minn. at 370–71, 38 N.W.2d at 841.

³¹See notes 13–15, *supra.* See also notes 19–30, *supra,* and accompanying text.-

³²See notes 13–15, *supra.*

³³Perhaps because the legal inquiry continues as an effort to refute the Holmes premise in *Dietrich* of the unity between mother and unborn child. See notes 19–23, *supra,* and accompanying text.

³⁴*Libbee v. Permanente Clinic*, 518 P.2d 636 (Ore. 1974); *West v. McCoy*, 233 S.C. 369, 105 S.E.2d 88 (1958); *Peterson v. Nationwide Mutual Insurance Co.*, 175 Ohio St. 551, 26 Ohio Op.2d 246, 197 N.E.2d 194 (1964); and *Gullborg v. Rizzo*, 331 F.2d 557 (3rd Cir. 1964); see also, *Shousha v. Matthews Drivurself Service, Inc.*, 210 Tenn. 384, 358 S.W.2d 471 (1962) (quoting Medical Dictionary); *State ex rel. Hardin v. Sanders*, 538 S.W.2d 336 at 336n.1 (Mo. 1976) (quoting Webster's Third New International Dictionary).

³⁵*Verkennes v. Corniea*, 229 Minn. 365, 38 N.W.2d 838, (1949); *Hale v. Manion*, 189 Kan. 142, 368 P.2d 1 (1962) and *White v. Yup*, 85 Nev. 527, 458 P.2d 617 (1969).

³⁶*Todd v. Sandidge Construction Co.*, 341 F.2d 75 (4th Cir. 1964); *Lawrence v. Craven Tire Company*, 210 Va. 138, 169 S.E.2d 440 (1969); and *Seattle—First National Bank v. Rankin*, 59 Wash.2d 288, 367 P.2d 835 (1962).

³⁷*Britt v. Sears*, 150 Ind.App. 487, 277 N.E.2d 20 (1971).

[38]*Maniats v. Grant Hospital,* 15 Ill.App.3d 903, 305 N.E.2d 422 (1973) and *Keyes v. Construction Service, Inc.,* 340 Mass. 633, 165 N.E.2d 912 (1960).

[39]*Rainey v. Horn,* 221 Miss. 269, 72 So.2d 434 (1954).

[40]*Kelley v. Gregory,* 282 App.Div. 542, 125 N.Y.S.2d 696, app. granted 283 App.Div.2d 914, 129 N.Y.S.2d 914 (1953) (quoting Barnhart, American College Dictionary).

[41]See, e.g., *Mitchell v. Couch,* 285 S.W.2d 901 (Ky. 1955); *West v. McCoy,* 233 S.C. 369, 105 S.E.2d 88 (1958); *Gullborg v. Rizzo,* 331 F.2d 557 (3rd Cir. 1964); and *Toth v. Goree,* 65 Mich.App. 296, 237 N.W.2d 29 (1975). But *cf. Smith v. Brennan,* 31 N.J. 353, 157 A.2d 497 (1960) stating that "age is not the sole measure of viability."

In *Roe v. Wade,* 410 U.S. 113, 159, 162–63 (1973), the United States Supreme Court in the landmark abortion decision divided pregnancy into trimesters, treating the fetus as "viable" in the third trimester, or after completion of the sixth month of pregnancy. *Roe* referred to viability as the point at which the fetus has the capability of meaningful life outside the mother's womb, *id.* at 163, and stated that "viability is usually placed at about seven months (28 weeks) but may occur earlier, even at 24 weeks." *Id.* at 160.

[42]415 Pa. 47, 48–50, 202 A.2d 9, 10–11 (1964) (a ten week old stillborn fetus).

[43]*Hale v. Manion,* 189 Kan. 142, 368 P.2d 1 (1962); and *Gullborg v. Rizzo* 331 F.2d 557 (3rd Cir. 1964).

[44]4 Misc.2d 283, 284–85, 156 N.Y.S.2d 49, aff'd 3 N.Y.2d 800, 166 N.Y.S.2d 3, 144 N.E.2d 644 (1956).

[45]252 Miss. 172 So.2d 186 (1965).

[46]175 Ohio St. 551, 197 N.E.2d 194 (1964).

[47]352 Mass. 446, 225 N.E.2d 926 (1967).

[48]175 Ohio St. 551, 197 N.E.2d 194 (1964).

[49]*Williams v. Marion Rapid Transit, Inc.,* 152 Ohio St. 114, 39 Ohio Op. 433, 87 N.E.2d 334, 10 A.L.R.2d 1051 (1949).

[50]175 Ohio St. 551, 197 N.E.2d 194 (1964).

[51]352 Mass. 446, 225 N.E.2d 926 (1967).

[52]See also *Smith v. Brennan,* 31 N.J. 353, 157 A.2d 497 (1960).

[53]See also *In re Logan,* 4 Misc.2d 283, 156 N.Y.S.2d 49, aff'd 3 N.Y.2d 800, 166 N.Y.S.2d 3, 144 N.E.2d 644 (1956); and *Presley v. Newport Hospital,* 365 A.2d 748 (1976). *Cf. Porter v. Lassiter,* 91 Ga.App. 712, 87 S.E.2d 100 (1955).

[54]See note 14, *supra.*

[55]*Stokes v. Liberty Mutual Insurance Co.,* 213 So.2d 695 (Fla. 1968); *Endresz v. Friedberg,* 24 N.Y.2d 478, 30 I.N.Y.S.2d 65, 248 N.E.2d 901 (1969); *Britt v. Sears,* 150 Ind.App. 487, 277 N.E.2d 20 (1971) (dissent); *Marko v. Philadelphia Transportation Co.,* 420 Pa. 124, 216 A.2d 502 (1966); *Todd v. Sandidge Construction Co.,* 341 F.2d 75 (4th Cir. 1964) (dissent); *Drabbels v. Skelly Oil Co.,* 155 Neb. 17, 50 N.W.2d 229 (1951); and *State ex rel. Hardin v. Sanders,* 538 S.W.2d 336 (Mo. 1976).

[56]*Smith v. Brennan,* 31 N.J. 353, 157 A.2d 497 (1960); *Sylvia v. Gobeille,* 101 R.I. 76, 220 A.2d 222 (1966); *Bennett v. Hymers,* 101 N.H. 483, 147 A.2d 108 (1958); *Kelley v. Gregory,* 282 App.Div. 542, 125 N.Y.S.2d 696, app. granted 283 App.Div.2d 914, 129 N.Y.S.2d 914 (1953); *Wolfe v. Isbell,* 291 Ala. 327, 280 So.2d 758 (1973); *Day v. Nationwide Mutual Insurance Co.,* 328 So.2d 560 (Fla. App. 1976); *cf. Kwaterski v. State Farm Mutual Automobile Insurance Co.,* 34 Wis.2d 14, 148 N.W.2d 107 (1967) (dictum); *Toth v. Goree,* 65 Mich.App. 296, 237 N.W.2d 29 (1975) (dissent).

[57]*State ex rel. Hardin v. Sanders,* 538 S.W.2d 336 (Mo. 1976); *Endresz v. Friedberg,* 24 N.Y.2d 478, 30 I.N.Y.S. 2d 65, 248 N.E.2d 901 (1969); *Drabbels v. Skelly Oil Co.,* 155 Neb. 17, 50 N.W.2d 229 (1951); and *Smith v. Brennan,* 31 N.J. 353, 157 A.2d 497 (1960).

[58]*Britt v. Sears,* 150 Ind.App. 487, 277 N.E.2d 20 (1971) (Hoffman, C.J., dissenting).

[59]*Stokes v. Liberty Mutual Insurance Co.,* 213 So.2d 695 (Fla. 1968); *Todd v. Sandidge Construction Co.,* 341 F.2d 75 (4th Cir. 1964) at 78–79 (Haynsworth, J., dissenting); *Kwaterski v. State Farm Mutual Automobile Insurance Co.,* 34 Wis. 2d 14, 148 N.W.2d 107 (1967); *Marko v. Philadelphia Transportation Co.,* 420 Pa. 124, 216 A.2d 502 (1966); *Gay v. Thompson,* 266 N.C. 394, 146 S.E.2d 425, 15 A.L.R. 3d 983 (1966); *Kelley v. Gregory,* 282 App. Div. 542, 125 N.Y.S.2d 696, app. granted 283 App. Div. 2d 914, 129 N.Y.S.2d 914 (1953); *Day v. Nationwide Mutual Insurance Co.,* 328 So.2d 560 (Fla.App. 1976); and *Sylvia v. Gobeille,* 101 R.I. 76, 220 A.2d 222 (1966).

[60]*State ex rel. Hardin v. Sanders,* 538 S.W.2d 336 (Mo. 1976); and *Endresz v. Friedberg,* 24 N.Y.2d 478, 30 I.N.Y.S.2d 65, 248 N.E.2d 901 (1969).

[61]*Sylvia v. Gobeille,* 101 R.I. 76, 220 A.2d 222 (1966).

[62]*Day v. Nationwide Mutual Insurance Co.,* 328 So.2d 560 (Fla.App. 1976). See also *Wolfe v. Isbell,* 291 Ala. 52, 265 So.2d 596 (1972) ("It is a biological fact that there is a living human being before viability.").

[63]*Day v. Nationwide Mutual Insurance Co.,* 328 So.2d 560 (Fla.App. 1976); and *Smith v. Brennan,* 31 N.J. 353, 157 A.2d 497 (1960).

[64]*Wolfe v. Isbell,* 291 Ala. 327, 280 So.2d 758 (1973); *Bennett v. Hymers,* 101 N.H. 483, 147 A.2d 108 (1958); and *Smith v. Brennan,* 31 N.J. 353, 157 A.2d 497 (1960).

[65]*Marko v. Philadelphia Transportation Co.*, 420 Pa. 124, 216 A.2d 502 (1966); and *Gay v. Thompson*, 266 N.C. 394, 146 S.E.2d 425, 15 A.L.R.3d 983 (1966).

[66]31 N.J. 353. 157 A.2d 497 (1960), overruling *Stemmer v. Kline*, 128 N.J.L. 455, 26 A.2d 489 (1942).

[67]See, e.g., *Sinkler v. Kneale*, 401 Pa. 267, 164 A.2d 93 (1960); *Sylvia v. Gobeille*, 101 R.I. 76, 220 A.2d 222 (1966); and *Bennett v. Hymers*, 101 N.H. 483, 147 A.2d 108 (1958).

[68]See, e.g., *State ex rel. Hardin v. Sanders*, 538 S.W.2d 336 (Mo. 1976); and *Endresz v. Friedberg*, 24 N.Y.2d 478, 301 N.Y.S.2d 65, 248 N.E.2d 901 (1969).

[69]365 A.2d 748 (R.I. 1976).

[70]See text accompanying notes 85–104, 138–143, 193–220, *infra.*

[71]See text accompanying notes 12–15, *supra.* For additional discussion of the live-birth criterion, see also notes 150–192, and 205–218, *infra,* and accompanying text.

[72]See note 12, *supra.*

[73]*Dietrich* itself is perhaps the best example of the short length of time which an infant must exhibit life signs in order to be deemed born alive. In *Dietrich,* Holmes treated the case as if the child was born alive because movement in its limbs was observed for up to 10 to 15 minutes after birth. 138 Mass. at 14–15.

  Also illustrative is *Wolfe V. Isbell,* 291 Ala. 327, 280 So.2d 758 (1973), in which an infant who lived for approximately 50 minutes was deemed born alive.

[74]See notes 8 and 10, *supra.*

[75]*Moen v. Hanson,* 85 Wash.2d 597, 537 P.2d 266 (1975); *Libbee v. Permanente Clinic,* 518 P.2d 636 Ore. 1974), rehearing denied, 520 P.2d 361; *Chrisafogeorgis v. Brandenberg,* 55 Ill.2d 368, 304 N.E.2d 88 (1973); *Hatala v. Markiewicz,* 26 Conn.Sup. 358, 244 A.2d 406 (1966); *Valence v. Louisiana Power & Light Co.,* 50 So.2d 847 (Louisiana App. 1951); *Baldwin v. Butcher,* 184 S.E.2d 428 (W.Va. 1971); and *Stidam v. Ashmore,* 109 Ohio App. 431, II Ohio Op.2d 383, 167 N.E.2d 106 (1959) (unjust and absurd). Most of the cases argue that the distinction is absurd because it allows the wrongdoer to completely escape liability in the situation where the harm is most severe – death. Eich v. Town of Gulf Shores, 293 Ala. 95, 300 So.2d 354 (1974); *Presley v. Newport Hospital,* 365 A.2d 748 (1976); *Mose v. Greyhound Lines, Inc.,* 331 N.E.2d 916 (Mass.Sup.Ct. 1975); *Baldwin v. Butcher,* 184 S.E.2d 428 (W.Va. 1971); *Todd v. Sandidge Construction Co.,* 341 F.2d 75 (4th Cir. 1974); and *White v. Yup,* 85 Nev. 527, 458 P.2d 617 (1969). In *O'Neill v. Morse,* 385 Mich. 130, 188 N.W.2d 785 (1971), the court argued that birth was an arbitrary point from which to measure life on the theory that "it is merely a change in the form of life" rather than "the beginning of life." In *Justus v. Atchison,* 53 Cal.App.3d 556, 126 Cal.Rptr. 150 (1975), the parents of the still-born child unsuccessfully argued that the live-birth distinction was so arbitrary as to deny them equal protection of the laws under the Fourteenth Amendment. See text accompanying notes 209–211, *infra.*

[76]See, e.g., *State ex rel. Hardin v. Sanders,* 538 S.W.2d 336 (Mo. 1976); and *Cardwell v. Welch,* 25 N.C.App. 390, 213 S.E.2d 382 (1975).

[77]In *Presley v. Newport Hospital,* 365 A.2d 748 (R.I. 1976), the plurality opinion argued that no line had to be drawn at viability or birth because medical science had established the separate existence of the unborn from the moment of conception. In *Bayer v. Suttle,* 23 Cal.App.3d 361, 100 Cal. Rptr. 212 (1972), the dissenting opinion based its rejection of the live birth requirement partially on the view that the line between death before birth and after birth is medically indecisive.

  The case of *In Re Estate of Irizarry,* 21 Misc.2d 1099, 198 N.Y.S.2d 673, 674–75 (1960), is a tragic illustration of the difficulty of proving live birth. The infant had died during or shortly after his delivery, which occurred at the mother's home because the hospital refused to admit her. The court denied recovery because of the lack of evidence of the infant's status between the time immediately after birth and the moment the ambulance arrived, at which time the infant was dead. The attending ambulance physician and the police sergeant testified that the infant was stillborn.

[78]Relevant life signs would include nonreflexive bodily movement, respiration, pulsation of the umbilical cord, heartbeat. Without attempting to provide precise definitions, several courts have referred to the foregoing signs in discussing live birth. See, for example, *Dietrich v. Northampton,* 138 Mass. 14 (1884) (movement of the limbs); *cf. O'Neill v. Morse,* 385 Mich. 130, 188 N.W.2d 785 (1971) (regulation).

[79]See *Appendix.*

[80]See notes 16–20, *supra,* and accompanying text.

[81]See, e.g., *Leal v. C.C. Pitts Sand & Gravel, Inc.,* 419 S.W.2d 820 (Texas, 1967); and *Magnolia Coca Cola Bottling Co. v. Jordan,* 124 Tex. 347, 78 S.W.2d 944, 97 A.L.R. 1513 (1935).

[82]See, e.g. *Smith v. Luckhardt,* 299 Ill.App. 100, 19 N.E.2d 446 (1939); *Newman v. Detroit,* 281 Mich. 60, 274 N.E. 710 (1937); and *Allaire v. St. Luke's Hospital,* 184 Ill. 359, 56 N.E. 638 (1900).

[83]See, e.g., *Squillo v. New Haven,* 14 Conn.Supp. 500 (1947); and *Woods v. Lancet,* 303 N.Y. 349, 102 N.E.2d 691, 27 A.L.R.2d 1250 (1951) (dissent).

[84]See *Drabbels v. Skelly Oil Co.,* 155 Neb. 17, 50 N.W.2d 229 (1951); and *Allaire v. St. Luke's Hospital,* 184 Ill. 359, 56 N.E. 638 (1900). *Smith v. Brennan,* 31 N.J. 353, 157 A.2d 497 (1960) (dissent). See

generally, *Comment*, "Recovery for Prenatal Injuries: The Right of A Child Against Its Mother," X *Suffolk Univ.L.Rev.* 582 (1972); and *Note*, "The Impact of Medical Knowledge on the Law Relating to Prenatal Injuries," 110 *U. of Pennsylvania L.Rev.* 583–586 (1962).

[85]See Lon Fuller. *Legal Fictions* (1–48) (Stanford 1967).

[86]*Id.* at 140, n.11 relying in part on Corner, *Ourselves Unborn* 69 (1944).

[87]*Id.* at 140–42.

[88]*Id.* Canada had decided thirteen years previously to recognize a cause of action in tort on behalf of the child injured before birth and after attaining viability. *Montreal Tramways v. Leville*, 4 D.L.R. 337, Can.S.Ct. 456 (1933).

[89]65 F.Supp. at 142–43, Judge McGuire also argued that the law, lest it be "an arid and sterile thing," *must* keep pace with medical science.

[90]See, e.g., *Woods v. Lancet*, 303 N.Y. 349, 102 N.E.2d 691, 17 A.L.R.2d 1250 (1951); *Mallison v. Pomeroy*, 205 Ore. 690, 291 P.2d 225 (1955); *Bennett v. Hymers*, 101 N.H. 483, 147 A.2d 108 (1958); and *Seattle–First National Bank v. Rankin*, 59 Wash.2d 288, 367 P.2d 835 (1962).

[91]See *Williams v. Marion Rapid Transit, Inc.*, 152 Ohio St. 114, 39 Ohio Ops. 433, 87 N.E.2d 334, 10 A.L.R.2d 1051 (1949); *Womack v. Buchhorn*, 384 Mich. 718, 187 N.W.2d 218 (1971); *Woods v. Lancet*, 303 N.Y. 349, 102 N.E.2d 691, 27 A.L.R.2d 1250 (1951); *Mallison v. Pomeroy*, 205 Ore. 690, 291 P.2d 255 (1955); and *Bennett v. Hymers*, 101 N.H. 483, 147 A.2d 108 (1958).

[92]*Woods v. Lancet*, 303 N.Y. 349, 102 N.E.2d 691, 27 A.L.R.2d 1250 (1951) contains an excellent discussion of the role of the doctrine of *stare decisis* in such a situation, where external developments render previous legal premises erroneous. See also *Tursi v. New England Windsor Company*, 19 Conn.Sup. 242, 111 A.2d 14 (1955); and *Mallison v. Pomeroy*, 205 Ore. 690, 291 P.2d 225 (1955).

[93]Most courts simply stated that ample precedent exists for recognition of a cause of action. See, for example, *Woods v. Lancet*, 303 N.Y. 349, 102 N.E.2d 691, 27 A.L.R.2d 1250 (1951); *Mallison v. Pomeroy*, 205 Ore. 690, 291 P.2d 225 (1955); and *Seattle–First National Bank v. Rankin*, 59 Wash.2d 288, 367 P.2d 835 (1962). See also *Torigian v. Watertown News Co.*, 352 Mass. 446, 225 N.E.2d 926 (1967); and *Daley v. Meier*, 33 Ill.App.2d 218, 178 N.E.2d 691 (1961).

[94]See, e.g., *Woods v. Lancet*, 303 N.Y. 349, 102 N.E.2d 691, 27 A.L.R.2d 1250 (1951); *Mallison v. Pomeroy*, 205 Ore. 690, 291 P.2d 225 (1955); and *Seattle–First National Bank v. Rankin*, 59 Wash.2d 288, 367 P.2d 835 (1962).

[95]303 N.Y. 349, 102 N.E.2d 691 (1951), overruling *Drobner v. Peters*, 232 N.Y. 220, 133 N.E. 567 (1921).

[96]*Id.*, 102 N.E.2d at 695.

[97]*Id.*, 102 N.E.2d at 695.

[98]282 App.Div.2d 542, 125 N.Y.S.2d 696, appeal granted 283 App.Div.2d 914, 129 N.Y.S.2d 914 (1953).

[99]*Id.*, 125 N.Y.S.2d at 698.

[100]125 N.Y.S.2d at 697.

[101]*Day v. Nationwide Mutual Insurance Co.*, 328 So.2d 560 (Fla.App. 1976); *Hornbuckle v. Plantation Pipe Line Co.*, 212 Ga. 504, 93 S.E.2d 727, (1956); *Daley v. Meier*, 33 Ill.App.2d 218, 178 N.E.2d 691 (1961); *Womack v. Buchhorn*, 384 Mich. 718, 187 N.W.2d 218 (1971); *Bennett v. Hymers*, 101 N.H. 483, 147 A.2d 108 (1958); *Smith v. Brennan*, 31 N.J. 353, 157 A.2d 497 (1960); *Sinkler v. Kneale*, 401 Pa. 267, 164 A.2d 93 (1960); *Labree v. Major*, 306 A.2d 808 (R.I. 1973); *Delgado v. Yandell*, 468 S.W.2d 475 (Tex.Civ.App. 1971), error ref. nre. 471 S.W.2d 569; and *Puhl v. Milwaukee Auto Insurance Co.*, 8 Wis.2d 343, 99 N.W.2d 163 (1959). See also *Jorgensen v. Meade Johnson Laboratories, Inc.*, 483 F.2d 237 (10th Cir. 1973) (by implication). In addition, those jurisdictions that have upheld wrongful death actions for children who survived birth but died from injuries inflicted before they were viable should be held, by implication, to approve suits for injuries regardless of the fact that they were inflicted before viability. See *Wolfe v. Isbell*, 291 Ala. 327, 280 So.2d 758 (1972); and *Torigian v. Watertown News Co.*, 352 Mass. 446, 225 N.E.2d 926 (1967). See generally, *Toth v. Goree*, 65 Mich.App. 296, 237 N.W.2d 29 (1975) (Maher, J., dissenting).

[102]See note 8, *supra*.

[103]See *Bennett v. Hymers*, 101 N.H. 483, 147 A.2d 108 (1958); *Daley v. Meier*, 33 Ill.App.2d 218, 178 N.E.2d 691 (1961); *Womack v. Buchhorn*, 384 Mich. 718, 187 N.W.2d 218 (1971); *Smith v. Brennan*, 31 N.J. 353, 157 A.2d 497 (1960); *cf. Toth v. Goree*, 65 Mich.App. 296, 237 N.W.2d 29 (1975) (Maher, J., dissenting).

[104]See *Note*, "The Impact of Medical Knowledge on the Law Relating to Prenatal Injuries," 110 *U. of Pennsylvania L.Rev.* 568–570 (1962).

[105]*Renslow v. Mennonite Hospital*, 40 Ill.App.3d 234, 351 N.E.2d 870 (1976); and *Jorgensen v. Meade Johnson Laboratories, Inc.*, 483 F.2d 237 (10th Cir. 1973).

[106]In *Jorgensen v. Meade Johnson Laboratories, Inc.*, 483 F.2d 237 (10th Cir. 1973), the United States Court of Appeals for the Tenth Circuit, applying Oklahoma law, held that a child afflicted with Down's syndrome (mongolism), allegedly the result of chromosome damage caused by birth control pills taken by the mother prior to pregnancy, could recover damages for its affliction from

the manufacturer of the birth control pills if it could establish a causal connection between the alleged defect in the pills and the injury. The court justified its holding in the *foreseeability* of the harm to an unborn child in the event that the woman taking the pills later became pregnant.

In *Renslow v. Mennonite Hospital*, 40 Ill.App.3d 234, 351 N.E.2d 870 (1976), a hospital was charged with negligently administering a transfusion of Rh-negative blood to a thirteen year old girl who had Rh-positive blood. The transfusion allegedly caused the "sensitization" of her blood, which was not discovered until eight years later, when the woman was being tested during pregnancy. When the condition of her blood was diagnosed, labor was induced because of fear for the child's life. The child was born prematurely and two complete exchange transfusions had to be administered, and the child suffered damage to its brain and nervous system. The court reasoned that the critical fact was not that the negligent conduct occurred prior to conception, but that it was *foreseeable* at the time of the transfusion that the girl might one day become pregnant and that the effects of the negligent conduct would harm her unborn child. But see *Morgan v. United States*, 143 F.Supp. 580 (D.N.J. 1956) (applying Pennsylvania law), which involved a similar factual situation as *Renslow* and reached the opposite conclusion on the grounds that the child was not in existence at the time of the harm-inducing conduct, and that, therefore, no duty was owed to it.

[107] See *Appendix*.

[108] See notes 111–114, *infra*, and accompanying text.

[109] See notes 115–123, *infra*, and accompanying text.

[110] 65 F.Supp. 138 (D.D.C. 1946). See text accompanying notes 24–30 and notes 79–97, *supra*.

[111] See, e.g., *Garfield Memorial Hospital v. Marshall*, 204 F.2d 721 (D.C.Cir. 1953); *Young v. Group Health Cooperative of Puget Sound*, 85 Wash.2d 322, 534 P.2d 1349 (1975); *Norland v. Washington General Hospital*, 461 F.2d 694 (8th Cir. 1972); *Sox v. United States*, 187 F.Supp. 465 (E.D. So.Car. 1960); *Wale v. Barnes*, 278 So.2d 601 (Fla. 1973); and *Reynolds v. West*, 237 Miss. 613, 115 So.2d 742 (1959). *Cf. Fallaw v. Hobbs*, 113 Ga.App. 181, 147 S.E.2d 517 (1966) (limiting discussion to whether the contributory negligence of the mother bars her child's suit also).

[112] Included among the cases that cited medical knowledge to refute the legal premise that the unborn viable fetus is a part of its mother are such early decisions as *Kine v. Zuckerman*, 4 Pa. D.&C. 227 (1924); *Couper v. Blanck*, 39 So.2d 352 (La.App. 1923); *Scott v. McPheeters*, 33 Cal.App.2d 629, 92 P.2d 678 (1939); *Lipps v. Milwaukee Electric R. Light Co.*, 164 Wis. 272, 159 N.W. 916 (1916); and *Bonbrest v. Kotz*, 65 F.Supp. 138 (D.D.C. 1946). See also *Woods v. Lancet*, 303 N.Y. 349, 102 N.E.2d 691, 28 A.L.R.2d 1250 (1951); *Shousha v. Matthews Drivurself Service, Inc.*, 210 Tenn. 384, 358 S.W.2d 471 (1962); *Mallison v. Pomeroy*, 205 Ore. 690, 291 P.2d 225 (1955); *cf. Verkennes v. Corniea*, 229 Minn. 365, 38 N.W.2d 838 (1949).

[113] See, e.g., *Bonbrest v. Kotz*, 65 F.Supp. 138 (D.D.C. 1946); *Amann v. Faidy*, 415 Ill. 422, 114 N.E.2d 412 (1953); and *Williams v. Marion Rapid Transport, Inc.*, 152 Ohio St. 114, 39 Ohio Ops. 433, 87 N.E.2d 334, 10 A.L.R.2d 1051 (1949).

[114] See, e.g., *Womack v. Buchhorn*, 384 Mich. 718, 187 N.W.2d 218 (1971); *Woods v. Lancet*, 303 N.Y. 349, 102 N.E.2d 691, 28 A.L.R.2d 1250 (1951); and *Williams v. Marion Rapid Transit, Inc.*, 152 Ohio St. 114, 39 Ohio Ops. 433, 87 N.E.2d 334, 10 A.L.R.2d 1051 (1949).

[115] As noted previously, eleven jurisdictions have upheld suits by or on behalf of children for injuries inflicted before viability. See note 101, *supra*. Many of these cases specifically relied on developments in medical science, both for evidence of the independent physiological existence of the unborn prior to viability and for increased assurance of the ability to determine the existence of a causal link between the injury and the alleged conduct. See *Sinkler v. Kneale*, 401 Pa. 267, 164 A.2d 93 (1060); *Smith v. Brennan*, 31 N.J. 353, 157 A.2d 497 (1960); *Torigian v. Watertown News Co.*, 352 Mass. 446, 225 N.E.2d 926 (1967); and *Bennett v. Hymers*, 101 N.H. 483, 147 A.2d 108 (1958). *Cf. Day v. Nationwide Mutual Insurance Co.*, 328 So.2d 560 (Fla.App. 1976).

[116] See, e.g., cases cited in note 103, *supra*.

[117] 93 S.E.2d 727, 728 (1951), conformed to 94 Ga.App. 328, 94 S.E.2d 523.

[118] *Id.*, 93 S.E.2d at 728–730 (Duckworth, C.J., concurring, and Almand, J., dissenting).

[119] *Id.*, 93 S.E.2d at 728.

[120] 401 Pa. 267, 164 A.2d 93, 93–96 (1960).

[121] *Restatement (Second) of Torts*, Explanatory Notes §869, at 174–175 (Tent. Draft No. 16, 1970). See also Prosser, *Law of Torts*, §55 at 337–338 (4th ed. 1971).

[122] *Id.*, Comment d at 177.

[123] 328 So.2d 560, 562–563, (Fla.Dist.Ct.App. 1976). See also *Puhl v. Milwaukee Auto Insurance Company*, 8 Wis.2d 343, 99 N.W.2d 163 (1959); and *Bennett v. Hymers*, 101 N.H. 483, 147 A.2d 108 (1958).

[124] Some statutory system permitting compensation for a wrongful death exists in each state, either allowing the survival of the deceased's claim against the wrongdoer or creating a new cause of action (derivative in nature) in certain designated beneficiaries, or both. The former system

affords a "survival action," the latter a "wrongful death" action. See *Appendix;* see also notes 8–10, *supra,* and accompanying text.

Interestingly, this is the fact pattern that confronted Holmes in the *Dietrich* case, where the child was born prematurely during the sixth month of pregnancy and died between ten and fifteen minutes after birth. See notes 16–18, *supra,* and accompanying text.

[125] See text accompanying notes 80–99, *supra.*

[126] See, e.g., *Evans v. Olson,* 550 P.2d 924 (Okla. 1976); *Hogan v. McDaniel,* 204 Tenn. 235, 319 S.W.2d 221 (1958); *Hall v. Murphy,* 236 So.Car. 257, 113 S.E.2d 790 (1960); *Leal v. C.C. Pitts Sand & Gravel, Inc.,* 419 S.W.2d 820 (Texas 1967); and *Steggall v. Morris,* 363 Mo. 1224, 258 S.W.2d 577 (1953).

[127] See notes 150–192, *infra,* and accompanying text.

[128] For the discussion of the trend to reject the viability requirement in the context of a child's suit for damages for its own prenatally inflicted injuries, see notes 115–123, *supra,* and accompanying text.

[129] See notes 140–146, *infra,* and accompanying text.

[130] 39 So.2d 352 (La.Ct. of App. 1923).

[131] See notes 24–27, *supra,* and accompanying text.

[132] *Verkennes v. Corniea,* 229 Minn. 365, 38 N.W.2d 838 (1949). See notes 29–30, *supra,* and accompanying text.

[133] 153 Ohio St. 529, 92 N.E.2d 809, 809–810 (1950).

[134] 152 Ohio St. 114, 87 N.E.2d 334, 340 (1949).

[135] 92 N.E.2d at 812–813. The defendants proposed a statutory construction argument that, since the statute had been passed in the nineteenth century, long before any American court had held that an unborn child had an independent legal existence for the purposes of recovering for prenatal injuries, and had been reenacted several times since then without any change in phraseology, the legislature could not have imputed to it an intent to recognize a cause of action in this situation. The court rejected this argument, stating that since the *Williams* case was the first case by the Ohio Supreme Court to decide the issue of the child's right to recover from prenatal injuries, it was to be presumed that the rule announced therein "had been the law at and since the time the wrongful-death statute was enacted."

[136] *Id.,* 92 N.E.2d at 810–812.

[137] That is, most states argued in favor of a cause of action in this situation on the ground that the independent legal existence of the unborn child had already been established by the cases that allowed the child itself to obtain damages for prenatally inflicted injuries. See, for example, cases cited in note 126, *supra.*

[138] *Kelley v. Gregory,* 282 App.Div.2d 542, 125 N.Y.S.2d 696 (1953). See notes 98–104, *supra,* and accompanying text.

[139] *Porter v. Lassiter,* 91 Ga.App. 712, 87 S.E.2d 100 (1955). In *Porter,* the analysis of whether the fetus was "quick" was pegged to the date of the stillbirth, which occurred when the mother was four and one-half months pregnant, rather than the date of the injury, which was three months earlier.

[140] 352 Mass. 446, 225 N.E.2d 926 (1967).

[141] *Id.*

[142] *Id.*

[143] See note 10, *supra.* For the cases on this point that arose in the context of the child's suit for injuries, see *Appendix* and note 8, *supra.*

[144] *Presley v. Newport Hospital,* 365 A.2d 748 (1976).

[145] See cases cited in note 155, *infra.* See also notes 181–186 and 202–281, *infra,* and accompanying text.

[146] 274 N.C. 152, 161 S.E.2d 531 (1968).

[147] See notes 150–192, *infra,* and accompanying text.

[148] See notes 193–222, *infra,* and accompanying text.

[149] See notes 223–225, *infra,* and accompanying text.

[150] See note 12, *supra,* and *Appendix.*

[151] *Padillow v. Elrod,* 424 P.2d 16 (Okla. 1967); *Kilmer v. Hicks,* 22 Ariz.App. 552, 529 P.2d 706 (1975); *Davis v. Simpson,* 313 So.2d 796 (Fla.App. 1975); *Stokes v. Liberty Mutual Insurance Co.,* 213 So.2d 695 (Fla. 1968); *Cardwell v. Welch,* 25 N.C.App. 390, 213 S.E.2d 382 (1975), cert. denied 287 N.C. 464, 215 S.E.2d 623 (1975); *Yow v. Nance,* 29 N.C.App. 419, 224 S.E.2d 292 (1976); *McKillop v. Zimmerman,* 191 N.W.2d 706 (Iowa 1971); *Lawrence v. Craven Tire Company,* 210 Va. 138, 169 S.E.2d 440 (1969); *Endresz v. Friedberg,* 24 N.Y.2d 478, 30 I.N.Y.S.2d 65, 248 N.E.2d 901 (1969); *State ex rel. Hardin v. Sanders,* 538 S.W.2d 336 (Mo. 1976); *Estate of Powers v. Troy,* 380 Mich. 160, 156 N.W.2d 530 (1968); and *Presley v. Newport Hospital,* 365 A2d 748 (1976) (Kelleher, J., and Joslin, J., dissenting).

[152] *Presley v. Newport Hospital,* 365 A.2d 748 (1976) (dissent); *Britt v. Sears,* 150 Ind.App. 487, 277 N.E.

2d 20 (1971) (dissent); *Keyes v. Construction Service, Inc.*, 340 Mass. 633, 165 N.E.2d 912 (1960); *Hogan v. McDaniel*, 204 Tenn. 235, 319 S.W.2d 221 (1958); *Kelley v. Gregory*, 282 App.Div. 542, 125 N.Y.S.2d 696, app. granted 283 App.Div.2d 914, 129 N.Y.S.2d 914 (1953); *Endresz v. Friedberg*, 24 N.Y.2d 478, 30 I.N.Y.S.2d 65, 248 N.E.2d 901 (1969); and *Carroll v. Skloff*, 415 Pa. 267, 164 A.2d 93 (1960).

[153]*Eich v. Town of Gulf Shores*, 293 Ala. 95, 300 So.2d 354 (1974) (dissent); *Presley v. Newport Hospital*, 365 A.2d 748 (1976) (dissent); *cf. Drobner v. Peters*, 232 N.Y. 220, 133 N.E. 567, 20 A.L.R. 1503 (1921).

[154]*State ex rel. Hardin v. Sanders*, 538 S.W.2d 336 (Mo. 1976); *Cardwell v. Welch*, 25 N.C.App. 390, 213 S.E.2d 382 (1975), cert. denied 287 N.C. 464, 215 S.E.2d 623 (1975); and *Endresz v. Friedberg*, 24 N.Y.2d 478, 30 I.N.Y.S.2d 65, 248 N.E.2d 901 (1969).

[155]*Graf v. Taggert*, 43 N.J. 303, 204 A.2d 140 (1964); *Gay v. Thompson*, 266 N.C. 394, 146 S.E.2d 425, 15 A.L.R.3d 983 (1966); *Muschetti v. Charles Pfizer & Co.*, 208 Misc. 870, 144 N.Y.S.2d 235 (1955); *In re Logan*, 4 Misc.2d 283, 156 N.Y.S.2d 49 aff'd 3 N.Y.2d 800, 166 N.Y.S.2d 3, 144 N.E.2d 644 (1956); *In re Bradley's Estate*, 50 Misc.2d 72, 269 N.Y.S.2d 657 (1966); *Endresz v. Friedberg*, 24 N.Y.2d 478, 301 N.Y.S.2d 65, 248 N.E.2d 901 (1969); *Berg v. New York Society for Relief of Ruptured & Crippled*, 136 N.Y.S.2d 528 (Sup. 1954), rev'd on other grounds, 286 Appl.Div. 783, 146 N.Y.S.2d 548, rev'd on other grounds, 1 N.Y.2d 499, 154 N.Y.S.2d 455, 136 N.E.2d 523; *Butler v. Manhattan Ry. Co.*, 143 N.Y. 417, 38 N.E. 454, 26 L.R.A. 46 (1894); *Britt v. Sears*, 150 Ind.App. 487, 277 N.E.2d 20 (1971) (dissent); and *Marko v. Philadelphia Transportation Co.*, 420 Pa. 124, 216 A.2d 502 (1966); *cf. Miller v. Highlands Insurance Company*, 336 So.2d 636 (Fla.App. 1976).

[156]*Todd v. Sandidge Construction Co.*, 341 F.2d 75 (4th Cir. 1964) (dissent). See also *Restatement (Second) of Torts*, §869, note 2 at 175–176 (Tent. Draft No. 16, 1970). But see *Eich v. Town of Gulf Shores*, 293 Ala. 95, 300 So.2d 354 (1974); *Moen v. Hanson*, 85 Wash.2d 597, P.2d 266 (1975).

[157]*Drabbels v. Skelly Oil Co.*, 155 Neb. 17, 50 N.W.2d 229 (1951). But see *Rainey v. Horn*, 221 Miss. 269, 72 So.2d 434 (1954) (rejecting the argument on the ground that state law prohibited a child from suing its mother).

[158]Perhaps the best example of this argument is the dissenting opinion of Justice Black in *O'Neill v. Morse*, 385 Mich. 130, 188 N.W.2d 785 (1971). See also *Presley v. Newport Hospital*, 365 A.2d 748 (Joslin, J., dissenting); and *Estate of Powers v. Troy*, 380 Mich. 160, 156 N.W.2d 530 (1968).

[159]See *Cardwell v. Welch*, 25 N.C.App. 390, 213 S.E.2d 382 (1975), cert. denied 287 N.C. 464, 215 S.E.2d 623 (1975); *Kilmer v. Hicks*, 22 Ariz.App. 552, 529 P.2d 706 (1975); *Lawrence v. Craven Tire Co.*, 210 Va. 138, 169 S.E.2d 440 (1969); *State ex rel. Hardin v. Sanders*, 538 S.W.2d 336 (Mo. 1976); *Padillow v. Elrod*, 424 P.2d 16 (Okla. 1967); *Estate of Powers v. Troy*, 380 Mich. 160, 156 N.W.2d 530 (1968); *Stokes v. Liberty Mutual Insurance Co.*, 213 So.2d 695 (Fla. 1968); *Baldwin v. Butcher*, 184 S.E.2d 428 (W.Va. 1971) (dissenting); and *Presley v. Newport Hospital*, 365 A.2d 748 (1976) (dissenting). But see *Baldwin v. Butcher*, 184 S.E.2d 428 (W.Va. 1971).

[160]See *Padillow v. Elrod*, 424 P.2d 16 (Okla. 1967); and *Estate of Powers v. Troy*, 380 Mich. 160, 156 N.W.2d 530 (1968).

[161]See, e.g., *McKillop v. Zimmerman*, 191 N.W.2d 706 (Iowa 1971); *Stokes v. Liberty Mutual Insurance Co.*, 213 So.2d 695 (Fla. 1968); *Britt v. Sears*, 150 Ind.App. 487, 277 N.E.2d 20 (1971) (Hoffman, C. J., dissenting); and *Presley v. Newport Hospital*, 365 A.2d 748 (1976) (Kelleher, J., dissenting); *cf. State ex rel. Hardin v. Sanders*, 538 S.W.2d 336 (Mo. 1976); and *O'Neill v. Morse*, 385 Mich. 130, 188 N.W.2d 785 (1971) (Black, J., dissenting). But see *Britt v. sears*, 150 Ind.App. 487, 277 N.E.2d 20 (1971).

[162]53 Cal.App.3d 556, 126 Cal.Rptr. 150 (1975).

[163]Cal. Civ. Code §26 (West 1973) (originally the California wrongful death statute in existence at the time of this suit was Cal.Civ.Pro. Code §377 (1968).

But *cf. Moen v. Hanson*, 85 Wash.2d 597, 537 P.2d 266 (1975), in which the court stated that "minor" was used to modify "child" solely for the purpose of marking the outer boundary of the parents' cause of action.

[164]53 Cal.App.3d 556, 126 Cal.Rptr. at 153–154 (1975).

[165]The amended statute has deleted the modifier "minor" and like most wrongful death statutes, simply uses the term "person." Cal.Civ.Pro. Code §377 (West 1975 Amendment).

[166]Cal.Civ. Code §29 (West 1973) (originally enacted 1872, amended in 1941 by Stats. 1941, c. 337, p. 1579, §1).

[167]126 Cal.Rptr. at 153–155. The court also analogized to the legislative history of a similar provision in the criminal code. 126 Cal.Rptr. at 155.

[168]This criticism should also apply to those decisions that justify the live-birth requirement by analogy to property laws, which protect the rights of a child *en ventre sa mere* to inherit property from the moment of conception, but condition that protection on the live birth of the child. See note 152, *supra*.

[169]See, e.g., *Evans v. Olson*, 550 P.2d 924 (Okla. 1976); *Baldwin v. Butcher*, 184 S.E.2d 428 (W.Va. 1971); *O'Neill v. Morse*, 385 Mich. 130, 188 N.W.2d 785 (1971); and *Kwaterski v. State Farm*

Mutual Automobile Insurance Co., 34 Wis.2d 14, 148 N.W.2d 107 (1967). *Cf. Jasinsky v. Potts*, 153 Ohio St. 529, 42 Ohio Ops. 9, 92 N.E.2d 809 (1950).

[170]See, e.g., *Britt v. Sears*, 150 Ind.App. 487, 277 N.E.2d 20 (1971); *Evans v. Olson*, 550 P.2d 924 (Okla. 1976); and *O'Neill v. Morse*, 385 Mich. 130, 188 N.W.2d 785 (1971).

[171]See *Britt v. Sears*, 150 Ind.App. 487, 277 N.E.2d 20 (1971); *Evans v. Olson*, 550 P.2d 924 (Okla. 1976); *Baldwin v. Butcher*, 184 S.E.2d 428 (W.Va. 1971); *Kwaterski v. State Farm Mutual Automobile Insurance Co.*, 34 Wis.2d 14, 148 N.W.2d 107 (1967); and *Jorgensen v. Meade Johnson Laboratories Inc.*, 483 F.2d 237 (10th Cir. 1973).

[172]410 U.S. 113 (1973).

[173]See *Kilmer v. Hicks*, 22 Ariz.App. 552, 529 P.2d 706 (1975); *Chrisafogeorgis v. Brandenburg*, 55 Ill.2d 368, 304 N.E.2d 88 (1973) (dissent).

[174]538 S.W.2d 336 at 337–340 (Mo. 1976).

[175]*Id.* at 339, quoting *Roe v. Wade*, 410 U.S. 113, 162 (1973).

[176]55 Ill.2d 368, 304 N.E.2d 88 (1973) (Ryan, J., dissenting).

[177]304 N.E.2d at 95 (Ryan, J., dissenting). See also *Toth v. Goree*, 65 Mich.App. 296, 237 N.W.2d 20 (1975).

[178]*Libbee v. Permanente Clinic*, 518 P.2d 636 (Ore. 1974), rehearing denied, 520 P.2d 361; and *Presley v. Newport Hospital*, 365 A.2d 748 (1976) (Bevilacqua, J., concurring).

[179]The implications of *Roe v. Wade* on nonabortion areas of the law is only beginning to receive the attention it deserves from legal commentators. See, for example, M. R. Levy and E.C. Duncan, "The Impact of *Roe v. Wade* on Paternal Support Statutes: A Constitutional Analysis," 10 *Family L.Q.* 179 (1976).

[180]See, e.g., *Toth v. Goree*, U.S. Mich.App. 296, 237 N.W.2d 297 (1975) (using *Roe v. Wade* to reaffirm rule permitting recovery for stillborn fetus in wrongful death action); *State ex rel. Hardin v. Sanders*, 538 S.W.2d 336 (Mo. 1976) (using *Roe v. Wade* to reaffirm rule denying recovery for stillborn fetus in wrongful death action).

[181]See cases cited in note 155, *supra.*

[182]See cases in note 155, *supra.*
 But see *Rice v. Rizk*, 453 S.W.2d 732 (Ky. 1970) (proof of lost earning power of stillborn fetus not required); *City of Louisville v. Stuckenborg*, 438 S.W.2d 94, 40 A.L.R.3d 1213 (Ky. 1968) (death after birth) (holding that evidence of earning capacity is not absolutely essential to a wrongful death recovery). See, generally, *Gullborg v. Rizzo*, 331 F.2d 557 (3rd Cir. 1964) (which upheld recovery and listed several factors from which an estimate of pecuniary loss could be made).

[183]See S. Speiser and S. Malawer, *An American Tragedy: Damages for Mental Anguish of Bereaved Relatives in Wrongful Death Actions*, 51 *Tulane L.Rev.* 1, 17–21 (1976), hereinafter referred to as "Speiser and Malawer," in which the authors call for the elimination of the pecuniary loss limitation on the damage award available to bereaved relatives under state wrongful death statutes.

[184]See *Delgado v. Yandell*, 468 S.W.2d 475 (Tex.Civ.App. 1971), aff'd., 471 S.W.2d 569; *Rice v. Rizk*, 453 S.W.2d 732 (Ky. 1970); *Evans v. Olson*, 550 P.2d 924 (Okla. 1976); and *Kwaterski v. State Farm Automobile Insurance Co.*, 34 Wis.2d 14, 148 N.W.2d 107 (1967).

[185]See *Marko v. Philadelphia Transportation Co.*, 420 Pa. 124, 216 A.2d 502 (1966); *Durrett v. Owens*, 212 Tenn. 614, 371 S.W.2d 433 (1963); *State ex rel. Hardin v. Sanders*, 538 S.W.2d 336 (Mo. 1976); *Endresz v. Friedberg*, 24 N.Y.2d 478, 301 N.Y.S.2d 65, 248 N.E.2d 901 (1969); *Occhipinti v. Rheem Mfg. Co.*, 252 Miss. 172, 172 So.2d 186 (1965); *In re Bradley's Estate*, 50 Misc.2d 72, 269 N.Y.S.2d 657 (1966); *Britt v. Sears*, 150 Ind.App. 487, 277 N.E.2d 20 (1971) (dissent); *Nelson v. Peterson*, 542 P.2d 1075 (Utah, 1975); and *Carroll v. Skloff*, 415 Pa. 47, 202 A.2d 9 (1964).
 The drafters of the tentative draft of §869 of the Restatement also apparently adhere to the position that permitting recovery in a survival action for the injury and death of a stillborn child involves the danger of duplicating the mother's damage award for her pain and suffering experienced as a result of the miscarriage. See *Restatement (Second) of Torts*, §869, note 2 at 175–176 (Tent. Draft No. 16, 1970).

[186]*Gay v. Thompson*, 266 N.C. 394, 146 S.E.2d 425, 15 A.L.R.3d 983 (1966).
 But see *Eich v. Town of Gulf Shores*, 293 Ala. 95, 300 So.2d 354 (1974), in which the court rejects the live-birth distinction and argues that any punitive effect which might accrue from the speculative nature of the recovery is perfectly compatible with the Alabama wrongful death act's purpose to punish the wrongdoer whose actions result in the loss of human life. See also *Huskey v. Smith*, 289 Ala. 52, 265 So.2d 596 (1972); and *White v. Yup*, 85 Nev. 527, 458 P.2d 617 (1969).

[187]See notes 76 and 154, *supra.*

[188]See notes 76–77, *supra*, and accompanying text.

[189]*Carroll v. Skloff*, 415 Pa. 267, 164 A.2d 93 (1960); and *Smith v. Brennan*, 31 N.J. 353, 157 A.2d 497 (1960).

[190]See notes 181–185 and accompanying text.

[191]See notes 73–74 and 124–129, *supra*, and accompanying text, which discusses the virtually unanimous recognition of the "personhood" of the child born alive for purposes of recovery under most wrongful death and survival statutes.

[192]See note 154, *supra*. For discussions of the major criticisms raised in opposition to the live-birth distinction, see note 75, *supra*, and notes 205–220, *infra*, and accompanying text.

[193]See notes 11–15, *supra*, and accompanying text.

[194]*Id.*

[195]See, e.g., *Mitchell v. Couch*, 285 S.W.2d 901 (Ky. 1955); *Libbee v. Permanente Clinic*, 518 P.2d 636 (Ore. 1974), rehearing denied, 520 P.2d 361; *White v. Yup*, 85 Nev. 527, 458 P.2d 617 (1969); *Seattle—First National Bank v. Rankin*, 59 Wash.2d 288, 367 P.2d 835 (1962); see also *Verkennes v. Corniea*, 229 Minn. 365, 38 N.W.2d 838 (1949); *Hale v. Manion*, 189 Kan. 142, 368 P.2d 1 (1962); and *White v. Yup*, 85 Nev. 527, 458 P.2d 617 (1969).

    See also historical discussion of the origins of the viability distinction in the text accompanying notes 20–26, *supra*.

[196]See *Baldwin v. Butcher*, 184 S.E.2d 428 (W.Va. 1971); and *Mitchell v. Couch*, 285 S.W.2d 901 (Ky. 1955).

[197]410 U.S. 113, 162–163 (1973).

[198]See *Libbee v. Permanente Clinic*, 518 P.2d 636 (Ore. 1974), rehearing denied, 520 P.2d 361; and *Presley v. Newport Hospital*, 365 A.2d 748 (1976) (Bevilacqua concurring) and *Eich v. Town of Gulf Shores*, 293 Ala. 95, 300 So.2d 354 (1974).

[199]*Libbee v. Permanente Clinic*, 518 P.2d 636 (Ore. 1974), rehearing denied, 520 P.2d 361; *Mallison v. Pomeroy*, 205 Ore. 690, 291 P.2d 225 (1955); and *White v. Yup*, 85 Nev. 527, 458 P.2d 617 (1969).

[200]See *Britt v. Sears*, 150 Ind.App. 487, 277 N.E.2d 20 (1971); *Evans v. Olson*, 550 P.2d 924 (Okla. 1976); *Baldwin v. Butcher*, 184 S.E.2d 428 (W.Va. 1971); *Kwaterski v. State Farm Mutual Automobile Insurance Co.*, 34 Wis.2d 14, 148 N.W.2d 107 (1967); and *Rainey v. Horn*, 221 Miss. 269, 72 So.2d 434 (1954).

[201]*Id.*

[202]See *White v. Yup*, 85 Nev. 527, 458 P.2d 617 (1969); *Todd v. Sandidge Construction Co.*, 341 F.2d 75 (4th Cir. 1964); *Baldwin v. Butcher*, 184 S.E.2d 428 (W.Va. 1971); *Moen v. Hanson*, 85 Wash.2d 597, 537 P.2d 266 (1975); and *Miller v. Highlands Insurance Company*, 336 So.2d 636 (Fla.App. 1976).

[203]See *Rice v. Rizk*, 453 S.W.2d 732 (Ky. 1970); *Libbee v. Permanente Clinic*, 518 P.2d 636 (Ore. 1974), rehearing denied, 520 P.2d 361; *Stidam v. Ashmore*, 109 Ohio App. 431, 11 Ohio Pos.2d 383, 167 N.E.2d 106 (1959); *Evans v. Olson*, 550 P.2d 924 (Okla. 1976); and *Pehrson v. Kistner*, 222 N.W.2d 334 (1974).

    See, generally, Speiser & Malawer, *supra*, note 183.

[204]*Eich v. Town of Gulf Shores*, 293 Ala. 95, 300 So.2d 354 (1974); and *White v. Yup*, 85 Nev. 527, 458 P.2d 617 (1969).

    See note 186, *supra*.

[205]See note 75, *supra*.

[206]See, e.g., *Eich v. Town of Gulf Shores*, 293 Ala. 95, 300 So.2d 354 (1974); and *Stidam v. Ashmore*, 109 Ohio App. 431, 11 Ohio Ops.2d 383, 167 N.E.2d 106 (1959).

[207]See *Eich v. Town of Gulf Shores*, 293 Ala. 95, 300 So.2d 354 (1974); *Presley v. Newport Hospital*, 365 A.2d 748 (1976) (plurality opinion); *Moen v. Hanson*, 85 Wash.2d 597, 537 P.2d 266 (1975); *Libbee v. Permanente Clinic*, 518 P.2d 636 (Ore. 1974), rehearing denied, 520 P.2d 361; *Hatala v. Markiewicz*, 26 Conn.Sup. 358, 224 A.2d 406 (1966); *Mone v. Greyhound Lines, Inc.*, 331 N.E.2d 916 (Mass.Sup.Ct. 1975); *Baldwin v. Butcher*, 184 S.E.2d 428 (W.Va. 1971); *Stidam v. Ashmore*, 109 Ohio App. 431, 11 Ohio Ops.2d 383, 167 N.E.2d 106 (1959); *Todd v. Sandidge Construction Co.*, 341 F.2d 75 (4th Cir. 1964); *White v. Yup*, 85 Nev. 527, 458 P.2d 617 (1969); *Valence v. Louisiana Power & Light Co.*, 50 So.2d 847 (Louisiana App. 1951); and *Bayer v. Suttle*, 23 Cal. App. 3d 361, 100 Cal.Rptr. 212, (1972) (dissent).

[208]See *Presley v. Newport Hospital*, 365 A.2d 748 (1976) (plurality opinion); *Eich v. Town of Gulf Shores*, 293 Ala. 95, 300 So.2d 354 (1974); *Kwaterski v. State Farm Mutual Automobile Insurance Co.*, 34 Wis.2d 14, 148 N.W.2d 107 (1967); *Mone v. Greyhound Lines, Inc.*, 331 N.E.2d 916 (Mass.Sup.Ct. 1975); *Baldwin v. Butcher*, 184 S.E.2d 428 (W.Va. 1971); *Todd v. Sandidge Construction Co.*, 341 F.2d 75 (4th Cir. 1964); *White v. Yup*, 85 Nev. 527, 458 P.2d 617 (1969); and *Bayer v. Suttle*, 23 Cal.App.3d 361, 100 Cal.Rptr. 212 (1972) (dissent).

[209]See note 75, *supra*.

[210]53 Cal.App.2d 556, 126 Cal.Rptr. 150, 155–158 (1975).

[211]293 Ala. 95, 300 So.2d 354 (1974). See also note 186, *supra*.

[212]385 Mich. 130, 188 N.W.2d 785 (1971). See also, for example, *Mitchell v. Couch*, 285 S.W.2d 901 (Ky. 1955); *Mone v. Greyhound Lines, Inc.*, 331 N.E.2d 916 (Mass.Sup.Ct. 1975); *Baldwin v. Butcher*, 184 S.E.2d 428 (W.Va. 1971); *Libbee v. Permanente Clinic*, 518 P.2d 636 (Ore. 1974), rehearing denied, 520 P.2d 361; and *White v. Yup*, 85 Nev. 527, 458 P.2d 617 (1969).

[213]385 Mich. 130, 188 N.W.2d at 787 (1971).

[214]*Id.*, 188 N.W.2d at 787.

[215]The cases which have analogized to property law's treatment of the unborn in favor of recognition of a cause of action for the wrongful death of a stillborn fetus include the following: *Libbee v. Permanente Clinic*, 518 P.2d 636 (Ore. 1974), rehearing denied, 520 P.2d 361; *Wolfe v. Isbell*, 291 Ala. 327, 280 So.2d 758 (1973); *Verkennes v. Corniea*, 229 Minn. 365, 38 N.W.2d 838 (1949); *Baldwin v. Butcher*, 184 S.E.2d 428 (W.Va. 1971); *Rainey v. Horn*, 221 Miss. 269, 72 So.2d 434 (1954); *Kwaterski v. State Farm Mutual Automobile Insurance Co.*, 34 Wis.2d 14, 148 N.W.2d 107 (1967); *Todd v. Sandidge Construction Co.*, 341 F.2d 75 (4th Cir. 1964); *Toth v. Goree*, 65 Mich.App. 296, 237 N.W.2d 29 (1975) (dissent); and *O'Neill v. Morse*, 385 Mich. 130, 188 N.W.2d 785 (1971).

Of these cases, the following reasoned that it would be unjust to protect the property rights of the unborn but not its health or life: *Baldwin v Butcher*, 184 S.E.2d 428 (W. Va. 1971); and *O'Neill v. Morse*, 385 Mich. 130, 188 N.W.2d 785 (1971).

[216]See, e.g., *Eich v. Town of Gulf Shores*, 293 Ala. 95, 300 So.2d 354 (1974); *Porter v. Lassiter*, 91 Ga.App. 712, 87 S.E.2d 100 (1955); *Libbee v. Permanente Clinic*, 518 P.2d 636 (Ore. 1974), rehearing denied, 520 P.2d 361; *Kwaterski v. State Farm Mutual Automobile Insurance Co.*, 34 Wis.2d 14, 148 N.W.2d 107 (1967); and *Britt v. Sears*, 150 Ind.App. 487, 277 N.E.2d 20 (1971).

[217]293 Ala. at 99, 300 So.2d at 356 (1974).

[218]150 Ind.App. 487, 277 N.E.2d 20, 25–27 (1971).

[219]*Id.*, 277 N.E.2d at 26, n.34, quoting Ind.Ann.Stat. §35–3801 (b) (Burns, 1971).

[220]See, generally, note 151, *supra*, and text accompanying notes 158–170, *supra*, which discusses other frequently urged arguments of statutory construction and legislative history in favor of the live-birth distinction.

[221]91 Ga.App. 712, 87 S.E.2d 100, 101–102 (1955).

[222]*Id.*, 87 S.E.2d at 102. The court relied in part on the previous decision of the Georgia Supreme Court in *Hornbuckle v. Plantation Pipe Line Co.*, 212 Ga. 504, 93 S.E.2d 727 (1956), which upheld a child's suit for prenatal injuries.

[223]See dissenting opinions of Kelleher, J., and Joslin, J., preferring live-birth requirement at 757–761.

[224]*Id.*, 365 A.2d at 754–756 (Bevilacqua, C.J., concurring).

[225]*Id.*, 365 A.2d at 753–754 (plurality opinion).

See also *Toth v. Goree*, 65 Mich.App. 296, 237 N.W.2d 29 (1975) (Maher, J., dissenting) (Maher also rejects the viability requirement in this situation).

JURISDICTIONAL TABLE ON LAW OF PRENATAL HARM*
(As of September 1, 1978)

*Grateful acknowledgment is given for substantial assistance in setting this table to Gary Dietsch, J. D., 1977, University of Iowa; Member of the Ohio Bar.

JURISDICTIONAL TABLE ON LAW OF PRENATAL HARM

(CA = Cause of Action; NCA = No Cause of Action)

	VIABLE FETUS					
	LIVE BIRTH				STILLBORN	
	LIVES		DIES			
	CA	NCA	CA	NCA	CA	NCA
ALABAMA			*Huskey v. Smith*, 289 Ala.52, 265 So.2d 596 (1972)		*Eich v. Town of Gulf Shores*, 293 Ala. 95, 300 So.2d 354 (1974)	
ALASKA						
ARIZONA					*Kilmer v. Hicks*, 22 Ariz. App. 552, 529 P.2d 706 (1975)	
ARKANSAS	*Norland v. Washington General Hospital*, 461 F.2d 694 (8th Cir. 1972)					
CALIFORNIA	*Scott v. McPheeters*, 33 Cal.App. 629, 92 P.2d 678 (1939), hearing den. by Sup. Ct. as reported in 33 Cal. App.2d 640, 93 P.2d 562 *Libby v. Conway*, 192 Cal.App.2d 865, 13 Cal. Rptr. 830 (1961)				*Justus v. Atchison*, 139 Cal. Rptr. 97, 565 P.2d 122 (1977)	
COLORADO			*Callaham v. Slavsky*, 153 Colo. 291, 385 P.2d 674 (1963)			

JURISDICTIONAL TABLE ON LAW OF PRENATAL HARM
(Continued)

PREVIABLE FETUS					
LIVE BIRTH				STILLBORN	
LIVES		DIES			
CA	NCA	CA	NCA	CA	NCA
		Wolfe v. Isbell, 291 Ala. 327, 280 So.2d 758 (1973)			
					Mace v. Jung, 210 F.Supp. 706 (D. Alaska, 1962)
		Justus v. Atchison, 139 Cal. Rptr. 97, 565 P.2d 122 (1977) (dictum)			*Norman v. Murphy*, 124 Cal. App.2d 95, 268 P.2d 178 (1954)

Table continued on following page

JURISDICTIONAL TABLE ON LAW OF PRENATAL HARM
(Continued)

	VIABLE FETUS					
	LIVE BIRTH				STILLBORN	
	LIVES		DIES			
	CA	NCA	CA	NCA	CA	NCA
CONNECTICUT	*Tursi v. New England Windsor Co.,* 19 Conn. Sup. 242, 111 A.2d 14 (1955); *Simon v. Mullin,* 34 Conn. Supp. 139, 380 A.2d 1353 (1977) (dictum)		*Prates v. Sears, Roebuck & Co.,* 19 Conn. Sup. 487, 118 A.2d 633 (1955)		*Gorke v. LeClerc,* 23 Conn.Sup. 256, 181 A.2d 448 (1962) *Hatala v. Markiewicz,* 26 Conn. Sup. 358, 224 A.2d 406 (1966)	
DELAWARE			*Worgan v. Greggo & Ferrara, Inc.,* 50 Del. 258, 128 A.2d 557 (1956)		*Worgan v. Greggo & Ferrara, Inc.,* 50 Del. 258, 128 A.2d 557 (1956) (dictum)	
DISTRICT OF COLUMBIA	*Bonbrest v. Kotz,* 65 F. Supp. 138 (D.D.C. 1946) *Garfield Memorial Hospital v. Marshall,* 204 F.2d 721 (D.C.Cir. 1953)				*Simmons v. Howard University,* 323 F. Supp. 529 (D.D.C. 1971)	
FLORIDA	*Wale v. Barnes,* 278 So.2d 601 (Fla. 1973) (dictum)				*Stokes v. Liberty Mutual Ins. Co.,* 213 So.2d 695 (Fla. 1968) *Stern v. Miller,* 348 So.2d 303 (Fla. 1977)	

JURISDICTIONAL TABLE ON LAW OF PRENATAL HARM
(Continued)

PREVIABLE FETUS					
LIVE BIRTH				STILLBORN	
LIVES		DIES			
CA	NCA	CA	NCA	CA	NCA
		Simon v. Mullin, 34 Conn. Supp. 139, 380 A.2d 1353 (1977)			
Day v. Nationwide Mutual Ins. Co., 328 So.2d 560 (Fla. Dist. Ct. App. 1976)				*Stokes v. Liberty Mutual Ins. Co.,* 213 So.2d 695 (Fla. 1968) (dictum); *Stern v. Miller,* 348 So.2d 303 (Fla. 1977)	

Table continued on following page

JURISDICTIONAL TABLE ON LAW OF PRENATAL HARM
(Continued)

	VIABLE FETUS					
	LIVE BIRTH				STILLBORN	
	LIVES		DIES			
	CA	NCA	CA	NCA	CA	NCA
GEORGIA	*Hornbuckle v. Plantation Pipe Line Co.*, 212 Ga. 504, 93 S.E.2d 727 (1956) *Tucker v. Howard L. Carmichael & Sons, Inc.*, 208 Ga. 201, 65 S.E.2d 909 (1951)					
ILLINOIS		*Rodriguez v. Patti*, 415 Ill.496, 114 N.E.2d 721 (1953)	*Amann v. Faidy*, 415 Ill. 422, 114 N.E.2d 412 (1953)		*Chrisafo-georgis v. Brandenberg*, 55 Ill.2d 368, 304 N.E.2d 88 (1973) *Pleasant v. Certified Grocers of Illinois, Inc.*, 39 Ill. App. 3d 83, 350 N.E.2d 65 (1976) *Maniates v. Grant Hospital*, 15 Ill. App.3d 903, 305 N.E.2d 422 (1973)	
INDIANA					*Britt v. Sears*, 150 Ind. App. 487, 277 N.E.2d 20 (1971)	
IOWA					*Wendt v. Lillo*, 182 F.Supp. 56 (N.D. Iowa 1960)	*McKillip v. Zimmerman*, 191 N.W.2d 706 (Iowa 1971) (dictum)
KANSAS	*Hale v. Manion*, 189 Kan. 142, 368 P.2d 1 (1962) (dictum)				*Hale v. Manion*, 189 Kan. 142, 368 P.2d 1 (1962)	

JURISDICTIONAL TABLE ON LAW OF PRENATAL HARM
(Continued)

PREVIABLE FETUS					
LIVE BIRTH				STILLBORN	
LIVES		DIES			
CA	NCA	CA	NCA	CA	NCA
Hornbuckle v. Plantation Pipe Line Co., 212 Ga. 504, 93 S.E.2d 727 (1956)				*Porter v. Lassiter*, 91 Ga. App. 712, 87 S.E.2d 100 (1955)	
	Renslow v. Mennonite Hospital, 40 Ill. App.3d 234, 351 N.E.2d 870 (1976) (dictum) aff'd in 367 N.E.2d 1250 (1977) *Daley v. Meier*, 33 Ill. App.2d 218, 178 N.E.2d 691 (1961)			*Renslow v. Mennonite Hospital*, 67 Ill.2d 348, 367 N.E.2d 1250 (1977) (viability rejected as a criterion)	
				McKillip v. Zimmerman, 191 N.W.2d 706 (Iowa 1971)	

Table continued on following page

JURISDICTIONAL TABLE ON LAW OF PRENATAL HARM
(Continued)

	VIABLE FETUS					
	LIVE BIRTH				STILLBORN	
	LIVES		DIES			
	CA	NCA	CA	NCA	CA	NCA
KENTUCKY			City of Louis- ville v. Stuckenborg, 438 S.W.2d 94, 40 ALR3d 1213 (Ky. 1968)		Mitchell v. Couch, 285 S.W.2d 901 (Ky. 1955) Rice v. Rizk, 453 S.W.2d 732 (Ky. App. 1970)	
LOUISIANA	Whatley v. Jones, 157 So.2d 351 (La.App. 1963)		Pan-Ameri- can Casualty Co. v. Reed, 240 F.2d 336 (5th Cir. 1957), cert. den. 355 U.S. 819, 78 S.Ct. 24, 2 L.Ed.2d 35		Valence v. Louisiana Power & Light Co., 50 So.2d 847 (La. App. 1951)	WASCOM v. American Indem. Corp. 348 So.2d 128 (La.App. 1977)
MARYLAND	Damasiewicz v. Gorsuch, 197 Md. 417, 70 A.2d 550 (1951)				State v. Sherman, 234 Md. 179, 198 A.2d 71 (1964)	
MASSACHUSETTS			Keyes v. Construction Service, Inc., 340 Mass. 633, 165 N.E.2d 912 (1960)		Mone v. Greyhound Lines, Inc., 75 Mass., Adv. Sh. 2326, 331 N.E.2d 916 (Mass. 1975)	
MICHIGAN					O'Neill v. Morse, 385 Mich. 130, 188 N.W.2d 785 (1971)	

JURISDICTIONAL TABLE ON LAW OF PRENATAL HARM
(Continued)

	PREVIABLE FETUS					
	LIVE BIRTH				STILLBORN	
LIVES		DIES				
CA	NCA	CA	NCA	CA	NCA	
		Torigian v. Watertown News Co., 352 **Mass.** 446, 225 N.E.2d 926 (1967)				
Womack v. Buchhorn, 384 **Mich.** 718, 187 N.W.2d 218 (1971)					*Toth v. Goree,* 65 Mich. App. 296, 237 N.W.2d 297 (1975)	
Dillon v. S.S. Kresge Co., 35 Mich. App. 603, 192 N.W.2d 661 (1971)						

Table continued on following page

JURISDICTIONAL TABLE ON LAW OF PRENATAL HARM
(Continued)

	VIABLE FETUS					
	LIVE BIRTH				STILLBORN	
	LIVES		DIES			
	CA	NCA	CA	NCA	CA	NCA
MINNESOTA					*Pehrson v. Kistner,* 301 Minn. 299, 222 N.W.2d 344 (1974) *Verkennes v. Corniea,* 229 Minn. 365, 38 N.W.2d 838 (1949)	
MISSISSIPPI	*Reynolds v. West,* 237 Miss. 613, 115 So.2d 742 (1959)				*Rainey v. Horn,* 221 Miss. 269, 72 So.2d 434 (1954)	
MISSOURI	*Steggall v. Morris,* 363 Mo. 1224, 258 S.W.2d 577 (1953) (dictum)		*Steggall v. Morris,* 363 Mo. 1224, 258 S.W.2d 577 (1953)		*State ex rel. Hardin v. Sanders,* 538 S.W.2d 336 (Mo. 1976)	
NEBRASKA					*Drabbels v. Skelly Oil Co.,* 155 Neb. 17, 50 N.W.2d 229 (1951) *Egbert v. Wenzl,* 199 Neb. 573, 260 N.W.2d 480 (1977)	
NEVADA					*White v. Yup,* 85 Nev. 527, 458 P.2d 617 (1969)	
NEW HAMPSHIRE					*Poliquin v. Macdonald,* 101 N.H. 104, 135 A.2d 249 (1957)	
NEW JERSEY	*Smith v. Brennan,* 31 N.J. 353, 31 A.2d 497 (1960)				*Graf v. Taggert,* 43 N.J. 303, 204 A.2d 140 (1964)	

JURISDICTIONAL TABLE ON LAW OF PRENATAL HARM
(Continued)

		PREVIABLE FETUS			
LIVE BIRTH				STILLBORN	
LIVES		DIES			
CA	NCA	CA	NCA	CA	NCA
Bennett v. Hymers, 101 N.H. 483, 147 A.2d 108 (1958)				*Poliquin v. Macdonald*, 101 N.H. 104, 135 A.2d 249 (1957) (dictum)	
Smith v. Brennan, 31 N.J. 353, 31 A.2d 497 (1960) (dictum)				*Graf v. Taggert*, 43 N.J. 303, 204 A.2d 140 (1964)	

Table continued on following page

JURISDICTIONAL TABLE ON LAW OF PRENATAL HARM
(Continued)

	VIABLE FETUS					
	LIVE BIRTH				STILLBORN	
	LIVES		DIES			
	CA	NCA	CA	NCA	CA	NCA
NEW YORK	*Woods v. Lancet*, 303 N.Y. 349, 102 N.E.2d 691, 27 A.L.R.2d 1250 (1951)					*Endresz v. Friedberg*, 24 N.Y.2d 478, 301 N.Y.S.2d 65, 248 N.E.2d 901 (1969)
NORTH CAROLINA	*Stetson v. Easterling*, 274 N.C. 152, 161 S.E.2d 531 (1968) (dictum)			*Stetson v. Easterling*, 274 N.C. 152, 161 S.E.2d 531 (1968)		*Gay v. Thompson*, 266 N.C. 394, 146 S.E.2d 425, 15 A.L.R.3d 983 (1966) *Yow v. Nance*, 29 N.C. App. 419, 224 S.E.2d 292 (1976), pet. for discretionary review denied 290 N.C. 312, 225 S.E.2d 833 (1976)
OHIO	*Williams v. Marion Rapid Transit, Inc.*, 152 Ohio St. 114, 39 Ohio Op. 433, 87 N.E.2d 334, 10 A.L.R.2d 1051 (1949)		*Peterson v. Nationwide Mutual Ins. Co.*, 175 Ohio St. 551, 26 Ohio Op.2d 246, 197 N.E.2d 194 (1964) *Jasinsky v. Potts*, 153 Ohio St. 529, 42 Ohio Op. 9, 92 N.E.2d 809 (1950)		*Stidam v. Ashmore*, 109 Ohio App. 431, 11 Ohio Op.2d 383, 167 N.E.2d 106 (1959)	
OKLAHOMA	*Jorgensen v. Meade Johnson Laboratories, Inc.*, 483 F.2d 237 (10th Cir. 1973) (Okla. Law) (dictum)		*Jorgensen v. Meade Johnson Laboratories, Inc.*, 483 F.2d 237 (10th Cir. 1973) (Okla. Law) (dictum)		*Evans v. Olson*, 550 P.2d 924 (Okla. 1976)	

JURISDICTIONAL TABLE ON LAW OF PRENATAL HARM
(Continued)

PREVIABLE FETUS					
LIVE BIRTH				STILLBORN	
LIVES		DIES			
CA	NCA	CA	NCA	CA	NCA
Kelley v. Gregory 282 App. Div. 542, 125 N.Y.S.2d 696, app. granted 283 App. Div. 914, 129 N.Y.S.2d 914 (1953)					In re *Logan*, 3 N.Y.2d 800, 166 N.Y.S.2d 3, 144 N.E.2d 644 (1956)

Table continued on following page

JURISDICTIONAL TABLE ON LAW OF PRENATAL HARM
(Continued)

	VIABLE FETUS					
	LIVE BIRTH				STILLBORN	
	LIVES		DIES			
	CA	NCA	CA	NCA	CA	NCA
OREGON	Mallison v. Pomeroy, 205 Ore. 690, 291 P.2d 225 (1955)				Libbee v. Permanente Clinic, 518 P.2d 636 (Ore. 1974), rehearing denied, 520 P.2d 361	
PENNSYLVANIA	Kine v. Zuckerman, 4 Pa. D&C 227 (1924)				Marko v. Philadelphia Transportation Co., 420 Pa. 124, 216 A.2d 502 (1966)	
RHODE ISLAND	Sylvia v. Gobeille, 101 R.I. 76, 220 A.2d 222 (1966)				Presley v. Newport Hospital, 365 A.2d 748 (1976) (dictum)	
SOUTH CAROLINA	Hall v. Murphy, 236 So.Car. 257, 113 S.E.2d 790 (1960)		Hall v. Murphy, 236 So.Car. 257, 113 S.E.2d 790 (1960)		Fowler v. Woodward, 244 So.Car. 608, 138 S.E.2d 42 (1964)	
TENNESSEE			Shousha v. Matthews Drivurself Service Inc., 210 Tenn. 384, 358 S.W.2d 471 (1962) Hamby v. McDaniel, 559 S.W.2d 774 (Tenn. 1977)			Durrett v. Owens, 212 Tenn. 614, 371 S.W.2d 433 (1963) Hamby v. McDaniel, 559 S.W.2d 774 (Tenn. 1977)
TEXAS			Leal v. C.C. Pitts Sand & Gravel, Inc., 419 S.W.2d 820 (Texas 1967)			

JURISDICTIONAL TABLE ON LAW OF PRENATAL HARM
(Continued)

PREVIABLE FETUS					
LIVE BIRTH				STILLBORN	
LIVES		DIES			
CA	NCA	CA	NCA	CA	NCA
Sinkler v. Kneale, 401 Pa. 267, 164 A.2d 93 (1960)				*Carroll v. Skloff*, 415 Pa. 47, 202 A.2d 9 (1964)	
Labree v. Major, 306 A.2d 808 (R.I. 1973) (dictum) *Sylvia v. Gobeille*, 101 R.I. 76, 220 A.2d 222 (1966) (dictum)				*Presley v. Newport Hospital*, 365 A.2d 748 (1976) (dictum)	
				West v. McCoy, 233 S.C. 369, 105 S.E. 2d 88 (1958)	
Delgado v. Yandell, 468 S.W.2d 475 (Tex. Civ. App. 1971), error ref. nre. 471 S.W.2d 569					

Table continued on following page

JURISDICTIONAL TABLE ON LAW OF PRENATAL HARM
(Continued)

	VIABLE FETUS					
	LIVE BIRTH				STILLBORN	
	LIVES		DIES			
	CA	NCA	CA	NCA	CA	NCA
UTAH						*Nelson v. Peterson,* 542 P.2d 1075 (Utah 1975) *Webb v. Snow,* 102 Utah 435, 132 P.2d 114 (1942)
VIRGINIA	*Bolen v. Bolen,* 409 F. Supp. 1371 (W.D. Va. 1975)					*Lawrence v. Craven Tire Co., 210* Va. 138, 169 S.E.2d 440 (1969)
WASHINGTON	*Seattle— First Na- tional Bank v. Rankin,* 59 Wash.2d 288, 367 P.2d 835 (1962)				*Moen v. Hanson,* 85 Wash. 2d 597, 537 P.2d 266 (1975)	
WEST VIRGINIA					*Baldwin v. Butcher,* 155 W.Va. 431, 184 S.E.2d 428 (1971) *Panagopoulous v. Martin,* 295 F.Supp. 220 (S.D.W. Va. 1969)	
WISCONSIN					*Kwaterski v. State Farm Mutual Auto- mobile Ins. Co.,* 34 Wis. 2d 14, 148 N.W.2d 107 (1967)	

JURISDICTIONAL TABLE ON LAW OF PRENATAL HARM
(Continued)

PREVIABLE FETUS					
LIVE BIRTH				STILLBORN	
LIVES		DIES			
CA	NCA	CA	NCA	CA	NCA

Puhl v. Milwaukee Auto Ins. Co., 8 Wis. 2d 343, 99 N.W.2d 163 (1959) (dictum)

INDEX

Page numbers in *italics* refer to illustrations; (t) indicates tables.